Birthing a Better Way

Birthing
a Better Way

12 Secrets for Natural Childbirth

KALENA COOK & MARGARET CHRISTENSEN, M.D.

Number 4 in the
Mayborn Literary Nonfiction Series

University of North Texas Press
Mayborn Graduate Institute of Journalism
DENTON

10 9 8 7 6 5 4 3 2 1

Permissions:
University of North Texas Press
1155 Union Circle #311336
Denton, TX 76203-5017

The paper used in this book meets the minimum requirements of the American
National Standard for Permanence of Paper for Printed Library Materials,
z39.48.1984. Binding materials have been chosen for durability.

Library of Congress Cataloging-in-Publication Data

Cook, Kalena.
  Birthing a better way : 12 secrets for natural childbirth / Kalena Cook &
Margaret Christensen; foreword by Christiane Northrup.
– 1st ed.
  p. cm. – (Number 4 in the Mayborn literary nonfiction series)
Includes bibliographical references and index.
  ISBN 978-1-57441-297-0 (cloth : alk. paper) –
  ISBN 978-1-57441-298-7 (pbk. : alk. paper)
  1. Pregnancy–Popular works. 2. Natural childbirth–Popular works. 3. Infants–
Care–Popular works. I. Christensen, Margaret, 1960- II. Title. III. Title: 12 secrets
for natural childbirth. IV. Title: Birthing a better way : twelve secrets for natural
childbirth. V. Series: Mayborn literary nonfiction series ; no. 4.
  RG525.C697 2010   618.4'5–dc22   2010016242

Birthing a Better Way: 12 Secrets for Natural Childbirth
is Number 4 in the
Mayborn Literary Nonfiction Series

Design and Illustrations: Kalena Cook
Cover Photograph: Digital Vision/Digital Vision/Getty Images
Kalena Cook's Photograph: John Payne Photography
Dr. Margaret Christensen's Photograph: Marla E. McDonald

Dedications

To our son William Franklin,
whose natural birth inspired this book,
and to Bill for his love and encouragement.

Kalena

To my children Caitlin, Austin, Michael and Madeline
and their father Jim for being a wonderful
supporter of unmedicated birth.

Margaret

Disclaimer:

Birthing a Better Way: 12 Secrets for Natural Childbirth offers information for your general knowledge and is designed for educational purposes only.

You should not rely on this information as a substitute for, nor does it replace, your health-care professional or other personal medical attention, advice, care, diagnosis or treatment.

This book is not intended to promote or endorse any medical practice, program, agenda, medical tests, products or procedures. If you have any concerns about your own health or the health of your baby, you should always consult with your provider—obstetrician or midwife.

The authors and publishers do not accept responsibility and disclaim any liability arising, whether directly or indirectly, from errors in text, or from the use, misuse or misapplication of material in this book.

Note: Most stories from moms, midwives, doctors, birth centers, hospitals, nurses and other professionals in the book were obtained by in person, one-on-one interviews. A few distance interviews were done by phone. Co-authors Kalena Cook and Margaret Christensen, M.D. wrote their own stories.

You can do it!

Usted puede hacerlo

Sie können es tun

Vous pouvez le faire

Puoi farlo

U kunt het doen

Você pode fazê-lo

Du kan gjøre det

Contents

by Christiane Northrup, M.D.

Author of *Women's Bodies, Women's Wisdom* and *Mother-Daughter Wisdom*

Deep inside each of us is the wisdom we need to give birth. We are born with these instincts; they are part of our collective psyche. For ages, women have given birth with relatively few problems. Yet, in recent times, we stopped believing in our own body's intelligence and turned to so-called "pregnancy experts" who rely on tests, machines, and surgical implements. As a result, modern obstetric practice is more invasive and more likely to lead to complications that will affect the health of the mother and her child, and even their relationship. Frankly, nothing is more important for a mother and baby than an *optimal* start in life.

As long as we receive the right medical and emotional support, our bodies can give birth normally (and respond naturally) with little intervention. My 90-pound, 4-foot, 11-inch maternal grandmother delivered my mother and my aunt at home. Both weighed over nine pounds. Good thing no one ever told her that her pelvis wasn't adequate. The key to an optimal outcome begins by examining your own beliefs about birth and updating the ones that don't serve you or your baby.

For example, I have seen countless times how *fear* impedes the process of natural childbirth:

Fear of the birth process: Most pregnant women have been told horror stories about labor and delivery. These stories work their way into the subconscious, becoming "self-fulfilling prophecies" that play themselves out according to what a woman believes will happen. They also affect the type of care she chooses.

Fear of pain: Giving birth is hard work. And it can also be painful. But it's a different kind of pain than the pain of being hurt or injured. Once you know that nothing bad is going to happen to you from the pain, you can deal with it. With labor pains you can *work* with them and *dive under* them into your calm center.

Fear on the part of one's caregiver: The combination of a fearful laboring woman and a fearful doctor can prevent the body from functioning normally. Any veterinarian (or midwife) will tell you that neither animals nor humans birth well when they are frightened or when skeptical strangers are around.

Birthing a Better Way gives voice to the following 10 natural principles which women have trusted to counter their fears (discussed further in my book, *Mother-Daughter Wisdom*).

1. Labor proceeds on its own schedule.
2. Childbirth by nature is a peak experience, characterized by joy, love and ecstacy. Women who have been in touch with their own wisdom during labor rarely develop the postpartum depression or other mood disorders that are so common in our culture.
3. Birth is sexual.
4. How we are born imprints both mother and baby.
5. Natural birth is safe.
6. What we believe affects how we give birth.
7. Who you choose to have with you in the delivery room can change your experience.
8. Who you choose to listen to (or read) about labor can change your experience.
9. Fear hurts.
10. Labor can be hard work. Labor can hurt. The rewards are worth it!

Right now, you are holding a book full of natural birth wisdom from mothers, midwives and physicians. It counters fear with faith. It shows you how to choose and be informed about your birth through inspiring stories of many women. It also shares what evidence-based medicine has *proven* is best for birth. May your courage be strengthened to carry you through the transforming journey of not only birth but motherhood.

Remember, "That which you are seeking is also seeking you."

PREFACE

by Margaret Christensen, M.D.

*"Now why do you want to go natural? You're kidding, you mean
you're not going to get an epidural!? Why would you want an
out-of-hospital birth? It's so dangerous! Why that's barbaric,
unmedicated women in childbirth are like animals!"*

These are the comments and questions I had to respond to when trying to enlighten my fellow physician colleagues and much of the Labor
and Delivery staff at my hospital on why I had birthed my four babies
unmedicated, why I supported the midwifery model of care, why I chose
an out-of-hospital birth center for my last birth, and why I had so many
patients who wanted to "go natural."

This book answers those questions by speaking to you through the
voices of many different women who've chosen this same path. Their
powerful stories speak to the truth of women's intuitive wisdom, the
sacredness of our bodies and our trust in the birth process. We need to
hear their stories. Unfortunately in our culture, we have been taught stories of fear and negativity surrounding the functions of our bodies as
women, especially of birth.

Our medical system supports this negative view. I was never taught
about the wonder of experiencing the tremendous power and strength of
my body, of the incredible sense of joy from completing such an arduous
task, of the access to transcendent states of consciousness during labor, of
the profound spiritual transformation possible in the process, of the lifelong well of courage available when one consciously chooses to face
pain, fear, and the unknown in laboring and birthing new life. I was only
taught that birth is a disaster until proven otherwise, best medicated, medicalized, managed and controlled. Having to listen to women give voice to
their pain was far too uncomfortable for physicians to bear. After all, "this
is the era of modern medicine, no one should have to suffer."

Yet, all the sacred wisdom traditions have told us for thousands of
years that to face fear and the unknown with trust, courage and faith in
oneself and in Spirit, and to find meaning in suffering opens us to greater
connection with the Divine. Because we have collectively refused to face
this reality, it is no wonder that we have such an epidemic of depression,
loss of moral values, and addictions in our culture. So how can we help to
heal women and our culture of the fear and negativity surrounding birth,

opening ourselves to the possibility of personal transformation and deepening our spiritual connection through birth?

Storytelling is among the most ancient forms of healing. As women living today, we need to hear more stories about the strength, power and sacredness of our bodies and the normalcy of the birth process. As an obstetrician, I am well aware of the complications and need for medical interventions, which can be lifesaving when used appropriately. I am proud of my training, and of the fantastic advances of modern medicine. However, Western medicine is finally coming to scientifically validate what midwives and many women have understood for centuries: that all physical processes, including birth, as well as disease processes have psychological, emotional and spiritual components that must be addressed. Outcomes are improved when a woman and her family are supported in a holistic manner.

Yet, too much dogma, rigidity and fear continues to exist around the disease-based medical model. The paradigm of birth as a healthy normal process is extremely threatening to the medical system. The reality of the threats of medical malpractice, diminished time for building relationships in a managed care system, and of the patient's abandonment of responsibility for their own health in this fast-paced, harried, just-give-me-a-pill-and-make-my-pain-go-away culture makes change challenging.

I was fortunate that as a third-year medical student, pregnant with my first daughter, I had an intuitive sense of the "rightness" of wanting to birth without drugs. Little did I know that this experience was to have such a profound impact on my personal sense of self, on my connection to God and on the work I have chosen to do. It was the many positive stories that I read and heard, as well as my spiritual connection to the feminine face of the Divine, which inspired me and gave me courage in my births and in my life's journey.

There is no one simple answer to the questions my colleagues asked or for those of you who are asking yourselves, *how do I envision my birth?* I hope these stories will inspire you to trust in your intuition, your body's power and in the Sacredness of birthing "naturally."

Dr. Christensen, a board certified obstetrician-gynecologist, owns Christensen Center for Whole Life Health, a holistic functional medicine practice in Dallas, TX.

INTRODUCTION

by Kalena Cook

If you are planning a family or you are pregnant, congratulations! Having a baby is the most amazing and memorable life event you'll ever experience. You are beautifully designed to give birth. Many women want pain relief during labor. But you owe it to yourself to be informed about *all* of your options—it can make a big difference in your birth experience. *Birthing a Better Way: 12 Secrets for Natural Childbirth*, shows you how to make choices for the safest, most positive and powerfully transforming moment for both you and your baby.

Through *12 Secrets*, you will learn step-by-step what to do to prepare mentally, physically and spiritually for the healthiest delivery along with the best proven, or "evidence-based" outcome for you. We go beyond the how-to of childbirth classes, although they remain a good starting point. The time has come for this much-needed book that marries *What to Expect* in Natural Childbirth with the comfort of *Chicken Soup* for the Natural Birthing Soul—the vital information you need with reassuring stories of encouragement.

Even if you aren't sure what kind of birth you want or you are simply curious, consider the statistics: With over 4.3 million births a year in the U.S., 90 percent of *healthy* women are considered low-risk candidates for natural birth without intervening.[1] However, nearly one in four pregnant women are artificially induced with Pitocin and one in three have a cesarean, an all-time high of 31 percent.[2] To compare, C-sections were only 6.6 percent in the 1960s.

My personal quest began with wanting to avoid a C-section, so I would not be weak *and* sleep deprived while caring for our newborn. (See my story "Birth Quest" in the first chapter.)

My natural childbirth empowered and inspired me enough to write this book. As a researcher with a background in communications, I sought out over fifty natural birth stories and professional perspectives. Dr. Christensen provides the latest medical information and also shares the story of her four natural childbirths.

Meet four other physicians who chose out-of-hospital births for their *own* babies. A tremendous circle of professional and stay-at-home moms reveal birth both ways—numb and natural, as well as births in hospitals, birth centers and at home. Discover waterbirths, quick second births, breech births, vaginal birth after cesarean (VBAC) and twins. Hear dads' perspectives. Learn about interventions and the alternatives. Read what the various birth experts say.

Do these doctors and moms know something that a growing number of natural birth women like Cindy Crawford, Joely Fisher, Ricki Lake, Jessica Alba and Gisele Bundchen know? Yes. Childbirth is not a disease. Plus, women simply want to birth where they feel the most comfortable.

You are invited to join the circle. If they can do it and I can, so can you. Although it doesn't take being an athlete, it does take more than a wish, more than being healthy or "low risk." It takes being *proactive*—preparing by absorbing positive stories, choosing the right obstetrician or midwife, getting informed, facing your fears, and using safe comfort measures. You can then begin to plan and communicate your birth preferences.

Why natural? For healthy[3] women, natural childbirth remains the safest type of birth for you and your newborn. One could think of it as less complicated. This book shares the benefits that may not be told to you: Your brain produces *endorphins* to help ease contractions naturally. Having continuous encouraging support can reduce your labor time. You eliminate side effects. You get instant recovery. It's the best brain start for your newborn for being alert to breathe and breastfeed—essential for survival outside of the womb. We list alternative comfort measures including Nitrous Oxides (N$_2$0) gas. Plus find out how to turn your fears around. This kind of birth empowers you for motherhood. And it's your choice.

Today, natural birth happens in about 3-4 percent of U.S. births. One percent, or 40,000 births were out of hospital,[4] either at home or at birth centers. About 11,000 midwives[5] deliver babies and there exist 200 birth centers. Doulas, trained birth attendants, total 6,500 with a 30 percent growth annually.

While writing this book, what I discovered is this: We grow up with scary myths and misinformation about childbirth, but we are stronger than we realize. *Birthing a Better Way: 12 Secrets for Natural Childbirth* leads to an alchemy of a *whole* birth approach—mind, body and spirit.

Birth is sacred. A newborn baby should see his mother and hear her voice first. Allowing parents to meet, hold and kiss their baby in an unhurried private moment is important.

Changes come from consumer demand and just as some women want an epidural, other women have the right to go natural. We serve as the *bridge* between healthcare institutions and providers to make natural birth more accepted, supported and accessible like it is in many first world countries.

This collection of women's experiences and their perceptions serve as a valuable focus group for health care.

For you, the benefits of this book include step-by-step chapters that show how to get the birth of your life. As a Birth Mentor, I remind parents, "You are already connected to natural childbirth from either your grand-mother or great-grandmother."

There's a reason you are reading *Birthing a Better Way*. You are intelligent and intuitive. Why wouldn't you want to be informed and empowered?

This book is a gift, a resource to arm you with knowledge. Enjoy. May your birth bring you much love and joy.

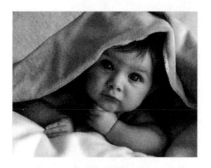

SECRET 1:

Read Positive Stories

The women you'll meet in this book, over fifty varied professionals, moms, executives, teachers, and even physicians—from Anglo, Black or African American, Hispanic, and Native American to Asian cultures—chose natural birth. Why did they make that choice in this day of epidurals, inductions, and cesareans? Along with sharing what birth is like, these moms reveal key *safety benefits* you need to know for you and your baby.

Why Women Choose Natural Birth

After tabulating the results from several years of more than fifty revealing one-on-one interviews, four main influences emerged for why healthy women wanted natural birth.

      1. Exposure to first-hand intimate stories,

      2. Getting informed about labor,

      3. Dislike of a medical environment or experience,

      4. Faith in one's own ability for the normal process of childbirth.

Exposure to First-hand Intimate Stories

A powerful incentive for some of the women interviewed was knowing that their *mother* birthed naturally. They grew up knowing their own birth was unmedicated: "I was born natural and my mother had good things to say about it. If Mom can do it, I can do it."

Influence can come from a sister or sister-in-law: "She talked about what a satisfying experience it was for her. The baby was alert, too," says Lee Ann.

Friends, or birth mentors, share their Birth Center pictures. "As I'm looking at these photos I'm thinking, gosh, this looks a whole lot more special than the hospital deliveries that I knew personally and as a resident. Hmmm, maybe I should think about this," one physician said.

Witnessing a hospital birth helps you see how an epidural and a continuous fetal monitor affects the mom's ability to push the baby out. Seeing an out-of-hospital birth, whether at a birth center or home, builds self-confidence.

Inspiration may even come from an experienced midwife, doula, or childbirth educator who looks you in the eye and says, "You can do this. You'll be fine."

Getting Informed About Labor

Most of the women read more than one book and searched for pregnancy or birth articles. Others listened to testimonials in group settings such as La Leche League for breastfeeding or prenatal yoga classes.

These women, reflecting a health and fitness market, enjoy learning. For example, moms-to-be become nutritionally-conscious of eating the best life supporting foods. Choosing a childbirth class that supports natural childbirth, such as Bradley or Birthing From Within, is important. And they begin to form some ideas of either what they envision or what they hope to avoid. An informed patient is a better patient for the caregiver.

Overall, more and more women these days desire a proactive approach to birth—being in partnership with their caregiver to openly communicate what they want.

Dislike of a Medical Experience

"The whole Obstetric practice seemed like a factory: We do this all the time, trust us, go along, you'll be fine. But no information was given about my gestational diabetes. No. I didn't want this," says Shelley, who switched to a birth center at thirty-two weeks of her pregnancy.

Grace recalls, "When I first went to the doctor's office, the waiting room looked like an assembly line. Fifteen women were waiting and the doctor left to deliver a baby. My intuition was telling me there had to be another way. I'm afraid of needles and I even break out in a sweat for blood tests. Unnecessary interventions could result in serious consequences. In a hospital, I felt I'd lose my rights."

"No needles," says Barbara, a Whole Foods buyer. "I wanted to avoid them because I had allergies all my life, which meant shots as a kid every single week. My older sister did water birth for the delivery of her baby.

My other sister had an epidural with her birth. I could compare and contrast their two experiences."

"For me, pregnancy or birth is not a disease. In a hospital it's like you're sick. I didn't want to be sick. I was looking through the paper for an alternative, a birth center, to have our first baby," says Melissa Crochet, an Obstetrician/Gynecologist.

A biology teacher, Kristen, watched birth shows on T.V. "I noted how many of those births ended up with C-sections which scared me. I started reading that some of the ways to avoid C-sections are to avoid interventions. I wanted to labor without anything to avoid surgery if possible."

Questioning the safety of drugs, Sherri says, "We grew up eating Ding Dongs, Twinkies, and Doritos. My mom got on a healthier path. She and I worked at a health food store while I was in high school. I went to college and majored in nutrition. I haven't taken an antibiotic since 1987. I found that God gave us food and herbs to heal our bodies, that there are other ways to balance whatever is imbalanced."

Faith in One's Own Ability for the Normal Process of Childbirth

"Women have been giving birth for thousands of years," becomes the mantra for natural birth moms. If it didn't work, we wouldn't be here. As far as body confidence, women range from warm receptivity with an inkling they want to try natural, to "I know I can do this." In between are surprising confessions: "I'm the biggest wimp for pain." Natural birth is not just for athletes, but ordinary women like you.

Women gain confidence in their bodies, sometimes like never before. "I had negative images of my body and never liked it. I wanted to conquer that and have *something else besides what my body looked like to feel proud of it.* That was a big attraction to me," says Jennifer.

Shelley, who had vaginal births after a cesarean (or VBAC), with one baby weighing 11 pounds, says, "I was afraid of the pain, yet it's amazing what labor feels like. It's nothing that you can't handle. It's instinctual. There was never a question whether or not I could handle it. Even in the midst of it I knew, like mountain climbing, it was something I could do. I *could* take one more contraction. I *could* deal with it. It's like having a bowel movement. You do that automatically, instinctually and there's nothing you can do to stop it. With birth, you know what to do. It's the most incredible feeling to me. I don't even use the word pain to describe it anymore. It's a process."

The natural process may be physical *and* spiritual. A chaplain at a hospital speaks about her sacred experience with a "Maternal" God. Others invoke marathon analogies. Women even use their intuition through their pregnancies. After birth many describe feeling empowered. "If I birthed this way, I can do anything."

In summary, these women varied in their initial reasons for choosing natural birth. However, each in her own way committed to a *whole birth* approach—mentally, emotionally, spiritually, and physically.

Learn to join mind, body and spirit by reading how other women prepared for birth through exercising, eating nutritiously, reading and taking classes, plus working through emotions to envision their own positive labor. You may even find a responsive chord when an idea becomes a personal spark for your own birth day.

Safety

On a cellular level, from our grandmother or great-grandmother, we are *all* connected to natural birth. Only about one percent of past generations experienced maternal death caused by poor diet, hemorrhage or infection. Today, a more natural method of delivery—eating nutritionally along with taking quality prenatal vitamins, avoiding early clamping of the umbilical cord, massage of the uterus, and other means—offers women a safe and rewarding alternative to clinical childbirth.

Many healthy women are discovering health benefits for their babies and themselves from natural childbirth. These women, whom you'll meet on the pages of this book, believe natural childbirth provides enormous inner strength that enabled them to transcend their fears and take command of their delivery.

Sheila Kitzinger
Anthropologist and Author

My mother was a midwife. I grew up reading her books and hearing her talk. I had no doubt that I could give birth with the power of my body.

Our five daughters were all born at home, all positive experiences. The most important event I've ever had is having babies myself. They were the high points in my life, both spiritually and psychosexually. Everything I've done has come out of my *joy* in birth. There wasn't any other way I wanted to go.

There is no such thing as *natural* childbirth. Birth without drugs is an oversimplified way of thinking of it. As a social anthropologist I study the culture of childbirth. All birth is a matter of culture. We create culture. We don't behave like the great apes.

In England, all women have midwives. Midwives do most of the births without a doctor present.

To compare, birth in the United States:
• has high intervention rates
• has high cesarean rates
• has been medicalized
• has become controlled by technology.

It's going that way in Britain. We do everything that the U.S. does, only a few years later. The cesarean rate is 21 percent, and rising. One in five women has her labor induced. Pitocin is used for inductions.

What is an alternative to Pitocin? Being embraced by your husband, being held and kissed by him, feeling loved and cherished, that's the real alternative to Pitocin to start labor.

Because my babies were all born at night, my older children came in right *after* birth.

But my daughter, Tess, has had three home waterbirths and had her older children present *during* her births. In fact, Sam, the older boy, made a birth plan for himself. He made a plan of what he wanted to do, how much he wanted to be involved. He wanted to cut the cord at the last birth, but decided against it. He wanted to make a cake for the midwives, which he did. He wanted Tess to hold the baby first, then me, and he would hold the baby. He was eight at the time.

The danger with home birth is not having a baby at home, but rather other people's *attitudes*. There's absolutely no evidence that for women who are in a low-risk category, birth at home is more dangerous than birth in a hospital. In fact, the opposite is true. After birth in hospitals, there is higher morbidity for mother and baby. They are more likely to have illnesses after a birth in a hospital than after a birth at home. In short, home births are *safer* than hospital births.

Also, it's *women* having the babies. It's their body, their birth, their babies. A man should support a woman's wants and needs.

Regarding husbands, I never talk about them as "coaches." It sounds as if it's an athletic competition. A woman needs to be in touch with the rhythms of her body, her spontaneous urges, to let the birth flow. If it's intellectualized, or if it's done on the basis of competition, labor is actually impeded. Even worse is the phrase, "failing to progress." The language of birth is appalling, isn't it?

The woman's in charge, not the support people. For example, my daughter, Tess, was going to have her first baby in Florida. She chose a female obstetrician, at a birth center, whom she was told would give her all she wanted. As soon as she met her, she realized that was not going to happen. There were going to be interventions which she couldn't control. She came back to England and had her baby in my house.

I was at Tess' first birth with two midwife friends. One was the senior midwife and the other was experienced, as the assistant. In the late first stage, Tess was having tremendous rushes of contractions and we were encouraging her saying, "Good, Tess. You're doing wonderfully!" Between contractions, Tess asked the midwife in charge, "Can I speak to you alone?"

When we came back in, Tess said, "You don't have to tell me I'm doing well. I know how I'm doing. So would you please shut up?" We shut up.

She had a waterbirth. She had a 10 1/2 pound baby without a tear, without drugs. It was exultant.

My main contributions to birth as an author are:
- Helping to give women a voice,
- Reassuring them to feel they have a right to speak out,
- Supporting them to communicate with their caregivers about what they want, and
- Encouraging their caregivers to communicate with them.

I began the Birth Crisis Network. Trained volunteer women make themselves available by phone for women who have been traumatized by birth so they can talk about it, when their families and their partners are fed up with hearing it. They validate their experiences and help them to find the power within themselves to cope.

What I earn from my books I put into the training of volunteers. The volunteers' own experiences are important but they must have worked through them. They can't come in immersed in grief about their own births. Some of them have been through terrible things. They need to have gotten to the other side before they can reach out and help other women. It's important for the trained ladies to know when to talk and when to stop talking, and to know how to listen in a reflective way.

A female priest emailed me because she is finding a lot of women who are seeking help with distress after childbirth. She hasn't had babies herself, but she wanted to help. She's in a poor area and is thinking of planning a Service of Healing in the church, which will be disturbing, I think, for the management of the local hospital. I could see this being organized all over the country. I'd love to do it.

I don't talk about "success" in birth. Some women have drugs and some women need them. It's not for me to judge. What is important are:

- Self-confidence,
- Having woman-to-woman help,
- Being in an environment which you control *yourself*, rather than one which is controlled by other people,
- Having a warm friendship with your caregivers, and having a one-on-one relationship with the midwife.
- Continuity of care, not having to meet a lot of different staff.

I like to tell stories because I have a wealth of experience of individual women and their births.

A great many women have suffered sexual abuse. There have been figures from a study published recently in the U.K.: One in twenty women has been sexually abused*. They bring this burden with them into childbirth. It's difficult to say to a woman, "Be in touch with your body, trust your body," when she's been exploited. She relives the memory, sometimes a vivid one, of sexual abuse in her birth experience. This is another area in which I work.

These women are not in a separate category of women. All of us know what sexual exploitation is like. It's not an illness. They can't be categorized as women who have been sexually abused, and treated differently. It is important for caregivers to understand how sexual abuse affects the experience of birth. When I gave a lecture on this subject in San Francisco, a lot of obstetric nurses, midwives, other nurses, and childbirth educators were present. What I hadn't reckoned with was the fact that a great many of the caregivers had been sexually abused, too. They were bringing *their* experience into the birth room. It affected how they behaved and their attitudes toward other women.

Penny Simkin, a dear friend, told the group that we could have a meeting of women who wanted to talk about their experiences in her hotel room afterward. You can imagine what happened. It was so crowded, it was standing room only. The experiences of caregivers needs addressing. This is another subject which I offer in my workshops.

My youngest daughter is Director of Communication and Media Studies at Brunel University in London, and she's done research on this, too. We're working closely together.

It's difficult for midwives sometimes. They're sucked into a big mechanistic system. But now they are challenging and asking the obstetricians questions. The obstetricians don't necessarily like it, but we have a lot of midwives who are doing research, and they are getting increasingly powerful, which is important.

I'm involved with teaching post-graduate midwives, too. I think it's great for midwives to go on and study and do research. This gives midwifery strength. We're starting a Multimedia Master's course run by The University of Sheffield. I'm teaching the module on Birth and Society. I've been teaching part of a Master's at Thames Valley University and had all-day workshops for midwives on this course in my own home.

If obstetricians or researchers say, "Women want this and women want that," I start to question. I need to know what the research was, the results, and the methodology—how good the research was. The important thing emerging from the research is that it's the *relationship* a woman has with her caregivers which is of primary importance in her feelings about the birth. A woman may have a cesarean section or an instrumental delivery, but this is less important than whether she has a good relationship with her caregivers, is able to *say* what she wants, can get the information she needs to make choices, and feels that they are her friends.

I think we'll start to see more home births because many more women are asking for them and insisting on them here in England. There are more midwives growing in confidence about assisting with home births. The British government has stated that women have a right to home births and they must be given that option.

Women are talking much more about their experiences in their *own* language, not medical language. Midwives are increasingly critical of the hospital system, and the midwives and the mothers are speaking out together. These are not midwives doing "alternative" births. They're mainstream midwives. That's a major difference between England and the U.S.

Wouldn't it be something if the United States followed *England's* lead on home birth?

---

* The National Center for Victims of Crime estimates that 1 in every 4 females and 1 in 6 males (or more) have been sexually abused before age 18 in the U.S.

Sheila Kitzinger authored many books including *The Complete Book of Pregnancy and Childbirth (revised)*, 2003; *The New Pregnancy and Childbirth: Choices and Challenges*, 2003; *Birth Your Way*, 2002; and *Rediscovering Birth*, 2001, *Birth Crisis*, 2006; and *The Year After Childbirth: Enjoying Your Body, Your Relationships, Yourself in Your Baby's First Year*, 1996.

A Birth Quest: Choosing a Whole Birth Approach
Kalena Cook's Story

In the dark stillness of 4 a.m., my eyes fly wide open in bed; my period is late. My husband, William, and I recently warmed up to the idea of having a baby. I felt reluctant because parenthood is such an enormous job. William said, "I don't want to be old someday, wondering if I missed out by not having a child." A window of time ... *"missed out."* The words resonated like a fine clock chiming the hour. We both did a few cleanses before conception. Surely, this would take a few months of *trying*.

Quietly, I feel my way to the bathroom to find the pregnancy test. Closing the door softly, I flip on the light, squint at the fine print and pee on a little plastic stick. Within a minute, it changes color and tests positive. Sometimes reality stares us in the face, yet we still try to focus in order to believe. Do I see this right? *Did we hit a home run on the first try?*

"What took you so long in there?" William asks. An invisible force seems to be working: It's Mother's Day.

Pregnant bellies of all shapes and sizes wait their turn in the doctor's reception room. As I'm sitting in the fluorescent lit examining room, the female obstetrician comes in briskly. She immediately hooks up the scanner without conversation. On a radar-type screen there's a little pulsing mass. "It's about the size of a piece of rice," she says. I don't think to question how this equipment works. But I wish she had at least asked my permission if it's okay to scan my womb. I go home with a polaroid of our fetus (visual proof for William), a pregnancy booklet and vitamin samples. I'm happy to let my belly out now. I feel excited, fertile and whole.

The next visit is a turning point. I'm told that I need an amniocentesis. The doctor recites her spiel, "You are over thirty-five. You need to get tested." Needles, amniotic fluid, chromosomes, percentage of Down Syndrome. I gasp.

"You need to call and set up an appointment with this other practice. All they do is amnioconteses." So unexpected; I felt quite healthy earlier today. But before I could think of what to ask, the meeting is adjourned. Reeling from the possibility I'm carrying an abnormal fetus, I watch the back of her white coat as she exits.

I cry all the way home. I pray, "Oh my God, do I need an amnio?" It was as if the baby was at risk unless proven otherwise. Is pregnancy a medical condition? Or, do we transform from maiden to mother in the natural course of life? What *do* I need? Information.

Think about a time you overcame fear. Facing the fear of pain, perhaps? Or defying death. I remember what it felt like on my first scuba dive in the ocean. Yes, I took a full-blown course practicing all the what-if's that could go wrong. Like running out of air under water...in which case you signal to your dive buddy a cut at your throat and try to calmly take turns breathing off your dive partner's regulator as you slowly ascend together. However, on that virgin day, I struggled with a leaking mask. Salt water stung my eyes. I landed on the sand floor and proceeded clearing my fogged-up mask while my so-called dive buddy took off. It felt like I could inhale water through my nose. All alone, I panicked. Forgetting the correct way to surface, I shot off like a rocket to the top. Some parrot fish took cover. It would have been more comfortable to get on the boat and never dive again. But with a little stubbornness and success, the beautiful and relaxing world under the sea opened to me. An angel fish looked me in the eyes, through a clear mask now, as if to say, "Relax and breathe."

At this point in my pregnancy, all I know is that I want to avoid a cesarean, which requires post-operative recovery. Caring for a newborn, not sleeping through the night, and the pain of surgery seems a bit much for this thirty-nine-year-old. I was born breech and my mother was, too. Yet, we were both delivered vaginally, unlike today when doctors perform C-sections for breech babies who cannot be rotated.

A neighbor, who used a birth center, recommends, *A Good Birth, A Safe Birth* by Diana Korte and Roberta Scaer. This book shares what women want—lots of contact with their baby, their partner present, cooperation along with support from the staff, and satisfaction in birth by actively making decisions. I discover how having a doula cuts down routine interventions like Pitocin and epidurals by more than half. Complications in 500 birth center births are significantly lower than in 500 hospital births. In the birth center, no IVs, monitors, or anesthesia were used. Only 6 percent had minimal pain drugs. The women ate, drank and moved about freely. In the hospital, all the women had IVs, 81 percent had electronic monitors, 70 percent had moderate to high doses of drugs for pain, and 30 percent had epidurals. Here are the differences[1]:

Complications	Hospital Birth %	Birth Center %
Mother		
Failure to progress	18.3	5.2
Labor augmentation	21.2	3.1
Cesarean section	9.2	2.8

Complications	Hospital Birth %	Birth Center %
Infant		
Fetal distress	5.3	.3
Meconium-stained fluid	11.9	2.3
Jaundice	12.6	2.4

An obstetrician's training is in surgery. Some obstetricians operate out of fear of malpractice. Use of one intervention can start a domino effect for more intervention. Epidurals bring risks and side effects including drugs crossing the placenta, diminishing the amount of oxygen to the baby's brain. These drugs can affect the baby's ability to breathe after birth. I was shocked to find that the FDA does not require drugs used in labor be proven safe for the unborn baby.

The authors offer a checklist on how to have a normal vaginal birth. Staying upright, changing positions and using water in the tub or shower helps in labor. Being upright helps for the pushing stage, too. Giving your baby good oxygen: push when needed for no more than six seconds and taking a deep breath after each contraction.

By reading other sources I found the *untold* story about amnios. Did you know that 85 percent of Down Syndrome babies are born to twenty year-olds? Down Syndrome may possibly be linked to accumulated radiation exposure (like from x-rays) over one's life. Robert Mendelsohn, M.D., and author of *Male Practice,* states that "an amniocentesis is a dangerous procedure that should be used sparingly, if at all to determine the abnormality of the fetus." Did you know that you could lose your baby from an amnio? It doubles the rate of spontaneous miscarriage. The amniotic sac gets punctured by a needle and therefore could leak. Even with ultrasound, the baby moves. Did you know that amnios are not entirely accurate? They can come back with a false positive. In other words, you carry a perfectly normal fetus, but you are told that something is wrong.

I make new decisions about what I want for my birth and form a positive image of my own health. I may be over thirty-five chronologically, but what about *biologically*? I'm at a healthy weight, don't smoke, have no health problems, and I keep up with my aerobics instructor in class.

Information brought me to the point where it's time to take a leap of faith. "Dear God, give me a sign of a rosebud if this baby is okay." Within a week, I walk by our buffet hutch one day and sense the sign is here. My aunt had mailed me a note card with a picture of a small baby rosebud attached to a beautiful full blossom. On faith, I decline an amniocentesis.

In finding Dr. Right, ask his or her cesarean rate, and the hospital's, too. If it is high, ask why. Sometimes it is the result of a large number of high-risk patients an obstetrician sees. Other times elective C-sections are requested by patients. Thinking a female obstetrician is the right choice may be presumptuous. Look for a provider, doctor or midwife, who listens to you and practices from a *holistic* birth model.

"What's your cesarean rate?" I ask the obstetrician. She couldn't tell me. I tour the hospital and ask again. "We are not able to give out that information." Isn't this public information? Like an investigative reporter, I go straight to this hospital's accounting office. "I'm wondering what does a normal vaginal birth cost on average?" The administrator says, "About $4,000 with no complications." A cesarean costs double; twice the income in less time.

I share my natural birth plan (see Appendix) with this doctor. "After doing some research, I'm leaning toward giving birth drug-free," I said. As a back-up plan, I had heard about a practice in town that includes midwives. She said, "You know, you may want to see Dr. Margaret Christensen who leans toward natural birth." It's the same one and we part ways.

Pregnancy is a watery time, the womb a small microcosm of the vast sea where my favorite animals, dolphins, live. Dolphins are intelligent, curious and playful mammals (born tail first, too). I feel passionate about protecting their oceanic world and enjoying them naturally (not in a concrete chlorine-filled prison). When I heard that you could swim with wild dolphins off of Key West, Florida, I found a way to go. One captain takes you out on his boat, spots the dolphins and encourages you to jump in the wide blue sea with your mask and fins on. You hang onto a ski rope with an oval board while being pulled slowly through the water. You can angle this board downward and upward to swim like a dolphin. It feels like you're flying through the water.

The first time, I watched dolphins at a distance. They're inspiring, but quite large. The second time, I worked up the courage to connect. I could hear them underwater by their clicks and high-pitched whistles. They could check me out with their echolocation sonar. Excitedly, I looked to my left, to the right, underneath me. Where were they? My heart was pounding. The water was crystal clear with white sand. I checked all over again. Nothing. But I could hear them closing in. Finally, I said out loud in my snorkel, "I can hear you, but I can't see you." Instantly, two dolphins appeared vertically before me mirroring each other. Did they understand or was it coincidental? We transcended an understanding higher than language. In that synchronized second, I *knew* that *they knew*. I had an intuitive knowing that's unexplainable, yet without a doubt. I thought I would swallow the ocean.

For the next appointment, I'm at a new unique practice led by an enlightened female obstetrician and gynecologist, Margaret Christensen, M.D., who supports a "midwifery model" of care. Natural birth is encouraged by using midwives with the doctor, who provides backup care for complications or high-risk moms. Dr. Christensen provides support as needed for an independent birth center near the hospital. Midwives stay throughout one's labor, whereas doctors usually come in at the end to deliver the baby. Because of a higher level of care, midwives provide great success helping moms deliver without drugs. The examining room displays beautifully framed art of women and babies.

I like Susan Akins, an experienced certified-nurse midwife, who spends time at each visit answering my questions with confidence, providing solid information and soothing reassurance. "There is no silly question," she tells me. "Because if you don't ask, that may be the one thing that gnaws at you. So ask." With her, my pregnancy feels back to normal. With a deep breath and a sigh of relief, I think, *oh this feels right*. My fear diminishes. I trust her and feel comforted under her wing. This switch to a midwife will prove to be one of the best decisions for my natural birth.

Still exploring all the options of where to birth, I visit a Victorian styled birth center. Inside are hardwood floors, lace curtains, candles, crocheted doilies and antique furniture (including a four-poster bed). It's like a bed and breakfast. The large jacuzzi tub looks like an inviting place to labor and possibly birth in. You can stay up to six hours after birth before going home. Two births can be accommodated at the same time. You could come here for prenatal visits, to give birth, to make footprints of your baby on the wall leading up the stairs and to attend a MaternaTea. This ritual is where you share your birth story (while holding or breastfeeding your baby) within a circle of other women who delivered the same month as you. Nice. This place offers a lot of appeal.

Contrast the quietness of the birth center to noisy remodeling going on in a hospital's labor and delivery hall. The fluorescent lights, the antiseptic smell of rubbing alcohol and the intrusion of the intercom calls does not feel relaxing. Suddenly, the fire alarms go off; lights flash and a siren sounds. Is it real or a false alarm? Burly men with hard hats and beer bellies walk around while nurses try to do their job in this crowded construction site. I see machines and carts everywhere. Some birthing rooms don't have windows. It's about as appealing as giving birth in a war zone.

A few days later, I tell Susan, my midwife, about the fire alarms going off. She laughs. "Oh, that construction should be done in about a week."

"What would be great is if I could have you at the Birth Center." We wish for the best of both worlds when faced with tough choices. However, the decision is made: our insurance doesn't cover the birth center, only the hospital. For me, good chemistry of the right birth attendant, with the same values, took priority over the place. Susan is respected at the hospital, yet I feel I could give birth *wherever* she is. Like a mentor, she tells me encouraging words throughout the pregnancy: "You'll do fine. You won't deliver a bigger baby than your body can handle. Yes, your baby is head down (remember the breach concern). You can birth drug-free at this hospital; they know you're mine." Susan has a personable way of being liked. She's experienced at delivering babies and even more exceptional at helping women become confident mothers.

I want a doula for our first birth because Susan may not be on call when I go into labor, and there's a possibility of getting another midwife I'm not as familiar with. A doula is a trained woman who helps during birth. A friend or a natural birth mom can be a doula, too. Doula means "mothering the mother." Doulas help the father with reassurance. She can provide emotional support as nurses come in and out and speak up for the wishes of the laboring mom if needed. I pray one morning for the right doula to be part of our birth team. That same day, at lunch, another pregnant woman sits at the table next to mine. We chat and she mentions using a doula, Mara Black. I get her phone number. Most prayers don't get answered within hours like that. Perhaps there's a Birth Angel that keeps pregnant moms from worrying. This doula happens to live close to our house, a plus for laboring at home.

William watches the expansion of my belly for nine months. His support means a lot: "I don't think most women put this kind of effort into researching their pregnancy and labor." Some younger women could say, "Oh well, my delivery wasn't quite what I had in mind. Next time I'll do things differently." Approaching forty, I didn't have that luxury of time. This may be my only childbirth.

Taking birth classes brought more focus to the labor process for the two of us as a couple. All the fathers-to-be could hear each other and laugh off their nervousness together. For example, when we found out some newborns have coneheads, one father asked, "What if the baby's head stays that way?" We all want our babies to be normal and sometimes birth presents surprises. Some of the visuals were graphic, even for me, although watching movies on natural birth helped ease our fears.

Experience teaches me to plan ahead and visit the director of LDR ahead of time with my birth plan. I want to go home after birth and avoid going upstairs to postpartum with its own set of rules. She's okay with it, no problem. I appreciate the flexibility of this hospital.

My womb is now a complete round swishy fishbowl. During lunch on my due date, contractions come every twenty minutes. I thought they were Braxton Hicks. I had prepared mentally to go into labor late to avoid anxiety if the due date passed. I dislike the term "false labor." Instead, I think of my body "tuning up for the symphony."

At 11 pm, we go to bed. The squeezing contractions keep coming. "William, let's time these." Although five minutes apart, they felt manageable, like cramps. I called the midwife who says, "Phone me when you can't laugh." I want her to sleep and be rested when we go into full action. I call our doula to come over while my husband takes the dog to the pet-sitters. She goes back home within an hour.

I can't sleep. It's 3 a.m. I feel uncomfortable and want to move around. I call the doula to come back over. Spontaneously, I ask her to give me counter pressure. We stand about the same height. When a contraction comes, she stands behind me and holds in my lower abdomen muscles on either side above the pelvis. I brace. I'm curious as to dilation. The contractions come now like waves of strong menstrual cramps. I'm fine in between. Talking to other moms who labored naturally has helped me to stay calm, stay home, and avoid rushing to the hospital too soon.

At 5 a.m., labor picks up. I call Susan but can't talk during a contraction. "I'll meet you at the hospital," she says. I ask her if all the pre-admission paperwork is done so I don't need to bother with it. She confirms and says, "I'll be at the hospital before you get there." I waddle in my nightie, robe and slippers. We pack the car and our doula, Mara, follows us.

We get to LDR at 6 a.m. The doors automatically fly open. At the end of a long hall, the staff seated at a desk stares at us. A contraction. I brace against the wall. Mara gets behind me and provides counter pressure. I'm sure it looks peculiar, even humorous. Who cares? I know what I want, and am ready to say "no" to hospital protocol. Nobody will take my newborn away from me. I am a protective mama bear.

The midwife, doula, and a nurse are in the room with William and me. "She's got a waist. From behind, you don't look pregnant at all," the nurse said. Suddenly, something snaps inside me like a rubber band. I could hear it but nobody else did. My water breaks. I don't look down. It's like riding on a roller coaster. I'm not sure what's around the curve, but a force moves this birth right along. I hang onto the bed.

I remember something important. The group watches as I pull an altar out of my suitcase. "Here's my grandmother's embroidered handkerchief." I laid it on the table. On top I put a silver cross, a small bowl of water, a feather for air, a leaf for the earth and a family stone sculpture. I'm wearing my mother's purple robe, a pin in the shape of baby's feet from my educator and a purple chiffon scarf, to tie my hair back, from my mother-in-law. These women's birth energy remains with me. I wouldn't be here without them. The energy shifts from medical to reverent.

Never lying down in the bed, I try different positions. I don't care for the birth ball because it's not stable. If it stayed put between a chair and the bed, it would work better. I feel extremely heavy, like an elephant unable to support its weight. I can squat if there's a person on each side of me helping to hold me up. The lights seem too bright, we dim them. Evoking the relaxation response, I listen to the heartbeat with music tape that I heard during prenatal massage. Enya's music sounds good, too.

I need something for relief. The sensations feel strong yet bearable, but the hot water bottles that I packed could be nice. They're not hot enough, so Susan gives William a job.

"Take these towels, wet them and put them in these bags. Go down the hall to the break room and microwave them." He relays back and forth between two sets. HEAT: A great relief. William provides the pain management. It's getting closer. The waves come; the ocean churns. This is when it gets a bit rough. I promise you that you won't drown. You do come out on the other side. *You can birth your baby.* Your body is working beautifully. Yes, it's intense squeezing. Some call it pain, but it's not even like when the dentist hits a nerve in your tooth with the drill. That's a sharp hurt that sends me through the roof. Still, I need a life ring to cope.

"Susan, I need something." I'm not asking for drugs, because I'm not suffering. Anyone else in her position with medical training might take over at this point and order pain medication. That could be a mistake. I want to keep from feeling overwhelmed by the strength of these high waves. And birth is close. Her response is the *heartbeat* of this story. "Kalena, what do you need?" *What do I need?* Anyone else, like an obstetrician, could have easily taken command and ordered an epidural. Instead I get to choose and decide, "A hot bath."

I get in the tub. Ahhh. After a short soak, I feel the urge to push. Given my affinity for the ocean, I would have liked a water birth. But, it's time to get out; the hospital doesn't like babies born in water. *Why not?* It seems like the perfect place to be in active labor. Comforting. A great entry for the baby. Yet, I want to get this baby out. *Now*!

The feeling to push is remarkable. It's as if there's this strong internal signal, "Get the baby out." All on board, in action, down the hatch. A bowling ball-type pressure is in my pelvis. It's uncontrollable. I need to push. I want to *puuush*. A tidal wave is coming. The amazing thing for me is my whole pelvis opens and it doesn't hurt to push. However, it takes enormous strength. No place to be dainty; something between a sumo wrestler and an Olympic weight lifter. The grunting sounds I make are from deep within me giving all I've got to push the baby down and out. It's okay to make noise in birth. Completely focused, I dive under. Beneath the surface of fluid comes fire. Like Kilawea on the Big Island of Hawaii, I become a volcano. From out of the depths I didn't know existed, I summon strength I didn't know I had to bring forth new life. It's like the energy bulges up out of the ocean. I'm barely aware that my husband gets behind me on the bed to push up on my back. Susan puts a sheet over a bar for me to pull on. I try it, but it's not quite manageable.

A team of female nurses appear and tell me to push in a chorus. Where did they come from? They vanish. The doctor over the midwives comes in and says, "Don't be afraid to push." I dislike the word "afraid" enough to correct her, "Say *be brave* to push instead." It's all a bit of a blur.

"Do you want to see the crowning?" Okay. I think they'll hand me a small mirror like a hairdresser does, but no. They roll in a giant chalkboard sized mirror. No. I can't look. I might freak out if the head comes out and the baby stays there for a moment and looks around.

The electronic fetal monitor is uncomfortable. "Get that thing off me. NOW! I mean it." It interferes. Although the hospital's protocol is to monitor the heartbeat of the fetus, many times this equipment gives false information and increases cesareans. I can feel it internally or maybe the baby can and is unhappy with it. (Don't let them strap that thing to you continuously...and it's required with an epidural.)

It's 9:00 a.m. This is the hardest work ever. Breathing. Pushing. Squeezing. Exertion. Pure raw natural power. I become a fiery force, transcendent of time. I need to fully *feel* from the waist down to push. I feel a connection to my mother, grandmother, all women around the world, back to the beginning of time. PUUUUUSSHHH. At 9:20 a.m., a baby son, William Franklin is born, weighing 8 pounds and 4 ounces.

I hold our newborn and study his scrunched-up face. He keeps his eyes closed. I'm waiting for him to look at me, like the videos we saw. My husband cuts the umbilical cord after it stops pulsing. After 20 minutes, I put him to my breast. His eyes remain shut. I hardly notice the placenta delivery. I tore. Susan stitches me slowly.

Bleeding. Blood is on the sheets, running down my legs, everywhere. It's the aftermath, like lava flowing after the eruption. I don't realize how winded I felt until I need to go to the bathroom. I could walk slowly. After an hour, Franklin gets weighed in the room and his meconium diaper gets changed by his dad. I feel weak yet exhilarated, quite winded and triumphant, like a marathon runner must feel. My lungs are exhausted from the natural grunting of pushing. After all the work researching and psyching up, I birthed our son. The endorphin rush is indescribable. A calm washes over me.

Looking at the face of this innocent, pink baby, his tiny fingers around mine, we are his protectors. I smell the newness of his velvety smooth head. It's a great start for him. I bring him to my breast. He's alert, breathing and sucking. I feel great too, satisfied at having a birth that I wanted. We did it. No one can take this experience away from me.

As I nurse our newborn contentedly, I look over at my husband. He is sitting on the sofa, looking quite dazed, staring straight into the empty wall. Not only has William been up for over 24 hours, he viewed birth as an emergency event. Even though the baby and I did fine, he had no idea how it would turn out. He doesn't realize that he's holding two open Dr. Peppers, one in each hand.

The hospital released us six hours afterwards. Of course, not until I signed reams and reams of documents.

Did it hurt? Birth is not suffering; I never felt tortured. If I had been numb with medication, I seriously doubt I could have pushed that big boy out. I could have felt a sense of disappointment with that outcome. However, the midwife asked me, "What do you need?" I was respected to make the *choice*. And that made all the difference.

At home the next day, William says, "I loved you before, but now after witnessing Franklin's birth, my love for you is deeper." His eyes water. We embrace as husband and wife transformed: the birth of parents.

I took the road less traveled in childbirth today, not knowing what lay ahead. *You can, too.* For thousands of years, women took the same path. All the searching...trusting one's intuition...the courage to make choices...keeping the faith and bringing a sacred element to the birth. Powerful and yet humbling. A moment of awe. Our midwife smiles. Her positive approach...she simply let me be in charge, waiting for birth to happen *patiently*, allowing me to get in the tub instead of ordering drugs. I've encouraged others, "You can do it..." and they did. They expressed incredible joy and highly recommend natural childbirth. You have the right to be satisfied with your own birth event.

Instead of success or failure, birth is all about facing our fears, owning our own health and acting on it. Get informed. Make choices. Take a whole birth approach; get committed mentally, physically, spiritually and emotionally. Our confidence can easily be shaken during labor. But that same confidence can strengthen us for the next step.

I challenge you to make your own Birth Quest. Whatever the outcome of your pregnancy and labor, feel proud that you participated actively, not passively. No matter what the journey holds for you, honor your body and love your baby. Parenting is by far a much longer and more challenging process than birth. May you feel on top of the world when you hold your newborn. May you be empowered for motherhood.

Note: The Birth Plan, a one page example, is in the Appendix.

A Physician Transforms Birth
Despite Repercussions
Dr. Margaret Christensen's Story

At age twenty-five and pregnant with my first daughter, Caitlin, I naively believed I'd be fine with a few "huff and puff" birthing classes offered at the hospital. But I ended up strapped to a tiny laboring bed with Pitocin dripping in my arm, cranking out powerful contractions for eighteen hours in a claustrophobic room, overwhelmed with pain that I could no longer bear and struggling to hold on. My husband, Jim, stayed with me, held my hands and urged me to breathe deep. When I felt ready to give up, he encouraged me.

Two weeks earlier I had been swimming off Galveston's beaches, floating weightlessly, moving up and down with the swelling and receding waves, surrendering to the rhythms of the tide. With that memory in mind, I let go to the swells of labor, floating on the tide of a powerful Birthforce, feeling the ancient rhythms of life and death, joy and pain, surrender and release coursing through my body. I felt connected to all the women who had labored before me, as if they were carrying me along the waves of labor.

Oblivious to the cold sterility of the delivery room, soon I became overwhelmed by the powerful urge to push, and I felt the searing heat of Caitlin's head erupting from me as though I were an ancient volcano bringing forth new life. As I held her against my breast, she stared at me with wide open eyes and in that moment, I found God.

Little did I know that this experience was about to change my personal sense of self, my spiritual connection and the work I have chosen.

In my third year of medical school, I read in a college psychology class the pioneering book of Klaus and Kennel, *Parent-Infant Bonding*. Its exploration of an unmedicated woman's brain chemicals and hormones in the early stages of infant attachment and breastfeeding affirmed what I felt instinctively.

As a medical student, I became a labor support person, or "doula," for indigent women at a large county hospital. I saw the tenderness and compassion the nurse-midwives at Ben Taub Hospital used to help comfort and encourage the birthing women. As a future obstetrician, I wanted to know what these laboring women, who did not have access to epidurals, were experiencing.

In each of my births it was as if a gift had been sent with each child. From reading the book, *Mind Over Labor,* I learned to use visualization and imagery to enter into a transcendent state for my second labor. To the pulsing rhythms of Pink Floyd, my body opened with courage and joy as I melted into the labor pain. My strength welled up to birth a calm and serene 9 pound, 11 ounce boy, named Austin.

Jim helped catch our son. His loving presence and confidence rallied me to trust my body. Holding and nursing baby Austin, I felt boosted with confidence. Our six-year-old daughter, prepared by reading books and watching stories about birth in animals and people, also stood by my side.

Four weeks after Austin was born, I had to return to work. Imagery of flowing rivers of milk helped encourage the letdown response as I ran into the women residents' closet-sized bathroom between surgery cases to pump breast milk.

I expanded my knowledge of women birthing from the book, *Spiritual Midwifery* by Ina May Gaskin, and the evidence supporting the safety and efficacy of midwifery care in *A Good Birth, A Safe Birth* by Diana Korte and Roberta Scaer. I took the time to witness several home births, but incognito. I worried that if I got caught, there would be severe repercussions from my medical peers. They frowned on home births.

Michael's birth, during my first year of practice, brought the insight of the importance of a relaxed and "homey" environment, in the concept of a one-room labor delivery and recovery (LDR), needed for women and their families, as well as the determination to provide this at our hospital. At that time we continued to have the out-dated model of a woman laboring in one tiny room, moving to deliver in a sterile operating room and having the baby whisked away to the nursery. The mom went off to a recovery room, separated by thin curtains from other exhausted women with no privacy to enjoy these sacred first moments.

I had considered having Michael at home, knowing I was a low-risk candidate with access to a competent and experienced nurse-midwife. However, I was fearful that I would lose my hospital privileges if my colleagues found out. Hostility existed towards out-of-hospital births among the hospital's superiors. Instead I insisted, as a consumer, on having my own LDR in the postpartum suite of the seventh floor of the hospital. At the minimum, I wanted a bathtub to labor in.

When I went back to work, I carried my baby in a sling at my office, nursing him on demand with the approval and support of my patients.

Into my second year of practice, I recognized that something was missing in the medical model of how I had been taught. Much of what patients were coming in for was in reality physical manifestations of the psychological, emotional, cultural and spiritual issues affecting them. What they needed as much as medicine was someone to hear their story. At the same time I realized how much *I* needed to have a spiritual core from which to practice medicine. I couldn't expect to be fully present for my patients if I couldn't refill my *own* well that was being drained daily.

One Sunday, I went to church after years of not going. When I heard the words "Mother-Father God," it blew my mind open. It confirmed to me the feminine spirit, women's bodies, and our physical processes as the embodiment of the Sacred in human form. This connection fueled my determination to bring nurse-midwives into my practice, get them hospital privileges, and serve as back-up for a nurse-midwife-run birth center, despite tremendous negative pressure from many of my colleagues.

During my fourth pregnancy I learned how to stand up for myself and to have the strength and courage to let go of what was not working for me in my life. By now I was into my fourth year of successful private practice with a strong sense of who I was and my mission in life. Yet there was a lot of fear around what others (my colleagues at the hospital and my then physician partner) would think. I felt protective of a sacred being growing within and I didn't let anyone outside of my family know I was pregnant until I couldn't hide it any more. This would be my last baby and this was a special opportunity for me. My daughter would be born at the Birth and Women's Center (a freestanding birth center) instead of at the hospital.

I had always enjoyed being pregnant once I got over the initial fatigue and nausea. I loved the feeling of this new life doing flips inside of me, fluttering and kicking to let me know she was present. That kicking was something I always missed after the babies were born. Yet this last pregnancy was definitely harder on me. I already had three children, a full-time practice and was struggling in an unhealthy relationship with my physician partner. I felt much more tired, both physically and emotionally. Thank God my husband was home full-time at this point, as the primary caregiver for our children. He took superb care of us all, allowing me to conserve my energies for my work.

At thirty-seven-and-a-half weeks pregnant, I was operating on a patient one morning at the hospital when I felt a trickle running down my leg. *Damn, I was not ready yet.* And my mom, whom I had wanted to participate in this birth, was still on a trip to Argentina, not expected to return for another four days. I was tired, having been up the previous night doing a delivery. Oh well.

Canceling my office appointments for the afternoon, I went home to bed, praying that this trickle was an overfull bladder and not amniotic fluid. I felt no contractions yet but only noticed mild cramping. I warned Jim that this was the real deal. He went into a flurry of activity, calling backup for the kids and whirling through the house, cleaning and preparing to welcome us back home when we returned with a new little one.

Hoping I could stave off the contractions for a while so I could sleep, I crawled into bed. Jim came beside me at midnight and we snuggled together, trying to get some rest. After many sleepless nights delivering other babies, I had learned how to nap in short little increments. By two a.m. though, real labor began. We took Caitlin, age ten, with us. Jim's mom had the two younger ones.

When we walked into the birth center at 3 a.m., lit candles gave a surreal glow to the Victorian-styled bedroom. Soft music played in the background, the covers of the lace canopy bed were turned down, and the Jacuzzi tub had been filled with warm water. I took in the pure beauty, a warm welcome by the midwives that touched my soul and brought me to tears. All of my births in the hospital had been good experiences, but something always seemed to be missing. That *something* was the acknowledgement that birth was more than physical, it was sacred.

First, I unpacked the things to create an altar, representing my family and friends who were with me in spirit, and honoring my ancestors. I brought tokens acknowledging the future and the strengths, gifts, and grace that I would need to face the challenges ahead. We said a prayer of gratitude for this place of holiness. I was able to fully focus on the powerful rhythms welling up within me.

I sat on a large yoga ball, Jim massaging my back, and Caitlin gently wiping my face with a washcloth. The certified nurse-midwives (CNMs) were quietly supportive, sensing that I needed their presence, yet allowing me to labor, and my husband and daughter to participate. I knew I was moving fast and started to feel overwhelmed. I had forgotten: this was hard work. I got into the tub and felt the soothing, calming water support me as Caitlin poured warm water over my belly with each contraction. This was her third birth to witness. What she was learning was that birth was a normal, healthy process, a joyful, sacred event, that women were strong and capable of bringing forth new life, that the pain involved was not insurmountable, and the belief in God's presence would carry us through our struggles.

At 5 a.m. I wanted to get in the bed; I knew things were close. Jim sat behind me, cradling my body with his strength and I focused with my eyes closed, connecting with this tiny being in my belly who was being swept forth into this world by ancient, primal forces. I opened up and let go of control and my fear.

I reached down and could feel her crowning. It felt like a fiery sensation. I held my hand there with warm washcloths that the midwives had provided and eased her out. The midwife said, "You do it, Margaret. You birth your own baby." And as her head and shoulders eased out, I reached down with both hands under her arms, as I had instructed many of my clients to do, and lifted her onto my belly. Jim held us both and Caitlin climbed onto the bed to kiss her newborn sister, Madeleine Celeste, meaning a "gift from Heaven."

After a warm herbal bath, we shared a sumptuous feast prepared by Mara, my wonderful doula. After birth, Grandma Dolly brought in Madeleine's two big brothers, ages six and four, to meet their new baby sister. We ate together as a family and the children went back home, Jim and I slept for two hours, nestled in the big canopy bed, while Madeleine nursed contentedly at my breast. By 11 a.m. we were ready to go. Outside the fog felt cool on that March morning. The whole experience had felt magical.

In giving birth to four amazing children, they each in turn brought important gifts to me which I'm thankful for. Finding God, visualizing and transcending during birth, bringing the one-room LDR for women and their babies to the hospital, standing up for myself and even letting go of what wasn't working helped me grow as a woman and mother. Discovering the missing piece—the sacredness of birth—complimented my training as a physician, especially as an obstetrician and gynecologist.

Express Delivery at the Hampton Inn
Shannon's Story

Shannon, a beautiful graphic designer with long, thick hair, is married to a commercial photographer, Jack. She had two babies and labored both ways, numb and natural.

In her first labor, her water broke and a doctor discovered that her baby was in the posterior position. Her dream of a natural childbirth disintegrated. She was transferred from the birth center to a hospital, enduring an epidural.

For her second birth, Shannon chose a midwife, who advised, "You have to make a decision: Do you think birth is *naturally* safe or unsafe?" Learn how Shannon's second labor happens even though it's unexpectedly at a hotel.

The girl next to me in Bradley class said, "Just hope you don't have *posterior labor.*"

"Oh, that won't happen to me," I vowed.

I was nervous about giving birth at home and went to a birth center.

During labor, I was having pain in my back. *I went somewhere else in my mind.* I was transferred from the birth center to the hospital at five a.m., and given an epidural.

The doctor told me my baby, Emma, is posterior and turned her half way. An hour later, the baby turned the whole way. I dilated to 10 centimeters. I was still under the influence of the epidural, yet I could push effectively.

My twin sister, Shelley, encouraged me, "You can do it." I delivered vaginally two hours later. I was happy that I didn't have to have a C-section. Everything was fine.

The staff took her away. At that moment, I wished I hadn't gone to the hospital. I felt strange. I was out of it. Shaking. I didn't feel connected to Emma. I *really* wanted that feeling. For nine months I carried her and I felt all of her movements. Then she was taken from me.

I felt like I didn't have anything to do with her birth. It was all sort of happening *around* me, rather than happening *in* me. When you are numb, you can push, but it's not nearly as rewarding. All these other people are doing stuff *to* you. Your baby's not doing it *with* you; you're not doing it *with* your baby.

I like natural things. Intervening deviates from the natural process. Birth is naturally safe. Complications happen. But many medical professionals make you feel you can't birth. They don't say "you're not quite good enough to bring a baby into the world," but they intervene a lot.

For my second birth, I became informed. I kept fit, walked and did squats. We lived in a third floor apartment and I always took the stairs.

I was thirty-eight when pregnant with Audry. We didn't have a home because we were moving. That caused lots of stress. I was sick as a dog with the croup and the flu. Emma had the croup and Jack had the flu. We were all sick. We ended up in the emergency room a week before we had Audry. I think that's why I developed high blood pressure.

I chose a home-birth midwife. But ten days before my due date, I went back to an obstetrical and gynecological practice. I felt more and more anxious and needed to know that I could go to the hospital *if* I needed to, where our first daughter was born. I wanted to go somewhere I had been, but I wanted it to be the birth I wanted. I had already delivered vaginally, so I think, *okay, one baby has gone down.* That was reassurance.

That's why we went with a certified nurse-midwife (CNM), who worked in a hospital. I had already seen her, talked to her, and knew her. She said, "We'll take you." I wanted to cry. I thought that was the nicest thing you could ever do. The lay midwife would be our doula if we went to the hospital. "Come over right now," she said. The doctor checked me out. I felt relieved. I needed to know that I was taken care of by the right people with a backup plan.

When I went into labor, we were staying at the Hampton Inn Hotel before moving into our new home. I called my parents, "You've got to come get Emma." In the bathtub, I visualized the pink turtleneck coming over the baby's head that we had learned in childbirth class. I moaned.

I got out of the tub and called my doula. The hospital midwife had said earlier, "When your contractions are three minutes apart, come in to the office."

"I have to push," I said to Shelley, who was with me. She immediately called Jack.

"Hurry up and get here!" she said. He made it in eighteen minutes. She called our family to bring the birth kit.

Susan, the home birth midwife, arrived. She calmly said, "You're letting your energy go out the top of your head. Let it push through your body and out your bottom." She was sure of herself, "You're doing great." Susan never asked me to move. My favorite position was to stay on my right side. She was quiet, never touched me, and was respectful. We didn't even have the birth kit yet.

I'd describe labor as menstrual cramps. My cervix opened, and all of a sudden, I had the urge to push. To me, it was painful. I pushed three times. Didn't like pushing, hated it. But my husband helped. He got behind me with one foot against the wall. It felt incredible this time. The baby was inside me and *I* pushed her out. Susan caught our baby, Audry. I held her and rubbed in the vernix. It was Jack and me, bringing our newborn daughter into the world.

Even though labor was hard, it was such a *better* experience. There wasn't anything bad about it. It felt *really* powerful, even overwhelming at times. But, it was this process. There was never anything about it that didn't seem like she was part of me and I was connected to her. It was my job to birth her. At 1 a.m., Audry Hampton, weighing 10 pounds, 4 ounces, slept on her dad's chest for three hours. Jack was in heaven.

Since the birth of Emma, I have felt more *sure* of myself. I feel more confident in *every* part of my life.

The number-one problem with birth is nursing afterward. You don't learn it from your sister or mother. It's hard. You can watch a mom nurse her baby and think, *oh yeah, I can do that*. Then when you have your own baby, you think you can't go through with it, or you don't get into it. Keep at it. I nurse on demand and I'm proud of nursing my babies.

(Shannon nursed Audry while sharing her birth story.)

Whoosh!

Michelle's Story

I was not opposed to natural birth, but had no conviction to do it. A friend had an epidural with her first, but did not with her other two. She advised me, "Focus on the end result; pain is moving the child to you. It's a finite period, with pain playing a purpose."

Let me tell you how my first medicated birth was compared to my second natural birth. With my first baby, Andrew, I had dilated to 3 centimeters the week before. When I first got contractions, I thought, *This is easy. What are people complaining about?* At 11:00 p.m. I awoke, and they were stronger. My water broke at home. We went to the hospital at 4 a.m. and I gave birth at 11:00 a.m., in seven hours' time. I considered myself strong and stoic, yet I was surprised how much the contractions hurt and knocked me off balance. The epidural was given to me at 8:30 a.m. and went into effect at 9:00 a.m. But I think I was already in the transition stage, throwing up.

If I had studied more, and knew what to expect naturally, perhaps I would know I was close to pushing. I felt like crying. "Get your shoulders away from your ears and relax," the nurse said. The epidural helped relax me. I could feel the contractions but without the pain, and I could still push.

My second son, Jack Henry, came two weeks early. I had a check-up that day, with a pelvic exam showing 2.5 centimeters dilated and 90 percent effaced. I called my mother-in-law, who was in Arlington, Texas, to stand by.

At 10:30 p.m., I felt bloated, like I had a lot of gas. An hour later, the contractions were eight to nine minutes apart and coming faster each time: seven minutes apart, six minutes, five minutes. Labor happened a lot faster this time. We called the hospital. "Stay at home as long as possible," the nurse said.

"I need to come now!" We flew out of our house at 12:50 a.m., arrived for admittance at 1:05 a.m., and delivered at 1:59 a.m. It was an exhilarating 54-minute experience at the hospital.

Nobody on staff seemed to realize it was happening as fast as I did. At first, it was as if they weren't taking me seriously. The nurse didn't help me. I had a lot of rectal pressure. The urge to push was *overwhelming*. It took over.

"I need to push like a bowel movement, *bad,*" I told my husband, "and I can't stop it from coming. Go, tell the nurse." He did.

"Okay," she said, running out into the hall hollering, "I need a doctor right now."

The anesthesiologist came in and started an IV. "I feel like pushing," I told him.

"You may be too far along for an epidural," he said. "You could have this baby in ten minutes. You may have to go naturally."

My first reaction was, "But I didn't do the *natural* childbirth classes." I panicked for a full minute. My husband was supportive and strong, with a calm look on his face. He looked me in the eyes and said confidently, "You can do this."

"I feel the baby's hair; the baby is about to crown," the nurse said.

I felt like a wild animal, making high pitched noises. I was told to concentrate, focus, pant like a puppy between pushes. Afterward, what hurt the most was the stitches. I had so much adrenaline that my legs were shaking when I had to put my legs up for the doctor.

I feel sorry for any birthing woman who doesn't have a supportive partner. For example, my mother, whom I have a great relationship with, was nervous and upset to see me in labor pain.

If I give birth a third time, I'd like to go natural. I felt powerful afterward. I feel confident in what my body can do—the wisdom it has at working the *miracle* of childbirth.

Note: A common problem in hospitals that are used to routine epidurals, is that the newer nursing staff may be inexperienced with the labor of unmedicated women. The nurses don't know how to support and calm the mothers and are unaware of the stages of natural labor.

A VBAC Waterbirth at Home

"Fear, through the attitude of the practitioner, causes the throat to close down. Trust, an attitude that a mom uses to relax herself, helps the throat open, then the cervix."—Robbie Davis-Floyd, Ph.D.

Robbie, a social anthropologist and author in Austin, Texas, experienced a cesarean with the birth of her first child, Peyton. Her second birth was a vaginal birth after cesarean (VBAC) waterbirth at home. "Laboring in water seemed like a good idea. *Intuition* told me that it would be three days, a long haul," Robbie recalled. Her time getting ready for her second birth paid off—physically, mentally, and spiritually—in the natural delivery of a 10-pound son, Jason.

Robbie encouraged author Kalena Cook to see a remarkable birth center in Taos, New Mexico.[1] She helped her to reconnect with an advocate of waterbirth and dolphins, Rima Star,[2] and inspired Kalena to make a difference by affecting twenty percent of all births toward natural—a difference she wanted to make through this book.

Studying birth from around the world, Robbie says that birth, a life passage, reflects a lot about the values of our society. In Polynesia, women are revered during pregnancy and birth, participating in special rituals, like rubbing coconut oil on the pregnant mom's belly. Contrast that to Bangladesh, where menstruation and birth are thought of as "dirty." Midwives don't exist in Bangladesh.

An ardent advocate for women's natural birth here in the U.S., Robbie helped draft the "Mother Friendly Childbirth Initiative" for the Coalition for Improving Maternity Services (CIMS).[3] One excerpt reads, "Current maternity and newborn practices that contribute to high costs and inferior outcomes include the inappropriate application of technology and routine procedures that are not based on scientific evidence."

CIMS promotes normalcy of birth, empowerment in a woman's confidence to birth and care for her baby, give birth as she wishes with respect, and more.

"Creating the initiative was marked by a comet traveling across the starry sky," Robbie says. It happened over their retreat that night on Mount Madonna, California.

Robbie has written several books including, *Birth as an American Rite of Passage*.[4] In her book she compares two kinds of *birth models* and below are a few examples:

Technocratic	Holistic
body = machine	body = organism
pregnancy/birth inherently dysfunctional	pregnancy/birth inherently healthy
mind is above, separate from body	mind and body are one
supremacy of technology	sufficiency of nature
importance of science, things	importance of people
institution = significant social unit	family = essential social unit
pain is unacceptable	pain is acceptable
labor = a mechanical process	labor = a flow of experience
time is important; adherence to time charts	time is irrelevant; the flow of a woman's experience during labor
the doctor controls	the midwife supports, assists
the doctor delivers the baby	the mother gives birth to the baby

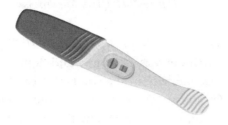

Get Informed and Shop Around

In a perfect world, you could trust that all things are safe for you. In reality, we have been blessed with a curious and discerning brain and a woman's remarkable intuition to help us make safe decisions for ourselves. You have a choice in pregnancy and birth: either get informed and make decisions or remain naive.

If you favor natural birth, do you want an experienced caregiver, personal service or straight-forward care? In selecting the right physician or midwife at the right hospital, birth center, or a home birth, consider the following questions.

Having a Baby? 10 Questions to Ask

Have you decided how to have your baby? The choice is yours.

First, learn as much as you can about all your choices. There are many different ways of caring for you and your baby during labor and birth.

Birthing care that is better and healthier for mothers and babies is called "mother-friendly." Some birth places or settings are more mother-friendly than others and that's important to your outcome. When you are deciding *where* to have your baby, you can choose from different places such as a:

- birth center,
- hospital, or
- home birth service.

In 2000, the Coalition for Improving Maternity Services (CIMS) came up with 10 things to look for and ask about, all supported by medical research. These are the best ways to provide mother-friendly care.

1. *"Who can be with me during labor and birth?"*

Mother-friendly birth centers, hospitals, and home birth services will let a birthing mother decide whom she wants to have with her during the birth. This includes fathers, partners, children, family members, or friends.

They will let a birthing mother have with her a doula, a person who has special training in helping women cope with labor and birth. A doula never leaves the birthing mother alone. She encourages her, comforts her, and helps her understand what's happening. Mother-friendly places have midwives as part of their staff so a birthing mother can have one with her if she chooses.

2. *"What happens during a normal labor and birth?"*

If caregivers give mother-friendly care, they will openly tell you how they handle *every part* of the birthing process. For example, how often do they give the mother a drug to speed up the birth? Or do they usually let labor and birth happen on its own timing?

Mother-friendly caregivers tell you how often they do certain procedures. For example, they will have a record of the percentage of C-sections (cesarean births) done annually. If the number is too high, you'll want to consider having your baby elsewhere.

Numbers we recommend you ask about.

- How frequently is Pitocin used? Oxytocin (a drug known as Pitocin) should not be used to start or speed up labor for more than one in ten women (10 percent).
- How often are episiotomies done? An episiotomy (ee-peezee-AH-tummy) should not be needed on more than one in five women, hopefully less. (An episiotomy is a cut in the opening to the vagina to make it larger for birth. It is not necessary most of the time.)
- What is their C-section rate? Ideally it should be no more than 10 percent if it's a community hospital. The rate should be 15 percent or less in hospitals for high-risk mothers and babies.

3. *"How do you allow for differences in culture and beliefs?"*

Mother-friendly birth centers, hospitals, and home birth services are sensitive to the mother's culture: differing beliefs, values, and customs.

4. *"Can I walk and move around during labor? What birth position do you suggest?"*

In mother-friendly settings, you can walk around and move about as you choose during labor. You can choose the most comfortable positions that work best for you during both labor and birth. (There may be a medical reason for you to be in a certain position.) Mother-friendly settings almost never put a woman flat on her back with her legs up in stirrups.

5. *"How do you make sure everything goes smoothly when my nurse, doctor, midwife, or agency need to work with each other?"*

Ask, "Can my doctor or midwife come with me if I have to be moved to another place during labor? Can you help me find people or agencies in my community who can help me before and after the baby is born?"

Mother-friendly places and people will have a specific plan for keeping in touch with the other people who are caring for you. They will talk to others who give you birth care. They will help you find people or agencies in your community to help you. For example, they may put you in touch with someone who can help you with breastfeeding.

6. *"What things do you normally do to a woman in labor?"*

Experts say some methods of care during labor and birth are healthier for mothers and babies. Medical research demonstrates which methods work best. Mother-friendly settings use methods proven effective by scientific evidence. But some birth centers, hospitals, and home birth services use unproven methods. For example, research has shown it's usually not helpful to break the amniotic sac.

That's why we recommend you ask about procedures that *should not be done.* Among them:
- They should not keep track of the baby's heart rate all the time with an electronic fetal monitor. Instead, it is best to have your nurse or midwife listen to the baby's heart from time to time.
- They should not break your bag of waters early in labor.
- They should not routinely use an IV to give you fluids.
- They should not tell you that you can't eat or drink during labor.

A birth center, hospital, or home birth service that does these things for most of the mothers is not mother-friendly. Remember, these should not be used without a special medical reason.

7. *"How do you help mothers stay as comfortable as they can be? Besides drugs, how do you help mothers relieve the pain of labor?"*

The people who care for you should know how to help you cope with labor. They should know about ways of dealing with your pain that don't use drugs. All drugs affect the baby. They should suggest "comfort measures" such as changing your position, relaxing in a warm bath, having a massage and using music. These comfort measures help you handle your labor more easily and help you feel more in control.

8. *"What if my baby is born early or has special problems?"*

Mother-friendly places and people will encourage mothers and families to touch, hold, breastfeed, and care for their babies as much as they can, even if your baby is born early or has a medical problem. However, in rare circumstances there may be a special medical reason why you shouldn't hold and care for your baby.

9. *"Do you circumcise babies?"*

Medical research does not show a need to circumcise baby boys. It is painful and risky. Mother-friendly birth places discourage circumcision unless there are religious reasons.

10. *"How do you help mothers who want to breastfeed?"*

The World Health Organization made the following list of ways birth services support breastfeeding:

- They tell all pregnant mothers why and how to breastfeed.
- They help you start breastfeeding within one hour after birth.
- They show you how to breastfeed, and how to keep your milk coming in if you have to be away from your baby for work.
- They encourage you and the baby to stay together all day and all night. This is called "rooming-in."
- They encourage you to feed your baby whenever he or she wants to nurse (feeding on demand), rather than at certain scheduled times.
- They should not give pacifiers ("dummies " or "soothers") to breast-fed babies.
- They encourage you to join a group of mothers who breastfeed and tell you how to contact a group near you.
- They have a written policy on breastfeeding. All the employees know about and use the ideas in the policy.
- They teach employees the skills they need to carry out these steps.
- Newborns should have only breast milk.

For more information visit: www.motherfriendly.org

Build Your Birth Team

Women are good at shopping. We buy based on the criteria of personal service, quality, safety, selection, convenience, timeliness and value or price. Why not shop around to find the right health provider for you? Visit caregivers and tour hospitals or birth centers. Even if you feel influenced by your insurance, know that some women have gotten coverage of their choice—like a birth center—by writing a letter.

"It is inherently unwise, and perhaps unsafe, for women with normal pregnancies to be cared for by obstetric specialists, even if the required personnel were available...Midwives and general practitioners, on the other hand, are primarily oriented to the care of women with normal pregnancies, and are likely to have more detailed knowledge of the particular circumstances of individual women."
—A Guide to Effective Care in Pregnancy and Childbirth

Who you feel safe with and supported best by is as important as where you birth. Interview: meet and greet. Then pick your team.

An Obstetrician-Gynecologist
If you select an obstetrician, their extensive training includes surgery. They typically come to assist at the pushing stage, before the delivery of the baby. Ask your physician, "How do you feel about natural birth?" Find out if the doctor is board eligible or board certified. Besides medical doctors and doctors of osteopathy who specialize in obstetrics and gynecology, some family physicians also provide delivery services.

A Midwife
• Certified Nurse-Midwives (CNMs) - have a nursing degree and midwifery education. The American College of Nurse-Midwives (ACNM) accredits the educational program and gives an exam. Currently there are over 10,700 members. Most CNMs practice in hospitals and birth centers with a C-section ratc of only 11.6 percent.

• Certified Professional Midwives (CPMs) - education may come through a variety of routes. The North American Registry of Midwives (NARM) evaluates skills and experience, with a written exam and assessment for certification.

• Direct Entry Midwives - are licensed in some states, like Texas, and are not required to become nurses first. The Midwifery Education and Accreditation Council (MEAC) accredits direct-entry educational programs and apprenticeships. They practice in home or birth center births.

A manager of a small Hawaiian hospital describes her two births with different providers. "My son was born with a physician in a hospital. I had an epidural which numbed me. It was exciting to have my son.

"My daughter was born with a midwife and the experience felt much better, less invasive. The midwives know what stage you are in by looking at your face. They don't check you so often for how effaced you are. They say, 'You're getting closer.' It was amazing, a real spiritual experience for me. Even though there was pain, it felt good because I had support."

One kind of training isn't necessarily better than another. Experience, where a midwife practices, and chemistry all play a part in choosing the right provider.

What is a Doula?

Doula, a Greek word, means a woman serving another woman. In labor, a **Birth Doula** is professionally trained to provide labor support. In ancient art, two women are shown with the birthing mom. One is the midwife and the other is supporting the laboring woman from behind or beside her as the doula.

A **Postpartum Doula** cares for the mom and newborn, gives breastfeeding support and advice, cooks, provides child care, runs errands and lightly cleans the home.

A Doula's View of Birth
Mara Black, Lay Midwife & Doula

Since 1975, Mara has been a founding member of the North Texas Midwifery Association. Her training included an apprenticeship with Barbara Cook for eighteen months, doing prenatals, clinicals, births, and postpartum. She became documented as a direct-entry midwife with the Texas Department of Health. She works at a birth center and has attended over 400 births.

I started helping friends with home births in the early 70s in Philadelphia. My mother had her babies at home and I continued the circle. A famous midwife, Lisa Goldstein, assisted the birth of my daughter, Lucia. I was in labor for eighteen hours. Two years later in Dallas, I had a son, Sammy. My third child was Joe. Their labors took six hours each.

Before, doctors resented direct-entry midwives, especially if a woman had complications and she had to be brought to the hospital. Their attitude has changed more favorably towards us now.

What I like best about my work is helping women with the joy and exhilaration of giving birth. Being part of a team works better for me versus being an independent midwife. I don't have the overhead expense and I do less paperwork. I'm instrumental in the childbirth itself, the spirituality of it, and the excitement. I like to give women encouragement for natural birth: the recovery is wonderful.

The most challenging aspect is managing my energy. If I've been up all night, I'm exhausted and barely have enough energy to take my contacts out.

Women seem to be compassionate in labor. They don't want to be too noisy, they're self conscious—excusing themselves and being apologetic. Sometimes it is hard for them to receive care. I compare a laboring mom to a three-year-old who doesn't know what she wants and is out of sorts. When I get a call from a client, I can tell in her voice if she needs me to be there with her.

Supportive things I share with expectant moms: Being awake and alert, it's courageous to have a baby this way. You feel strong. Pushing a baby out, feels soooo good. All the senses are there. No matter how tired one is, it's euphoric and better than any orgasm.

I do support women who have to have C-sections or epidurals. They want doulas, too. Some are tightened up like a lock and they need an epidural to relax.

The difference with induced labor is the birth process is done *to* you, someone *else* is working on your body as opposed to *you* doing it. For natural labor, listen to your body wisdom. It knows what to do.

Birth works by instinct. It's intuitive. Hispanic women that I've seen know how to let go. Whereas Anglo women read, but they need to understand that they need to allow the natural process to happen.

All births are awe inspiring. If they weren't, it would be boring to have to stay up all night for.

Take Childbirth Classes

Childbirth classes will help you network with others who are on the same journey, perhaps for the first time. The following classes include techniques and methods for having natural childbirth:

Bradley Husband-Coached Method

Classes are usually taught outside of the hospital. The husband plays a role in the birth by actively supporting his wife. Most attendees (over 90 percent) birth drug-free. Instructors cover natural childbirth, nutrition, relaxation and natural breathing, tuning in to your body, the husband as a coach, immediate contact with your new baby and breastfeeding starting at birth.

Birthing From Within®

Before her cesarean, Pam England (author and founder) believed women could avoid cesareans and other interventions by arming themselves with information, a positive attitude and a birth plan. Now she offers a multi-sensory approach to childbirth preparation including doing artwork.

Mentors believe that childbirth is a profound rite of passage, not a medical event (even when medical care is part of the birth). They teach parents the power of birthing-in-awareness, even when their birth experience is not what they had anticipated. They create a safe, nurturing class environment which invites parents to discover their personal strength and wisdom. They balance practical, useful information with introspective, multi-sensory experiences.

Birthing From Within teaches about birth from four perspectives: mother, father, baby and culture. Mentors help parents build a pain-coping mindset so they may fully participate in birth's rite of passage. Birthing From Within classes are not the end, but the beginning of a parent's journey.

Women state their top four favorites from this method are:
1. Telling them birth hurts,
2. Suggesting make noise like a coyote,
3. Creating art—most couldn't wait to try, and
4. Reading stories helps make them see birth personally.

Lamaze or Hospital Classes

Started by Dr. Lamaze, this method teaches breathing techniques to use during labor. Lamaze is usually taught in a hospital setting. Their philosophy of birth includes:

- Birth is normal, natural and healthy.
- The experience of birth profoundly affects women and their families.
- Women's inner wisdom guides them through birth.
- Women's confidence and ability to give birth is either enhanced or diminished by the care provider and place of birth.
- Women have the right to give birth free from routine medical interventions.
- Birth can safely take place in birth centers and homes.
- Childbirth education empowers women to make informed choices in healthcare, to assume responsibility for their health and to trust their inner wisdom.

However, depending on the hospital and who is teaching these philosophies, points may or may not be supported. Many hospital classes specifically prepare you for and are oriented towards epidurals and interventions.

Hypnotherapy

Women have benefitted from hypnotherapy for childbirth. Bette Epstein, a Hypnotherapist and trainer, shares in Chapter 11 how she works with clients. Hypnobirthing by Maria Mongan teaches relaxation techniques to eliminate fear, tension, and pain (although they avoid using that "p" word, pain). However, one mom who gave birth after taking Hypnobirthing said, "When contractions came right on top of each other in active labor and began to hurt, I felt I was doing something wrong."

Birth Works

For prior vaginal or cesarean births and VBACs, these classes help women gain confidence in their ability to birth. Classes help birth companions become aware of ways they can make labor safer and more comfortable. They are interactive and provide both a physical and emotional preparation for birth. Their program is suitable for parents planning a hospital, birthing center or home birth.

Due Dates

Did you know there is more than one way to predict an estimated due date (EDD)? The date was never meant to be cast in stone as "the" day. At best, it is a "guesstimate" even if you know your last menstruation. Average gestation of a baby happens over forty weeks, so caregivers know there may be reason for concern if labor happens either more than two weeks prior to the due date or up to two weeks past the date.

If you are healthy and have a normal pregnancy, your baby will trigger a chain reaction to set off labor. Michel Odont, M.D., calls it a "hormonal cocktail" that allows a bonding process to take place between mother and child. However, when delivery dates are preset with inductions or scheduled cesareans, the normal birth process is short-circuited.

Towards the end of nine months, with extra weight gain and extra fluids, you feel ready to be done with your pregnancy. We recommend you mentally prepare to use your due date as the beginning point of a within-the-week target. In other words, *don't sweat the due date.* Instead, enjoy your naps. Read up on breastfeeding. Babies arrive anywhere from 38 to 42 weeks which is considered normal.

Following are seven ways to calculate your due date. Ovulation occurs about 14 days before bleeding. However, not all women have 28-day cycles. When calculating your due date, consider the following:

1. What is the average length of your cycle?
2. Is your cycle regular?
3. What is the first day of the last two normal periods?
4. What date do you think you conceived?
5. Do you use contraceptives?
6. Ovulation can occur with orgasm and you may sense when you got pregnant.

Ways to Calculate Your Due Date:

1. Gestation Wheel
   a. Pointer on inner wheel on the date of last normal menstrual period (LNMP). The forty week pointer will fall on the expected date of birth.
   b. Conception date - ovulation pointer is placed on the probable fertilization date.

2. Naegele's Rule: A formula from 1709, but predicts using a 28-day cycle

From date of last menstrual period   _____

- subtract 3 months =   _____

+ add 7 days   =   _____ EDD

iPhone apps also predict due dates based on Naegele's rule.

3. Lunar Cycle: The phases of the moon, occurring within twenty-nine days, were used by women for thousands of years. Counting gestation at 290 days or from last menstruation, ten lunar months. (When using last day of menstruation, to Naegele's formula above, the date is similar to lunar months of 29 days.)

4. Wood's Method: A nurse-midwife professor saw flaws in due dates and came up with a more accurate way to consider varied cycles of women.

+ Add one year to first day of last menstrual period   _____

First time moms:

subtract 2 months and 2 weeks (or 14 days)   _____

Multiparas (has more than one child) subtract two months
and 2.5 weeks (or 18 days)   _____

+ Add or subtract the number of days her cycle varies
from 28 days.   _____

5. Simple Math

Add 266 days (38 weeks x 7 days) to date of conception,
or add five months to date of first definite quickening.

6. Mittendorf's Study: from thirty-one first-time uncomplicated pregnancies and eighty-three multiparas, length of pregnancy from first day of last period:

288 days for first time (note two days shorter than Lunar)

283 days for multiparas

7. Other Factors: Studies show that black or African American women tend to have 8 1/2 days shorter gestation than Caucasians.

Due Dates

Table 1: Estimated Due Dates from *Spiritual Midwifery*

Find the month and first day of your last menstrual period. Circle it. The date below, on *indented line* is the EDD.

Month	1	2	3	4	5	6	7	8	9	10	11	12	13	14	15	16	17	18	19	20	21	22	23	24	25	26	27	28	29	30	31	
Jan.	1	2	3	4	5	6	7	8	9	10	11	12	13	14	15	16	17	18	19	20	21	22	23	24	25	26	27	28	29	30	31	Jan.
Oct.	8	9	10	11	12	13	14	15	16	17	18	19	20	21	22	23	24	25	26	27	28	29	30	31	1	2	3	4	5	6	7	*Nov.*
Feb.	1	2	3	4	5	6	7	8	9	10	11	12	13	14	15	16	17	18	19	20	21	22	23	24	25	26	27	28				Feb.
Nov.	8	9	10	11	12	13	14	15	16	17	18	19	20	21	22	23	24	25	26	27	28	29	30	1	2	3	4	5				*Dec.*
Mar.	1	2	3	4	5	6	7	8	9	10	11	12	13	14	15	16	17	18	19	20	21	22	23	24	25	26	27	28	29	30	31	Mar.
Dec.	6	7	8	9	10	11	12	13	14	15	16	17	18	19	20	21	22	23	24	25	26	27	28	29	30	31	1	2	3	4	5	*Jan.*
Apr.	1	2	3	4	5	6	7	8	9	10	11	12	13	14	15	16	17	18	19	20	21	22	23	24	25	26	27	28	29	30		Apr.
Jan.	6	7	8	9	10	11	12	13	14	15	16	17	18	19	20	21	22	23	24	25	26	27	28	29	30	31	1	2	3	4		*Feb.*
May	1	2	3	4	5	6	7	8	9	10	11	12	13	14	15	16	17	18	19	20	21	22	23	24	25	26	27	28	29	30	31	May
Feb.	5	6	7	8	9	10	11	12	13	14	15	16	17	18	19	20	21	22	23	24	25	26	27	28	1	2	3	4	5	6	7	*Mar.*
June	1	2	3	4	5	6	7	8	9	10	11	12	13	14	15	16	17	18	19	20	21	22	23	24	25	26	27	28	29	30		Jun.
Mar.	8	9	10	11	12	13	14	15	16	17	18	19	20	21	22	23	24	25	26	27	28	29	30	31	1	2	3	4	5	6		*Apr.*
July	1	2	3	4	5	6	7	8	9	10	11	12	13	14	15	16	17	18	19	20	21	22	23	24	25	26	27	28	29	30	31	July
Apr.	7	8	9	10	11	12	13	14	15	16	17	18	19	20	21	22	23	24	25	26	27	28	29	30	1	2	3	4	5	6	7	*May*
Aug.	1	2	3	4	5	6	7	8	9	10	11	12	13	14	15	16	17	18	19	20	21	22	23	24	25	26	27	28	29	30	31	Aug.
May	8	9	10	11	12	13	14	15	16	17	18	19	20	21	22	23	24	25	26	27	28	29	30	31	1	2	3	4	5	6	7	*June*
Sept.	1	2	3	4	5	6	7	8	9	10	11	12	13	14	15	16	17	18	19	20	21	22	23	24	25	26	27	28	29	30		Sept.
June	8	9	10	11	12	13	14	15	16	17	18	19	20	21	22	23	24	25	26	27	28	29	30	1	2	3	4	5	6	7		*July*
Oct.	1	2	3	4	5	6	7	8	9	10	11	12	13	14	15	16	17	18	19	20	21	22	23	24	25	26	27	28	29	30	31	Oct.
July	8	9	10	11	12	13	14	15	16	17	18	19	20	21	22	23	24	25	26	27	28	29	30	31	1	2	3	4	5	6	7	*Aug.*
Nov.	1	2	3	4	5	6	7	8	9	10	11	12	13	14	15	16	17	18	19	20	21	22	23	24	25	26	27	28	29	30		Nov.
Aug.	8	9	10	11	12	13	14	15	16	17	18	19	20	21	22	23	24	25	26	27	28	29	30	31	1	2	3	4	5	6		*Sept.*
Dec.	1	2	3	4	5	6	7	8	9	10	11	12	13	14	15	16	17	18	19	20	21	22	23	24	25	26	27	28	29	30	31	Dec.
Sept.	7	8	9	10	11	12	13	14	15	16	17	18	19	20	21	22	23	24	25	26	27	28	29	30	1	2	3	4	5	6	7	*Oct.*

Sutter Davis Hospital
Leon Schimmel M.D. and Barbara Boehler, C.N.M.,
with Ellen Kassing, R.N.

On the family farm in Iowa, eleven-year-old Leon greased up and reached into the fattened laboring pig to help pull the piglet out. His hands were much smaller than his dad's, who looked on with approval, his breath visible in the chilly barn air at dawn.

Little did the boy know that he began a life path with all of its challenges and rewards. He would even curiously watch artificial insemination of the cows. "I liked working with animals, but not the conditions of twenty degrees *below* zero."

Later in college, an interest in biology shifted towards pre-med. During his internship, he liked a broad base, yet wanted a beginning and end to cases. That left the choices of internal medicine, pediatrics and obstetrics. "That's when the reproduction experience kicked in. I liked it. If I had an elective with obstetrics, I would do it. Anybody who wanted to trade out of obstetrics, I'd take it." It was during the Vietnam War, though, and Leon was sent overseas.

Two years later, Dr. Schimmel returned and completed his residency at the Medical College of Virginia. His son was born after he and his wife took the first Lamaze Prepared Childbirth class in Richmond. "There was a lot of pressure. It was a real frontier-breaker for the residency program. Somebody *inside* the system actually did it instead of some weirdo from the outside," Dr. Schimmel recalls. Everything was routine then—routine shaving, enemas, and routine IVs. Trying to affect change during residency brought controversy. For example, when Dr. Schimmel was in charge, he said, "No, we're not shaving this woman." The change didn't make sense to the other staff.

"We had a friend giving birth and she didn't have as much success because her baby was bigger. After hours in labor, her doctor became angry and refused to support her. He came in the next morning with an attitude asking, '*Now* what do you think of natural childbirth?'"

Under bright lights in a different hospital, Barbara Boehler had a typical birth thirty-two years ago. She was a prepared mother. Yet, it turned out to be exactly the kind of birth that Suzanne Arms wrote about in her book, *Immaculate Deception*. This first birth was traumatic for her, especially when Barbara's newborn was taken away from her.

When she got pregnant with her second child four years later, she decided to birth at home. After the type of hospital birth Barbara experienced before, she could never go through that again. "I knew intuitively that hospitals were not good places to have my babies. I was planning a home birth having no idea what that meant, though."

Barbara's husband at the time was a family practice doctor. They moved to a small town to start a clinic that would serve poor people. Their lab tech practiced as a lay midwife. One night, the midwife asked the physician to come help her with a birth. Barbara, pregnant with her second son, tagged along.

"That's when I had an epiphany, a calling. During that birth, I had this revelation, that this is what I was meant do. It felt like the voice of God. I saw a birth happen the way it's suppose to happen and I knew down in my bones that that was what I was to do for the rest of my life," Barbara says. She was only two weeks away from getting an Elementary Teaching Credential, but she quit because she *knew* she was meant to be a midwife. She began the journey the next day.

"What I wanted to do was take this wonderful birth that I'd seen at home, this beautiful, transcendent kind of experience, and bring that to poor women. They weren't going to have the economic means to pay out-of-pocket like my home birth clients. I wanted to take what I learned at home and bring it into an institution. I believed that was possible."

Barbara started delivering babies as a lay midwife in California. She got arrested for practicing medicine without a license once, but wasn't prosecuted. Now midwives are legal in California.

She decided to go back to school to get certified as a nurse-midwife. She worked two jobs: at night in Labor and Delivery and during the day in a free clinic with Hispanic farm workers, who had no insurance. "I decided poor women needed midwifery services. And more importantly, their babies needed to be born the way I saw babies born at home: respectfully, lovingly, with Spirit surrounding them. It seemed burningly important to me that their babies be born like that, not the way my oldest son was born, under glaring lights, with rough towels, and taken away from me. In order to do that, I had to go into the system and change it."

After becoming a certified nurse-midwife, she set up the first MediCal (or Medicare) obstetrical service in Yellow County, California. It began as a free clinic and became a community clinic. She worked for 20 years at

Memorial Hospital, a hospital surrounded by a community of farmers. Barbara says, "We did as close to home birth as you can have in an institutional setting."

"It's not about the room you're in. It's the *heart* in which that care is given. It's the intention and the attitude of the caregivers. I don't care if it's a fancy room. Because now, as a marketing tool, babies are born in fancy rooms in almost every major hospital across the country. I'm unimpressed with that. If babies are yanked out of their mothers by vacuum or forceps, if you've got a 25 percent C-section rate, if the babies that *do* make it out vaginally, their first introduction to the planet is a harsh and bright light, with people screaming at the mother, what have you gained? Nothing. Because the baby is born in a nice hotel-like room. Who cares?"

Memorial Hospital had tiny rooms, no wallpaper anywhere, and green metal cabinets. But a tremendous nursing staff, including Ellen Kassing, understood birth: that babies could come out, that babies were born healthy, and that babies had a mechanism in which they could breathe. Ellen and Barbara understood the necessity of getting women on their feet, out of bed, and into water. Barbara recalls, "We had these showers, and oh-my-gosh, you had to go down the hall and around the corner but we *used* them. We used every little piece of those rooms."

Babies were born in dimly lit rooms. Nurses and midwives knew to keep their mouths shut and tell the labor support people, "This is a *Holy* moment. We're going to act like we're in church." That was Barbara's theory for staff: if you don't scream and holler, if you act like you're in a sacred place, you can't go wrong. Your attitude is going to be just right. These babies were born into that kind of an atmosphere.

By 1979, Dr. Schimmel had read more about midwives, but hadn't met any yet. The concept of the nurse practitioners in the out-patient setting seemed to make total sense for midwives in the in-patient setting. He hired the first midwife in the area that year. This came about in the private practice before moving into the public sector, the reverse of what usually happens. Dr. Schimmel points out, "Usually midwives are okay for the poor people, Medicaid, the uninsured, because there's not much money for obstetricians. What does that say?"

Midwives taught Dr. Schimmel even more than he had already sensed. They taught the nursing side of medical care: understanding, flexibility, individualization, respect and mostly, faith that the perineum will be okay or "preservation of the perineum."

After adding midwives to his practice, some other family practice doctors stopped sending gynecological referrals to him. "I was told by mutual friends that when some doctors who had been in practice a while started talking about my having nurse practitioners and midwives, they felt so emotional they wouldn't be able to finish their sentences. They became irate," Dr. Schimmel recalls. The threat is to their ego and finances. They think, *we've paid our dues. How can nurses come in and deliver babies or see patients when they've spent only four years doing this and we had to grind in all those years?*

Three midwives and two nurse practitioners worked in Dr. Schimmel's practice. Barbara was hired as a part-time midwife and insurance was sought for her to do some of their births in the public sector. They got paid peanuts for these births. "If we had to cancel our office for a few hours, and not make anything on the birth, we lost money. Barbara would do births at the hospital during the day and it wouldn't interfere with our office.

"When we called the insurance company, they said, 'We're getting to it.' They later said, 'We're reevaluating your entire practice.' After their underwriting committee met, they told us, 'We've cancelled it.'" This was even a doctor-owned insurance company that Dr. Schimmel and his partner helped capitalize.

Dr. Schimmel filed a lawsuit which went on for several years. Finally, he went to court. He recalls, "The committee got the local medical society to sign off that we were an 'unacceptable risk.' The chairman of the underwriting committee, who was an obstetrician, lost patients because they transferred to our practice. These women wanted our kind of prenatal care with midwives." Dr. Schimmel got a different insurance but it was a major hassle.

Seven years later, Dr. Schimmel joined Sutter, another medical group. Sutter was building a big hospital in Davis, California, about twenty minutes down the road. Dr. Schimmel and Barbara Boehler became part of a team to set up what they call a birthing center. "It's like the birthing centers all through the nation in hospitals, they're not stand alone 'Birthing Centers.' It's another marketing tool."

Barbara recalls that Dr. Schimmel withstood incredible slings and arrows, but persevered. The doctors attacking Schimmel when he left Memorial to join Sutter Hospital changed their minds. They quickly started a midwifery service that's been going strong ever since.

Today if one tours Sutter Davis Hospital it's not only what you see, it's what is invisible: the philosophy of the founders and the staff at work. The rooms got bigger and prettier. "We lobbied hard to keep TVs out of rooms and we succeeded. That was our biggest victory as far as I'm concerned. We got water in every room. Now they have tubs in a couple of the rooms. We had to *fight* for these things, as you can imagine," Barbara says.

A culture exists in Yellow County of not expecting epidurals. From women with Ph.D.s from the University of California to farm workers in the fields who speak no English, natural birth has become *normalized*, an event in a woman's life. It's a *huge* event, yet it's normal for a woman's body. Barbara says, "We're fortunate that we've had hard-headed midwives and doctors who understood what we did. Dr. Leon Schimmel, is certainly a big part and he absolutely backed us up. He has a *feel* for birth. His wife at that time was a Nurse Practitioner. I think she influenced him, too."

"Anesthesiologists were not interested in doing epidurals. It took away from their other business. They didn't want to come in the middle of the night, especially. They were happy that we did not require it. They had enough business, so we didn't have that pressure.

You can have all those other components, but adding midwives brings personal support. Midwives at Sutter tell women in labor, "You can get up and I'll walk with you down the hallway. We'll walk together." Midwives say, "I promise you: your baby can come out. I promise you: your baby can come out without an epidural. I've seen it happen hundreds of times. It will happen for you, too."

Dr. Thomas H. Strong, Jr., author of *Expecting Trouble: The Myth of Prenatal Care in America*, makes a case for using the midwifery model with using obstetricians for fetal-maternal specialty, versus referring high-risk moms out. Obstetricians want low-risk patients where they only have to spend five minutes on prenatal visits and they come in to deliver when the baby's head is on the perineum. "It's all about time and money, after ego. I don't mean to be blatant about it, but it's a fact," says Dr. Schimmel.

Over half of the babies at Sutter Davis are delivered by midwives, as much as 60 percent and sometimes close to 70 percent. If you took a survey across the U.S., you'd only find a dozen hospitals like Sutter. When women talk to each other in their apartments in Yellow County, they aren't asking each other about when they got their epidural. Instead, they say, "Oh, yeah, I had my baby. The midwife walked the halls with me." Barbara would go outside with the women and walk in the grass, up and down stairs, and go everywhere. It became the community expectation that when you had a baby, the midwives delivered most of the babies. Barbara calls it a Birthing Island of Sanity.

"Birth is like jello: it has no boundaries and it doesn't have a certain shape, this soft squishy, lovely, juicy thing got put into a box. 'This is what it will look like. This is how it will graph. We'll take this amount of pain away. We'll pull the baby out.' We've mechanized something that ought *not* to be mechanized. I don't know what the long-term effects of that are. Will we pay the price some day?" Barbara wonders.

Dr. Stice, the first obstetrician in Yellow County, was an older doctor who shifted his viewpoint. He went from, "No, we don't need midwives," to seeing the benefits of midwives. He was one of Barbara's two most influential mentors.

"He taught me how to be a good midwife. He was seasoned enough. He had total faith and love for me. He believed that babies could be born without a whole lot of falderal (nonsense). He felt that if you waited long enough and you kept a good watch on things, that if the baby was a nice sturdy baby and the mom was a nice sturdy mom, the baby would be born without a lot of whoop-de-do around it. I loved that. Lovely patience. He was absolutely not afraid of birth, which is unusual today."

Dr. Schimmel says, "Labor support means *respect* for the way things usually go. The vast majority of births go fine. They need emotional support. They need physical support. But, that's not to say you don't keep a watch on them. Let people do their birth *their* way, *empower* them to do it their way. Give them a lot of support that 'it'll be fine,' even when it seems like it isn't to them." The keys are: giving support, allowing communication to calm fears, knowing how to deal with fear of pain or the unexpected, and being close enough to it without interfering yet still keeping birth safe.

All too frequently, obstetricians, family practice doctors and even some midwives take an alarmist approach, which is contradictory to a good outcome. For a first-time mother to feel comfortable in having her baby, she needs to *know* she's going to be all right, the baby is going to be all right, what's going on is within the range of "normal," the staff will keep things safe and be supportive.

For example, women in labor at Sutter Davis choose what position they're in. They choose whether they get up and move around. They choose if everything's fine, whether they even have an IV or not.

"If you get ready for a bicycle tour, it would help to prepare yourself that during the hardest part—the last five miles—*you* are going to finish versus someone's going to drive you or give you a rope tow. Giving birth is the most physically demanding project you'll ever undertake. You need good nutrition, a support system, sound advice, and good people to be sure you're safe. If natural birth doesn't work out, though, you're not a failure. You did everything you could to make it happen," Dr. Schimmel says.

Labor takes a whole team. Everyone has to be on the same page. The staff at Sutter Davis Hospital supports the mom who asks for a drug-free birth. Most do birth naturally and only 10 percent receive an epidural, usually because they are frightened. Recommendations include taking prepared childbirth classes, reading Sheila Kitzinger's books, and even using midwives in the practice to support moms in their labor and birth process. Obstetricians, while they're trained in birth, aren't *dedicated* to be with the laboring woman like midwives are.

The nurses that understood about birth in their hearts joined the Sutter Davis team. Barbara says, "We continued what we'd done before. Now, we have a little more room to work in. What I was the most intent on preserving was that babies are born in a church-like atmosphere. That idea survived." Nurses, like Ellen, support this philosophy.

Many other LDRs elsewhere work with interventions like IVs and fetal monitors. Only periodically do the nurses go into the room and check the mothers. If a mother is asking for help, they call her a "troublesome *demanding* patient," instead of offering support.

Ellen confirms the care women get at Sutter. "We don't rush the IVs. We do intermittent monitoring. We offer Telemetry where women are monitored while walking the halls. A lot of hospitals don't: once they're on monitoring, they stay on. Our's is intermittent, as long as we check that baby. It's okay. It works. We use a Doppler or we have the moms step back in the room and they get a little strip (from the monitor). They go through a contraction and we assess the contraction afterwards. If the baby tolerated the contraction, the mom goes back to walking around. We don't have the belt on her the whole time. It's a huge discomfort for some women. We monitor intermittently as long as the mom is doing well and the baby is doing fine. Moms shouldn't be strapped to the bed. They should be up walking in the hall or walking outside and getting fresh air.

"We make sure they drink and stay hydrated. That keeps them from having an IV. If the mom is comfortable with eating, that's okay, too.

"I'm with the mom one-on-one. I sit with her, offer water, offer a doula and even educate the family, encouraging the men to step in and watch. With the couple together, we discuss what's going to happen."

Dr. Schimmel says, "The single best thing about obstetrics is to provide the kind of support that enables the woman with the most fear of the birth process. Frankly, those who have the most fear of all are women who have been sexually abused. They transition from their anxiety in early pregnancy of not wanting an exam by even a woman provider. To follow and support that woman through a successful vaginal birth...[a pause of silence as he fights back emotion] ...then that woman thanks you. Those moments...are the most powerful."

Unfortunately in this country, women are often faced with a system and method of care that doesn't help them. It makes them more *dependent* on technology and on other people. They come out as new mothers who are dependent. Everyone has something in their past that didn't go well for them, whether it's sexual abuse or harassment. What better way to keep women down than to make them dependent on you? Dr. Schimmel says, "Barefoot and pregnant in the kitchen is one thing, but dependent on epidurals, C-sections, forceps and vacuums? How does that impact a mother?"

For Dr. Schimmel, the most difficult thing about obstetrics is the unrelenting pressure from all directions including the way people don't want to leave you alone. For example, if the water breaks, families ask, "When are you going to *do* something, doctor?"

The C-section rate in the U.S. in the early 1970s was under 10 percent. Now C-section rates have climbed to 30+ percent. Obstetricians weren't trained for 25 percent; they were trained for closer to 5 percent. " They basically allowed the pressures of work, lifestyle and finance to dictate how they did birth. Birth in this country is not evidence-based. In most diagnostic subgroups, it's the antithesis," says Dr. Schimmel.

"Doctors may use litigation fears as an easy way to justify doing C-sections, but it's a smoke screen." Dr. Schimmel explains that a doctor may say, "I'd like to do my C-section between the end of office hours at 4:30 and before dinner time at 7 or 8." That's the reason for the C-section rate. They are done at convenient times. C-sections between midnight and 8 a.m. are extremely rare. What does that tell you about the necessity of this intervention?"

Some hospitals have 60–75 percent C-section rates. ACOG (American College of Obstetricians and Gynecologists) comes to investigate and to find out what's wrong. "What's wrong" is busy practices. Labors that aren't spontaneous are induced in the morning and if the mother has not delivered by late afternoon, they do a C-section.

Barbara adds, "When I had my son, we fought to *not* get medicated. Now I see women coming in wanting to *schedule* their C-sections, feeling like they don't get good care unless they can have an epidural. An actress reportedly scheduled a C-section because of her husband's sports schedule. What in the world? Her doctor is consenting to do *that*? That's malpractice. I've been around long enough to know what adhesions look like. A C-section is not like getting a pedicure or a hair appointment. It's **major** surgery. You have to cut through *seven* layers before they get to the baby. Seven layers to heal."

A friend of Barbara's immigrated to the U.S. from Italy. He told her his first impression of America was in New York City: a big bustling city with tremendous amounts of advertisements to get rid of *pain*. Only someone coming from the outside can see that.

Barbara quit delivering babies after her name was on the chart of a Cerebral Palsy patient whose case went to court. "I sat in a courtroom for a two-month trial. I learned a lot about CP. I was found not guilty for the outcome." Now she manages nurses in a teaching hospital. "I'm in the belly of the beast. I'm watching people get trained in an obstetrical gynecological department. I have oversight of the nurses. I'm now asked to come and teach normal birth to the residents, which I'm delighted to do."

When Barbara taught nursing students, she showed a snippet from the Monty Python film, *The Meaning of Life*. At one point you see this woman in labor on a gurney. They push her through five doorways—"ba-boom, ba-boom." The woman exclaims, "Ah, ah!" After going down a long hallway, they get her in this room and bring in six machines. They lose the woman. "Here I am," she says. You see only her hand wave above the sea of machinery. The obstetrician rushes in, "The administrator is coming. Where is the machine that goes *ping*?" They say, "Oh, we've got it right here." You hear the sound "ping." The administrator smiles.

Barbara says, " I instruct the nursing students, 'Okay now we're going to Kaiser [the teaching hospital]...what I want you to do is look for that machine that goes *ping*.'" At the end of the semester the nurses said, "Barb, we thought you were nuts with that movie, you wild-eyed radical midwife. But, it was REAL. It was true."

It's supposed to be a satire, but Barbara thinks it's way too close to what's happening. "We have a mass delusion about birth. As a culture, we have been so protected from birth. Who sees a baby's birth? It's obscure: a woman is pregnant one day and she comes back five days later, holding a baby. The act of giving birth is not part of our culture. We have all this confusion and delusion about the safety of birth. People think it's a train wreck waiting to happen.

Barbara says, "My belief about birth is birth works: you can *count on it*. It is normal. It's designed to be a normal part of what women do with their bodies. I don't even want to say 'natural.' It's simply *normal*. It's a normal event in a woman's life. I have seen all the things that could go wrong, including the few babies who die, and I can still look anybody in the face and say, 'Birth is normal.' It's what defines us. It's why we are women. It's not like that's the only thing a woman should do. I'm not saying anything like that, but that's why our bodies are made the way they are: to give birth," Barbara says.

Sutter Davis Hospital completed the first Pregnancy and Delivery Initiative with women having their first baby, at term, head down with a homogeneous population not influenced by high risk factors. They put together evidence-based measures and spent a year collecting and fine tuning clean data.

In 2002, Sutter Davis won the best overall performance in a large health care system of twenty hospitals. Now a protocol for labor and delivery exists including:

- Avoid coming to the hospital too early and needing more intervention.
- Come at least three or four centimeters dilated.
- Wait for an epidural until you're at least in the active phase of labor.
- Let women move around while in labor.

Within an established medical system grows a model like the one Sutter Davis pioneered. After three years, early statistics show decreases in episiotomies, in third- and fourth-degree laceration rates, and in inductions overall.

Dr. Schimmel recommends requiring *every* residency program in the U.S. to work side-by-side with a midwifery program. Midwife faculty and obstetrician and gynecologist faculty working together means that the physicians who come out of that exposure are farther along in their education. Meshing the model in training makes a good start.

He recommends reducing the chance for anesthesiologists to approach a low-risk mother to talk to them about their services or market drugs. If a woman asks for it, that's a different story. But a woman's most vulnerable time is when she's dilated to four centimeters in labor for several hours and she's about to kick in and wrap this up. She's almost done. She doesn't need someone to come in and say, "I can take the pain away."

It is important that large health care systems acknowledge the value of non-physician providers, especially midwives.

Barbara sums up, "What captured my heart as a midwife—what I'm passionate about—is how babies are born and their experience. That is important to our understanding and embracing of normal birth."

Back in a labor room, a newborn begins to emerge from his mother's body. Nurse Ellen helps the father catch his child. "Do you want to cut the cord?" she asks him gently. "Why don't you give your baby to your wife." The husband, overwhelmed with emotion, places his tiny infant on his wife's belly. In that tender moment, mom, dad, and baby see each other's faces and their lifelong bond begins.

Chief Residents at Vanderbilt Choose
Midwife Ina May Gaskin at The Farm
Heidi Rinehart, M.D.'s and Rudolph Fedrizzi, M.D.'s Story

"Anything can happen. You know a lady gave birth and her baby had bilateral pneumothoraxes [air in the pleural spaces near the lungs]. And if she hadn't had access to medical care, her baby could've died. Are you sure you know what you are doing?"

My former supervising resident, who was now on the faculty at Vanderbilt, was questioning me. He took me to lunch because he was concerned about why Rudy and I, chief residents at the hospital, chose a birth center named The Farm for our upcoming birth of our first baby.

"I want a midwife-attended natural birth." I said. " And these midwives have four times as much experience attending births as Rudy and I put together. How can you argue that? They publish their statistics. And other statistics show that I'm making a very safe choice. I am much safer with a midwife than having a typical hospital birth." It gave me an opportunity to articulate my thoughtful choice. I *do* know what I'm doing.

Growing up, my mom talked about birth as a *good* thing. "It's physical, and yeah, it hurts, but when you're done you have this baby as a reward." What's the big deal? She worried about me in high school, though, because I was reading Masters and Johnson. I became interested in women's reproductive health, genetics, and sexuality. I had no personal experience, but I knew everything about family planning.

I believed I was going to medical school to promote women's health. Every year I considered quitting because medicine defines health only as the *absence* of disease. I thought health had many more facets.

Rudy Fedrizzi and I met in college. As first-year medical students, we heard Stan Sagoff, M.D., from Boston and Ina May Gaskin from The Farm speak about home birth. I listened to them talk about the midwifery model of care: promoting *health* in childbearing. This is not disease care in childbearing. *This makes sense.* I thought an effective way to change childbearing was from within the system. Not anymore. Now, I believe consumers, even renegades...people *outside the system* change the system by putting pressure on it.

As a fourth-year medical student, I spent two weeks with Ina May at The Farm, on my own time. Previously, the hospital births I'd witnessed had this limited view. Yet, I still studied midwifery by reading every book that I could get my hands on. The Farm is a soy bean farming commune in rural Tennessee where their birth center, staffed by midwives, serves their members and outside prenatal clients for natural childbirth. I saw videos and three births. The midwives showed me that birth could be a much wider spectrum.

Going into residency, I resolved that because I was going to be in the hospital one hundred hours a week, I was not going to be indoctrinated through sleep deprivation and intensity to ever forget this experience. *I saw natural birth.*

I kept trying to bring elements of midwifery care into Vanderbilt's hospital, like not doing episiotomies, not making women lie flat on their backs, and encouraging movement. A lot of ritual I couldn't impact, though; I was still a resident. I didn't have the ability to influence but, I kept chipping away at it. They thought I was a little weird, trying to do all this goofy stuff in birth, but they knew I was a reasonably good doctor and I earned the respect of other people.

By the time Rudy and I became chief residents, we married and became pregnant with Julianna. Rudy was the strongest physician in our residency class, and I was not at the bottom. When we chose to go to The Farm for our childbirth [she moves down from the sofa onto the floor criss-cross style] this was a personal choice. I wasn't doing it to make a statement to anybody else. I was doing it because it was the right thing for me. I wanted a natural birth. I *really* wanted one-on-one support of women during my labor. I didn't want to feel self-conscious in labor or worry about being uninhibited. I didn't want to be concerned about my performance or medical technologies hovering and used inappropriately. I wanted it to be an intimate family experience.

My dad, a commercial airline pilot, flew to Nashville to visit us. When he drove to our house, he found our note: "We've gone to have the baby."

The birth cottage at The Farm is in the middle of the woods— simple and rustic. If you think about the kinds of places people go to at Cape Cod or in mountain cabins, that's what it feels like.

I had an ordinary labor, yet it was extraordinary for me and Rudy. We left the culture of disease behind for a life-embracing environment for the birth of our child. The midwives encouraged me to spend extra time at The Farm before and after the birth. At the time, that didn't seem like the right thing to do. We drove down while I was in early labor. We arrived at 8 a.m. and Julianna was born at 8 p.m. that same day.

"I don't want to be your doctor," Rudy said. "I have to do that all the time with a lot of other people. I don't want to do it with my wife, too." But he had to shed expectations about the conduct of birth because none of the cues were the same as in the hospital. He couldn't figure out the progress. After they checked my dilation, Rudy asked, "Where is she?"

"Oh, she's *squishy*. It's *groovy* now," the midwife said. That's how they talk on The Farm. We're not groovy-hippy people.

No connection. The cues that Rudy could use to evaluate the progress in labor were absent. Dilation. Effacement. Contraction frequency. He heard foreign words in a midwifery context. In some ways, it was harder for him. I was busy in labor. But we both had fears.

Nobody told me how much it would hurt. I had back labor. I read every book on the shelf. I had been to 250 births. I had no clue what birth *felt* like. Photographs of me in labor show that my back was red from the rubbing. Pressure helped the most, where the hips and spine come together.

At one point, Rudy broke down and had to check me. He thought, *I don't know how far she has progressed. Is this baby ever coming? Should we get in the car and drive the 35 minutes to the nearest hospital or is this baby going to come? I have no idea anymore.* I could feel that he was scared and couldn't get his bearings. He checked me and I was eight or nine centimeters, minus one station.

"Bear down," he told me. The baby swooped down to plus one station. I still had a little dilating to go. This baby's going to come out. *Okay.* He relaxed, understanding that however "squishy" it gets, the baby will come out. He went back into the father role. Maybe that was *his* transition. He needed something that would help him feel like he could be confident, because the midwives spoke a language that he wasn't fluent in.

I had no concept when people talked about the hard part of transition. A lot of it was fear and confusion about how to cope with the *power* of labor—feeling like the lid is about to blow off the top of your head. Your energy expands. It's going to have to come out somewhere. It comes out as a baby.

From my experience of seeing hospital births, I noticed that women who eased the babies out tore less. They wanted their bottoms to be in good shape. When I pushed, I was determined that I wasn't going to *spit* this baby out. I was going to *ooooze* my baby out. I didn't realize how long I was taking, because I lost track of time.

Our baby was crowning for a while. Ina May thought that the tissues were not yielding because her head was half out for so long. I was going to inch her out millimeter by millimeter. And Rudy meanwhile worried about how many I.Q. points Julianna was losing. Ina May picked up the scissors to do this trivial episiotomy. She cut me a quarter inch, but that would be a half inch more circumference to get the baby out. The fact that she got the scissors told me that people got concerned that the baby had not been born yet. Because I could tell that everyone was getting anxious, I pushed her out in the next contraction. I had no more tear beyond that quarter inch.

Afterwards, I felt triumphant, floating, ecstatic. My birth was intimate and tender, a life-changing and empowering experience.

A full moon hung in the sky. My dad drove from our house an hour and a half into the night. When he arrived at The Farm, he said it was like going to the stable in Bethlehem— an unassuming cabin in the woods, to witness a miracle. He saw his new granddaughter, Julianna, and stayed a couple of hours. My mom came the next day.

Birth is like a volcanic earthquake happening inside your body. During labor, I thought I had to try to control that power. It was like I was running down railroad tracks. A big steam locomotive came bearing down on me and I had to run faster and faster to stay ahead of it. The tracks shook, the ground trembled. What I didn't realize was that I rode on the cow catcher. Yes, I was in the midst of all that tremendous power, but I could not fall off and all I had to do was hang on for the ride. It would carry me to where I wanted to go. The unleashing of that power carries you to your birth.

After finishing residency and taking eight months off, I returned to work much *calmer* in helping women with labor. I would say, "I've been where you've been. It feels overwhelming and you are doing fine. This is normal. Keep going, keep going...everything's fine."

When women want natural birth, we have this agreement: we won't give them pain medication unless they ask *three* times. The reason comes from my own labors. If I birthed in the hospital, I would be asking for the epidural NOW. Which is saying, "I'm struggling to cope and need an extra measure of support or reassurance right now to get me through."

Here's what blows my mind: Have you noticed that the people who complain about the pain of childbirth are the ones who have had pain medication? The women who do the work and are rewarded with an alert baby and the *ecstasy* that comes after birth know that the pain is a piece of the experience. Childbirth has many vivid sensations—the pressure, how wet you feel, the head-rushes as the blood flow surges with each contraction, everything getting loose. The only feeling we seem to be able to articulate is pain. It hurts. But what about all those other sensations, feelings and the *change in your state of consciousness?*

When I do prenatals for women who are afraid of childbirth, I say, "Okay, here's what you need to know: When you have a baby, you temporarily lose your mind. I don't mean in the screaming psychotic way. Your *consciousness* changes during birth. It's similar to your state of consciousness when you're making love and approaching an orgasm. Time fades away. Modesty, too. The particulars of what's going on outside of your immediate experience become unimportant. *You are a mass of feelings and sensations, with virtually no intellect.* Labor is the same. When you are in active labor, usually past four centimeters, that intellectual ability to analyze, keep track, and think goes away. *You become sensation and feelings. It's okay."* I see some women struggle at transition between because it's the place where they lose their mind. They feel this *undertow* of labor. They think they are losing their grip on reality.

I tell my prenatal ladies, "You know, when you're having a baby, you're not sick. But, it's a good rule of thumb that what you like when you have the flu or bad menstrual cramps are the same kinds of things that you'd like in labor. If you want somebody to fuss over you, pull your blankets up, brush your hair and rub your feet, that's what you're going to want in labor. And if you want to pull the covers up over your head and groan, *woooaa*, until you feel better, that's how you will be in labor, too. So *you can start to ask for what you need.* You don't know what you're going to want in labor, but I think that's a good rule of thumb.

During labor I ask a mom, "Would you like to go in the shower or would you like to stand up?" And they think, *Wow, those are brilliant suggestions. I'm glad you came up with those.* Even though they write on their birth plan that they want to stand up or shower during labor, they forget. It's *okay* to have that change in consciousness; that's a *normal* sign in labor. It's a part of the experience other than pain.

My goal as an obstetrician is to use technology judiciously. I want to minimize interference with the natural process. I utilize medical tools and pain medication, but minimally. For example, we had a VBAC last night, who had a long, slow gentle labor. She didn't get any Pit [Pitocin]. Her labor certainly did not conform to Friedman's curve*, not even close. She had one dose of Nubain, which is an intravenous narcotic. That's all.

The hospital staff seems confused. We provide medical care when it is required, but we do it with a philosophy of midwifery care which includes empowerment, informed choice, trust of the physiological process, and judicious, careful use of technology.

I find ways to change unnecessary hospital rituals. For example, the nurses snatch the babies and take them to the warmer as soon as the cord is cut, as if somehow measuring the length of the baby was more important than the mother greeting her child. Those tasks had to be completed before the mother could hold her baby.

"Can't it wait?" I would ask. "I think the baby is crying for his mother." You know what had impact? *Not cutting the cord*. The tendency among some of the nurses is still to grab the babies when the cord is cut. Some are itching for the baby. But if I can wait five, ten, fifteen minutes, it's time that the mother and the baby wouldn't have otherwise had.

Hospitals are set up to provide efficient care to many people. The rules and rituals that evolve around that goal make it difficult for them to have the flexibility to respond to individual needs. I recommend home birth; it ranks as my first choice. Birth centers rank second. Both are able to provide the individual responsive care that consumers want.

---

* Friedman's curve is an approximate dilation of 1/2 to 1cm per hour for first labors. It is meant for more of an average rather than an ideal, researchers note.

Unplanned Home Birth
April's Story

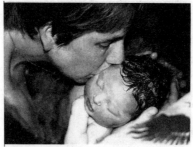

Photo: Chris Royce

I'm the last of four girls in my family to give birth. I witnessed two births—one standard birth in a hospital and one in a birthing facility, apart from Labor and Delivery where one could be as loud as you wanted to be.

The first birth was my sister's VBAC and I was her doula. I saw how disconnected she was when she got the epidural. She talked on the phone with her job during labor. I know she was scared about the VBAC because she had such a bad experience with her first child born by cesarean. Her first birth was scheduled because her doctor was going out of town. She got sick and the baby wasn't ready to come out. The baby was jaundiced so she couldn't nurse him right away. She felt guilty over not having the motherly bond with him. "I realized my doctor had some other agenda," she said. That wasn't the case with her second doctor. Her second birth went well, but she couldn't feel where to push. She had a seven pound baby and tore quite a bit.

I went to a friend's birth, who had two previous home births. But because her last baby was ten pounds, this was her third baby, and she was thirty-seven years old, she wanted to play it safer by choosing a birthing room inside the hospital. Her doctor was as close to a male midwife as I've ever seen. But when the nurses changed shifts, she ended up getting Pitocin. I could see the difference between her labor before and the level of pain that she was in after she received the Pitocin. She didn't have any pain meds. She pushed twice and her 8 1/2-pound son was born.

I'm not into hospitals because I've had to be in one due to ulcerative colitis. That was before getting pregnant.

My pregnancy was good even though I was nauseous for four months. I called different birth centers, went to tour a nice one and signed up. During my prenatal care, the midwife reprimanded me about not eating enough. At the next visit she said, "This is a big baby." I felt apprehension after hearing that.

During pregnancy I was busy planning our wedding. Mark and I became engaged and we moved the wedding up six months. At our wedding I met Mara, a childbirth educator and lay midwife, who came with a friend of mine. I started seeing Mara and she asked, "Would you like me to be your doula?"

"Sure." She got me together with different pregnant women. She took me swimming and gave me nutritious food. I started swimming on my own every day, laps, at six weeks before my due date.

Feeling good and strong, never swollen. I craved Thai food once a week. I used visualization tapes. I felt confident that I could give birth naturally. My sisters have all done it. I can do it too. I trusted my body to do what it was supposed to do.

"You're a perfect candidate to have your baby at home," Mara said.

My husband was supportive and eager for a home birth. He thought I could do it. He's into organic food and has a pregnancy-is-not-an-illness attitude. We went to birth classes with five other couples taught by Mara at a birth center. I knew her because of my friends who went to her.

I trusted the midwife at the first birth center I signed up with because of her experience. But she wasn't taking any new *home* birth clients. I still wasn't sure if I wanted to be at the birth center or at home.

I called the other midwife, Barbara, to ask if she would be willing to attend my birth at home.

"Yes, but how does the other midwife feel about it?" she asked. I told her I was all paid up until the birth. Both charged the same amount. I called the first midwife to ask her about the switching and she was okay with it. I felt fortunate to live in a community of experienced and capable midwives who are supportive of each other's work.

On Friday, I swam and felt a huge burst of energy. I swam farther and faster than I had the whole time for twenty minutes. I could have kept going. I realized, *something's up*. I started having contractions at midnight. But I didn't tell anyone until 8 am.

Mara came over and checked me out. I was only at 1 centimeter. She said, "Do whatever you want. Go to the grocery store. Take walks. Eat." I walked up and down the stairs. I saw the midwife at 9 that night. She checked me, still at one dilation. She gave me some herbal tinctures to make my labor stronger.

I didn't sleep Saturday night because I had contractions five to ten minutes apart. I was in labor all day Sunday. My pains became stronger. By Sunday night, I had tightening contractions for twenty-four hours.

Mara assisted with four births between Saturday night and Monday at the birth center. I kept in touch with her by phone. She came and checked me on Sunday and said, "Go about your day and keep taking baths." I became tired, distressed. It seemed like it was going on forever.

I knew that when you give birth at a birth center, you need to bring supplies like the Chux pads and olive oil for your perineum. I had a few supplies ready.

My neighbor brought over a good dinner for us on Sunday night, but I couldn't eat much. I was tired.

At 11:30 p.m. Mara and I talked. She told the first midwife what was going on. It was off the record because at this point she wasn't my midwife anymore. But, because she was a certified nurse-midwife (CNM) and could dispense drugs and Barbara couldn't, she knew she could make the difference in my birth by giving me a shot of Stadol, a muscle relaxer. It didn't stop my contractions, but it made me relax enough to rest. She gave me some encouragement, that the forty-eight hours is not for nothing. I slept for eight hours. I could feel the contractions but didn't care. I felt like a horse after gaining fifty pounds and now weighing 180 pounds.

I had no fear of the pain, even though one friend said birth felt like sitting on a camp fire!

By Monday morning, I felt rested. My contractions continued the same. I ate yogurt and called Mara and Barbara about 10:30 a.m. Barbara said, "Go on about your day. Pretend it's any other day." Barbara knew about the Stadol and was grateful. She thought it was a great idea. My water hadn't broken, there was no need to do anything else.

"I had two births last night, and I've got to get some sleep," Mara said. She came over, though, and after checking said, "You're softening up, but not dilating."

I became hysterical. I told my husband that I wanted to be alone, to leave. He had been with me this whole time and never left the whole two-and-a-half days except to get something to eat. He was ready to take a break and go somewhere else.

While in the bathtub, I called my sister, crying. She said, "Okay, I'm going to come over and I'll fix lunch." I called one of my friends who I had asked to attend my birth. I stayed in the tub. They came over, cleaned my home and brought loads of flowers into the house. They made my bedroom look beautiful and inviting, even changing the sheets. I hadn't done anything for two days. I felt better and calmed down.

Around 2:00, I had a couple bites of yogurt. I threw up. I lay down on the bed and my water broke which helped my birth along. In birth class, anything like coughing or throwing up pushes your diaphragm down and helps labor. They called Barbara who said, "Meet me at the birth center."

Within five minutes, I was having such active labor, that I couldn't even talk. I didn't have any clothes on. The idea of getting dressed made me nervous. I resisted walking *down the stairs* and getting in the car. At this point I was having fast, hard-hard-hard contractions. I went from going twenty miles-per-hour to going seventy in ten minutes."

They called Barbara back. "She doesn't want to get in the car."

"Great, tell her to stay put. I'm actually closer to your house than I am to the birth center." She came over, checked. "Oh, you have a cervical lip. Here are your choices: you can push through it for about three hours, or, in two contractions, I can move it with my fingers, but it's going to hurt."

"Go ahead and do it," I said. If you've been in labor for two-and-a-half days, you are not going to let anything slow you down. It did hurt. My husband said that was the only screaming I did.

I moaned during active labor. On my hands and knees, I felt like a wolf panting to get through those contractions.

Barbara checked again and said, "You're at 8 1/2 centimeters, you can start pushing."

I felt confident with Barbara. I knew from her track record and from other people's birth stories with her that if I followed everything she said to me during my birth, I wouldn't tear. That's how good she is. I was prepared to be focused on her. Mara came, even though she had been asleep and never heard the phone ring.

My husband came and he reminded me to breathe while my sister massaged my back. He straddled behind me. My sister was pushing on one leg and Mara on the other. I pushed for twenty minutes on my back. I remember feeling that I had this strength to do it. I did what they said and I maintained the pushing for the count. My husband was telling me when to breathe and when to push.

When the baby's head crowned, they said, "Oh, look at all that hair." They got the mirror and showed me. At that point, I focused intently on what Barbara was saying, "Okay, give me two little pushes. Now a long push. If I put my fingers down on your perineum, does that feel better or without?" That helped me focus on where to push.

Our baby was born. I felt great.

"See what flavor of baby you have," Barbara said.

It was a girl and we named her Francesca. I saw that she was all pink. They wrapped her up in a towel and laid her on me. I felt exhaustion and elation. I felt relieved to hear her crying and see her, that was all that mattered. The whole time I was pregnant, I was sure I was going to have a long, skinny bald-headed boy the way Mark was. But Francesca had dark wavy hair and this big round moon face. Her head was 14 1/2 inches.

The reason I dilated slowly is that I needed all those contractions to open up my hips. The baby weighed almost 10 pounds. My mom's labors went quickly after her water broke and that's what happened with me, too. Francesca didn't drop until the last day or two.

I nursed her immediately while they cleaned me up.

"You have some scrapes inside," Barbara said, "More like skid marks, not like tears, as if you skinned your knee and I want to stitch them up."

"Okay." But, I panicked and started crying. Here I had given birth to a big baby but I was not going to stand stitches because I was afraid that it would hurt. I was at my limit. "What would you do?" I asked.

"I'd stitch it up because it will heal faster," she said. With lidocaine, I couldn't feel a thing.

Because I didn't tear on the outside, I never had any discomfort. I heard from others that tearing was the worst part. It was important to me to maintain the integrity of my body.

They weighed our newborn and inked her feet while she screamed.

The placenta was big and I kept it. What I didn't know at the time was that I had lost quite a bit of blood. I found out from my birth chart later.

The midwives encourage you to drink juice and eat. My husband's brother and family came with home-made garden-fresh tomato sauce, meatballs and pasta. We had a feast for everyone including my stepson, all of the the midwives and their assistants. I was in bed with the baby. Nothing ever tasted so delicious.

It was neat to be home. Barbara made an herbal tea bath and after the meal, I got up and took a bath with Francesca. The herbs help heal the vagina and reduce swelling. I love the sweet picture of us bathing. Francesca had this beautiful head. While I was in the bathtub, everyone cleaned the meal up. My sister-in-law, bless her, did all the laundry from the birth. I wasn't planning on having birth at home and it used all my towels and sheets.

For a home birth, you need to have a high comfort level with yourself because it is not the norm in our society. People have many fears of things going wrong. That was one thing about Mara's birth classes, she did not bring up anything that could go wrong unless a couple asked. That gave me a lot of self-confidence.

If you get the chance, attend a birth, no matter what kind, so you can see what's going on. You can decide if you don't want to be attached to monitors so you can walk around, take a bath, and do whatever you want. The best thing about home birth was not having to get up and get in a car. At the birth center, you don't stay, you leave after six hours.

To have all my family around and be hospitable felt good. That's a real concern because some people aren't comfortable in their homes. They focus on everybody *else* being comfortable instead. Some women may not choose a home birth for that reason. But like any woman who gives birth will tell you, once you go into active labor anything could be happening around you and you wouldn't know it.

Read everything you can about both sides. Talk to other women who have given birth both ways. Once you get enough information, you figure out what you want.

I would have a home birth again. I think women could unless they had a physical problem. If our society would treat birth as normal, we would have the confidence and knowledge that we can do it. Women have been doing it for a while. My grandmother birthed five kids at home.

Praying to trust my body and trust my baby was important. Trusting that the baby knows when it's time to come was one reason why I didn't want a hospital birth. I wanted my baby and my body to choose the time and not a doctor.

When I dreamed of giving birth, I was at home. I couldn't have planned it any better because what I *had* planned was different than the birth we had.

Barbara was thrilled that I birthed at home and how smoothly it went. She was happy for me and remains a big champion of home birth.

Routine Fetal Photos May Be Unsound

Prenatal ultrasound is a diagnostic imaging technique using high-frequency sound waves and a computer to create images of blood vessels, tissues and organs of the fetus. Primarily, this procedure is performed to determine abnormalities, intrauterine growth retardation (IUGR), the age of the fetus, if multiples exist, and sometimes the sex of the child. But does ultrasound produce *accurate* results *without* risk to your baby?

Marsden Wagner, author of *Pursuing the Birth Machine*, says that ultrasound safety compares to assuming x-rays, routinely used for almost 50 years on pregnant women, presented no danger to the fetus. However, unrestricted use of x-rays on fetuses caused childhood cancer.

In a healthy woman with a normal pregnancy, routine ultrasound should be avoided. Scientific studies are finding new evidence that suggests caution. Exposure of embryonic tissues to radiation is critical because the cells are rapidly proliferating, and because of the potential developmental changes it may cause. Radiation exposure of fetal bone can result in secondary warming of adjacent soft tissues, of particular importance to the brain and spinal cord, especially with high-intensity Doppler beams.[1]

What You're Not Being Told About Ultrasound: Studies Raise Safety Concerns

Caution About Early Scans

Routine Ultrasound Scanning in the First Trimester: What are the Risks?

This study confirms that knowledge is incomplete, particularly in human studies of tissue. Ultrasound-induced heating can cause significant problems in later pregnancy. Yet, uncertainties remain for effects in early pregnancy where shear stresses from radiation pressure may be an important factor. Caution should be applied to the scanning in the early first trimester of an uncomplicated pregnancy.[2]

Lower Birth Weights or Growth Restriction

Effects of Frequent Ultrasound During Pregnancy: A Randomized Controlled Trial

From a study of 2,834 pregnant women, 1,415 received ultrasound at 18, 24, 28, 34 and 38 weeks gestation, for a total of five times (intensive group), while 1,419 received a single ultrasound at eighteen weeks (regular group). The intensive group showed one-third more IUGR babies.[3]

Marsden Wagner points out, "Ironically, it is now likely that ultrasound may lead to the condition, IUGR, that it has for so long claimed to be effective in detecting."

Heating of Tissue and Bone

"There is a need to investigate the thermal (heat) effects of diagnostic ultrasound (US) to assist the development of appropriate safety guidelines for obstetric use."[4]

Adverse Effects Need Research

The Safety of Prenatal Ultrasound Exposure in Human Studies

According to the FDA, there have been some reports that there may be a relation between prenatal ultrasound exposure and adverse outcome. Some of the reported effects include growth restriction, delayed speech, dyslexia, and an increase in non-right-handedness (especially in boys) associated with ultrasound exposure. Continued research is needed to evaluate the potential adverse effects of ultrasound exposure during pregnancy.[5]

Effect on Cell Division

Scientists found that ultrasound can stop cells from dividing normally. Patrick Brennan, head of the research team from University College of Dublin, Ireland, studied the changes in the cells of mice. With an 8 megahertz scan for 15 minutes, the cell division was 22 percent lower than normal. The rate of cell death doubled. Hospital scans use frequencies between 3 and 10 megahertz, lasting up to an hour. Ultrasound affects cells, possibly damaging DNA, yet implications for humans need further investigation.[6]

Effect on a Newborn's Brain

Brain development for a male fetus happens during a longer period compared to females, leaving a wider window for external influences. Scientists in Sweden studied Swedish men born between 1973 and 1978. Almost 7,000 received ultrasonic scans in the womb, 170,000 had not. They found that 32 percent of the men born between 1976 and 1978 were left-handed. Normally, only about nine percent of men are left-handed. Beginning in 1976, it was common for pregnant women to have two ultrasounds, one after seventeen weeks and another after thirty-seven weeks. Neuropsychiatrists suspect that right-handed people can become left-handed after suffering slight brain damage. A process called cavitation, where small bubbles in the body fluids vibrate from the ultrasonic waves, could influence brain development.[7]

Fetuses Hear Ultrasound As Loud

By inserting a tiny hydrophone inside a woman's uterus, researchers at the Mayo Foundation picked up a hum similar to the highest notes on a piano. When the ultrasound probe pointed right at the hydrophone, it registered 100 decibels, as loud as a subway train coming into a station.[8] Is it a wonder that fetuses move so much during ultrasound?

Training and Equipment Safety Indexes

According to Francis Duck, Chairman of the British Medical Ultrasound Society (BMUS) Safety Group, a trainee needs the supervision of a tutor to avoid excessive use and inappropriate exposure levels in obstetrics. Currently, there is no certification of ultrasound operators.

The ultrasound equipment needs two safety displays: a Thermal Index (TI) and a Mechanical Index (MI). The meanings and function of these indices help the trainee to be aware of safety management.

Thermal Index

To reduce the risk of thermal hazard, special care should be taken with sensitive tissues of the fetus such as an embryo less than eight weeks after conception, the head, brain or spine of any fetus or neonate or an eye at any age. A temperature elevation of 4°C, maintained for 5 minutes or more, is considered to be potentially hazardous to a fetus or embryo. Some diagnostic ultrasound equipment, operating in spectral-pulsed Doppler mode, can produce temperature increases in excess of 4°C in bone, with an associated risk of high temperatures being produced in adjacent soft tissues by conduction. Below is a table for safety exposures:

Table 1

Temperature elevation (°C)	Maximum exposure time (minutes)
5	1
4	4
3	16
2	64
1	128

Table 2

Thermal Index (TI)	Maximum exposure time (minutes)
2.5	1
2.0	4
1.5	15
1.0	30
0.7	60

Maximum recommended exposure times for an embryo or fetus.

TI>0.7 The overall exposure time (including pauses) of an embryo or fetus should be restricted in accordance with Table 2.

TI>1.0 Eye scanning is *not* recommended, other than as part of a fetal scan.

TI>3.0 **Scanning of an embryo or fetus is not recommended, however briefly.**

Mechanical Index

If the MI is greater than 0.3, there is a possibility of minor damage to neonatal lung or intestine. If such exposure is necessary, try to reduce the exposure time as much as possible.

If the MI is greater than 0.7, there is a risk of cavitation if an ultrasound contrast agent containing gas microspheres is being used. There is a theoretical risk of cavitation without the presence of ultrasound contrast agents. The risk increases with MI values above this threshold. [9]

Doppler for Fetal Heart Monitoring

The power levels used for fetal heart monitoring (CTG) are sufficiently low that the use of this modality is not contra-indicated, on safety grounds, even when it is to be used for extended periods.

Womb with a View

Is it necessary to do routine ultrasound for no medical reason? Is it accurate? Or do women sometimes get false positives and a misdiagnosis. The psychological stress to a pregnant woman is a consideration because it may lead to unnecessary worry. In addition, ultrasound does not detect Down Syndrome. Even with an amniocentesis, some people confess, "What difference is the outcome? I'm not going to give up my baby."

An alternative to an ultrasound for a healthy mom-to-be is to view photos in books or on the internet that show the stages of growth.

Conclusion

Ultrasound should never be used as a keepsake or souvenir such as 3-D videos. The FDA recommends avoiding unnecessary ultrasound videos because of radiation exposure, changes in the tissue and fluid of the fetus, time of exposure—over an hour, and without medical oversight, raising potential harm to the fetus.[10]

The embryonic period is known to be particularly sensitive to any external influences. Until further scientific information is available, ultrasounds should be carried out with careful control of output levels and exposure times. With increasing mineralization of the fetal bone as the fetus develops, the possibility of heating fetal bone increases. The user should prudently limit exposure of critical structures such as the fetal skull or spine during Doppler studies.[11]

Why take a chance? Could it lead to learning differences? You would not know until six years after birth, when your child is in first grade. Given that these studies recommend using caution, the need for more research is warranted. No absolute safety is stated nor guaranteed.

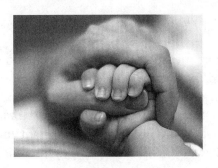

SECRET 3:

Turn Scared into Sacred

One of the most daunting hurdles facing women before birth is fear. Especially for the first time, some expectant mothers may burden themselves with concerns that may never happen. Sometimes negative feelings from a previous labor linger. Whereas animals rely on instinct or whether they can see, smell or hear danger, women tend to worry needlessly. Negative thoughts can grow into a dragon with several heads—anxiety, panic, and dread.

But hope exists. By looking at the ways you get scared, you can learn how to turn that energy into the sacred. *Turn Scared into Sacred* is the third natural birth secret: taking your darkest fears and facing them with faith in your own way. Frances Moore Lappe, co-author of *You Have the Power: Choosing Courage in a Culture of Fear,* says fear is an energy— an energy you can use to your advantage. Instead of freezing up, you can move through the stages of birth naturally by designing your "shield of courage" ahead of time.

According to a study[1] of fears among 329 pregnant women attending childbirth classes, their foremost fears include:

1. Pain
2. Prolonged labor
3. Panic during childbirth

These fears stemmed from a negative attitude and horror stories. Positive birth stories, the driving energy of this book, provide a powerful antidote for the deepest anxieties surrounding natural childbirth.

By the end of this chapter, we hope the fear dragon will dissolve into a puff of smoke replaced with faith in the natural birth process.

Regarding pain, the next chapter reveals Secret 4: *Don't Take Labor Lying Down*. No matter if you are athletic or a "wus" (as some moms admit in their stories), you will learn how to cope with labor pain by using proven comfort measures. Relaxation techniques keep your muscles from tensing up, freeing them for the hard work of pushing.

Prolonged labor, known in medical terms as dystocia, happens due to many factors. You will learn about the three "P's" traditionally known in medicine for dystocia. You will learn an important fourth "P" never discussed in a hospital, which is *psychological* dystocia. By asking questions, you or any caregiver can identify sensitive issues and overcome mental inhibitions.

During labor the most common question for first-time moms is, "Is what I'm feeling normal?" At no other time in her life is a woman feeling this vulnerable. She looks for feedback, especially encouragement.

Here's where Secret 2: *Get Informed and Shop Around* is critical. An unsupportive caregiver's negative response could be, "If you don't progress, we'll have to operate." The caregiver's fear transfers to the laboring mom.

Fear begins in the amygdala, a cluster of cells deep in the most primitive part of the brain that weighs information for emotion and threat. If a threat is sensed, the amygdala sends out immediate signals, triggering a jump, a shout or some other reflex action. The adrenal glands on top of the kidneys begin pumping adrenaline and noradrenaline, two chemicals that act as messengers to trigger reactions all over the body. This chemical rush causes the heart to race, breathing to quicken, pupils to dilate and saliva to dry up. In the extreme, it is common to experience hyperventilation, dizziness, trembling and even nausea.[2]

However, a caregiver's positive response, "You are doing great. Keep at it. What do you need?" puts fears to rest. The woman, in the midst of contractions, feels confident energy.

An example is the story about Lee Ann, a chaplain who panics because she thinks her fetus has died. Note how she copes. Plus, look at how her midwife reassures her.

At the end of this chapter, work out your own vision of how you want your birth to happen through a guided worksheet. Yes, your day is as important as a wedding day for celebrating a new stage in life. What if it could be your way? Your *birth* day!

Psychological Dystocia in Birth

"Dystocia" is a technical term that's used to describe a labor that is stuck for whatever reason. There exist three "P's" in obstetrics to explain dystocia: the *power,* the *pelvis* and the *passenger*. Commonly, dystocia is used to explain when the mother's labor is not going well and the baby is stuck because the mother is not having adequate contractions. That is the *power.*

The next way of looking at dystocia is the *pelvis*. The pelvis might be contracted or too small for this particular baby.

The third "P" is the *passenger*, the baby's position. For example, if the baby is posterior, the knobby part of the head toward the mother's back, labor often becomes long, slow, and painful. Or the baby is too big or the position or the head size is preventing passage through the birth canal.

An important factor that's overlooked is a fourth "P," *psychological dystocia*, which is seldom addressed in medical situations. From a holistic model, it can explain why labor may not be progressing.

The first and most common reason has to do with unspoken fears of *relationship issues* with your current partner or previous partners, perhaps with your own mother or other parenting issues, or relationships with those who are in the birthing environment. Unresolved anger is an example. Unresolved issues from childhood may also come up.

The second reason is fear regarding the *environment* that you are in or the caretaker you are with. For some women a hospital is a scary environment. Sometimes going to the hospital will slow down contractions. For others, the out-of-hospital birth—at a birth center or at home—even though that's what was chosen to begin with, doesn't feel safe or comfortable. Contractions may slow down because the mother feels hesitant. This is a basic animal response. When mammals fear that a predator might attack and harm their babies—their labors will stop. They will relocate to a place of safety before the labor can progress.

The third concern is about not having enough self or *enough love* to go around, especially for women who have other children. They worry about bringing another child into the world not only out of concern for how this will affect their other children, but about bringing a baby into a world that is dysfunctional.

The fourth issue causing fear and hesitation relates to *previous trauma*. A previous birth that has issues may need resolving. For example, women having a VBAC may have unresolved issues surrounding the need for a C-section the first time around. Or, they may get stuck in the exact same place as a previous labor. That's because our culture and the medical system creates underlying fear around the possible *risks* of VBAC.

Another form of trauma that may surface during labor is from *physical abuse or sexual abuse*, stemming from childhood or as an adult. It may come from a previous abortion.

If your labor is not going well, if you're not dilating, it's important to look at the three medical "P's" about the power of the contractions, the pelvis and the passenger—the baby itself. You need someone to ask, *"What is the matter? What is the matter from an emotional, psychological, or spiritual standpoint?"*

- Are you holding on for the right person to come—your spouse, your mother, or someone else you wanted at your birth?
- Are there cultural issues regarding the sex of the baby? For example, Asians wanting a boy and knowing they have a girl.
- Affairs and other relationship issues can compromise labor.
- VBACs: Are there concerns regarding previous experience, getting stuck at the same place versus fear of complications?
- Do you feel depressed?
- Are you worried about not enough love for the child?
- Do you worry over mothering and parenting skills?
- Are you reliving sexual/physical trauma?
- Are there too much dysfunctional family dynamics?
- Do you feel safety concerns about the environment?
- Is there a lack of trust in the caregiver?
- Are you mentally rebirthing bad experiences?
- Are you dealing with sexual abuse or incest?

Whatever the issue, when you are in the midst of labor the best solution is to *release* it. Don't expect immediate results. But over time, you can learn to release your fears and free your mind and body through calming, yoga-like breathing methods.

Is There a Heartbeat? Yes.
Rev. Lee Ann Rathbun's Story

As a chaplain for Baylor Hospital's Intensive Care Unit (ICU), I would trade Fridays with my co-worker who served as the chaplain for Labor and Delivery (L&D). It was hard when I was pregnant because when L&D calls, it's usually because of fetal death, or an anticipated one. At times it was painful to read the log of L&D cases. It skewed our view of normal birth because we knew about the pregnancies that go bad—even though most are normal and work out okay.

One day, I was with a family whose baby had been in intensive care and died. I took it personally. It was early in my pregnancy before I could feel the baby kicking. Had my baby died inside me? I called my midwife, Susan. "I've got to come over and hear his heartbeat because I know that he's not alive."

My undergraduate degree is in social work from Baylor University. I took a year to go to college in Australia, where my parents lived. I had grown up overseas because my dad worked in offshore drilling. Australia was the most spiritually *apathetic* place. I got out of the "Baylor bubble" and away from where you're expected to go to church.

Some Australians would ask me, "You believe in God? Why?" I got into these wonderful talks about spirituality and religion. It was stimulating. I thought, I've got to do something *mainstream* where I'm able to connect with people around spiritual things on a deeper level, with people who aren't going to be in a church.

I knew that my ministry was to be *outside* the walls of the church. When I finished college, I went to seminary at Southwestern in Fort Worth, Texas. I started doing an internship at John Peter Smith Hospital as a chaplain in 1986 and realized *this* was the place. I loved ministry in a hospital setting. It's different everyday, you encounter people at a crisis time in their lives where they are trying to make decisions about what is important, what's meaningful for them, and how their faith comes to bear. It was a great place to be where I felt *faith meets life*.

When my sister-in-law became pregnant, she talked about becoming an active consumer. She researched and learned that a midwife would serve as a partner with her, helping her have the kind of "natural birth" she wanted. As it turned out, she ended up having back labor for a long time and an epidural. But her second one was *everything* she hoped for. When I became pregnant, I was inspired by hearing her stories.

Another influence came from my friend who had a midwife, but the other midwife in the practice, Susan, was on call that weekend. She had a long labor and came close to getting a C-section. Susan did one more thing to change her position and she had a natural birth. She had such a great partner with Susan helping her do what she wanted.

I didn't know if I wanted to go natural as much as I wanted to do what was *best* for my baby and me. I wasn't adamantly against taking drugs. I thought, *if I can do it without, great. If it can happen naturally, wonderful. If I need meds, that's okay, too.* I didn't know what to expect. I didn't know how I would tolerate the pain or the whole experience.

My mom had good pregnancies and enjoyed them. My sister birthed her daughters overseas naturally, too—that's the way they birthed in Malaysia and in Singapore. She had quick labors, within six hours. Of course, she was twenty-something and I was thirty-eight. My mom and sister showed support for my choice of natural birth.

My husband, Rich, though, was nervous with a midwife. I had raved about Susan. "Let's go check out an obstetrician, too," Rich said. We interviewed a female doctor highly recommended by L&D. There was a patronizing way about her. "You probably don't want to go to those classes," she said to my husband. "Don't worry about it because we've got it all taken care of. We're going to take care of this whole thing. If you spend time reading books, read about child rearing. Don't worry about reading about birth because we'll get you through it." I thought, *you're not seeing us or hearing us both here, both interested. We want to be involved and want information.* Rich concluded that he didn't feel comfortable with this physician.

"When do you show up at the time of birth?" we asked her.

She said, "When you're dilated to around 7 centimeters."

I thought, *gosh, you're not going to be there, basically.* She was only on call one weekend a month, so the probability of having her at the birth was not high.

Rich went with me to meet Susan on my next visit. He liked her easygoing manner, her medical competence and protocols. Susan explained that she would use the same blood tests and prenatal screenings as an obstetrician. After that, he was on board.

On one occasion, I grew panicky about wanting to hear my baby's heartbeat. I walked over to her office and we listened to the heartbeat.

She gave me a big hug. "It's okay, Lee Ann," she reassured me. "I understand. Come over anytime you want."

I bought a prenatal yoga video that was calming. It helped me to focus on my inner strength. I read pregnancy meditations from a little pink book with a lotus on the front that came with a CD. It had beautiful meditations about the *sacredness* of this time. It reminded me of this huge event that was happening and to create the space emotionally, too.

Susan suggested reading Carl Jones' *Mind Over Labor*. I liked the recommended exercises. *Birthing From Within* by Pam England talked about how medication interrupted your body's own natural anesthesia. Sometimes the external medication would confuse you more so that you couldn't use your own coping capacities.

We did the regular childbirth class at Baylor Hospital. I had read *Birthing From Within* and was intrigued with going to those classes, but they were too far away. Out of seven couples in our hospital class, we ended up the exception about doing natural childbirth [laughs]. The class was more geared towards epidurals and pain medicine. The one thing that was reassuring was to know that I could get an epidural all the way up to birth, almost. They did not have a cut-off.

My mom, sister and sister-in-law came to the birth. The midwife functions as the doula, too. Rich's first wife died of cancer and all his hospital experiences have been filled with anxiety. He was open about how the hospital might be scary for him. He managed beautifully, though.

Rich and I had been involved in the practice of meditation, as part of our spirituality. That was important to me to center and focus. We learned to use a mantra from Father Lawrence Freeman, a Benedictine priest and the director of the World Center for Christian Meditation. He teaches using one word: *Maranatha* (mar'uh-NATH-uh) which means *Jesus comes*. It is rhythmic with four syllables. To meditate, you repeat the word, or mantra, in your mind over and over. When your mind strays, bring it back and start over with that word in your mind. If your attention strays, don't beat yourself up. Simply return to that word. We did a centering prayer for twenty minutes in the evenings.

I knew I didn't want anything to distract me from my daily meditation. That meditation became my motivation, if I did not want medication. *Meditation* instead of medication.

Even though I tell people about Ryan's birth, "It's still the most pain I've ever felt in my whole life. But it *was* great." They kind of look at me puzzled and say, "Okay, whatever."

Contractions started on a Sunday night and went away. I woke up Monday, called in, and Susan said, "Oh, I'm sure you'll be here soon enough." I ended up going on to work.

I showed up at my regular appointment on Thursday, the 27th of June. I wasn't actually due until the following Thursday.

I should have known something was happening. At 2:00 I went in for my yearly performance appraisal. I walked in and cried the whole hour. Two of my supervisors that I work with, both male, glanced at each other and said, "We've never seen you like this before." I couldn't stop.

I went to Susan's office and said, "I've been crying, but nothing's happening." Sure enough I was dilated to 2 centimeters. She said, "I thought I'd see you delivering before today, who knows if I'll see you next week or not."

At home, the contractions started again at 3 a.m. I didn't wake up because they felt more like menstrual cramps. They did not go away when I woke up at 7 a.m. I had already negotiated to work at home on Friday. I wasn't going to be going in to work.

"This is happening today," I told Susan over the phone. Contractions kept coming twenty minutes apart and seven minutes apart, all day long. Rich was at home, too, timing my contractions with his sports watch. We watched a couple of movies—all the while wondering, *is this going to get anywhere?*

I kept in touch with Susan. Finally at 5:00, I called her, frustrated. She suggested, "Why don't you go into the bath and do some nipple stimulation." I did. A real *shift* happened. I could tell the intensity had increased.

We had already called my mom, his sister and my sister all in other Texas cities. They got on planes. I was still in the bathtub when a friend picked them up at the airport.

When I talked to Susan again, I was hoping she'd say, "Come on in." But instead she said, "If I can talk to you like this, you're not ready." *Oh shoot,* I thought.

I got out of the tub and they stopped again. This went back and forth, but it wasn't for long. The contractions started up again. We got to the five-minute-apart time and called Susan before going to the hospital. We arrived at 9:00 p.m.

The nurse checked me and I was at 4cm. We started on a walk. We did one lap around the unit. Susan came after that. She said, "Keep on going." We did another lap, it was evident that something had changed. I thought,

My gosh, how am I going to get back to the room? I have to walk? The intensity increased. I had to stop, feeling like I'm folding up right now.

After I managed to return to my room, Susan checked and I had opened to 6 centimeters. She said, "Okay. Why don't you rest a bit."

As soon as she left, my water broke. She came back in and stayed with me. Susan got the labor ball out and I sat on it, which was helpful. I was on the ball next to the bed with my elbows resting on the mattress. I could rock back and forth. Rich rubbed my lower back. Susan guided him how to do that. That was helpful, too.

We brought in *Secret Garden*, an instrumental music CD. The lights were lowered. It was a beautiful, warm atmosphere. It helped me to center my thoughts and emotions on the wonder of the moment.

My nurse was attentive and caring. I thought I needed to stop so she could check the heartbeat. She said, "Keep doing what you are doing." She would bend down and connect the monitor on me without intrusion. Susan was glad to get her and wanted her as a nurse. Later the nurse said, "Anytime I get to work with Susan on a birth, I try to." They worked wonderfully in sync.

Suddenly, I got nauseous and threw up. That's when I heard Susan telling Rich, "You know that transition you heard about in class? We're in that transition now."

All the time she was whispering these things in my ear, "Think about all the women that are laboring with you now. Use their strength to help you through. You're doing beautifully." She was supportive, "This is going great." Encouraging...a lot about that power that is within you.

One contraction at a time. I remember telling myself as I was measuring up each one, *okay, we made it through that one.* If I started doubting, *I don't know if I can do the next one.* Stop that. I would resume my mantra in the midst of my fear: *Maranatha.*

During labor, I felt like I was surrounded by this experience of Mother God, and sitting in the lap of God. It was my most pure experience with the feminine side of God I'd ever had in my life. It was pure nurturing from a feminine side—comforting to me. I kept thinking with each contraction, *this is intense. I don't know if I can do it again.* Then it was over. I had a sense of "It's okay, I'm with you." When I went down underneath the waves, I relaxed into God's lap more and more.

I knew I was working hard but didn't realize that I was pushing. Susan said, "Keep on, you're pushing, that's good. Maybe now would be a good time to move up onto the bed." It was *seamless.*

There was no, "You can't push now until you are at the right stage." Instead, she kept saying, "Do what your body is telling you to do." I was not even conscious that I was grunting.

I got on my knees and draped over the ball on the bed. I could still rock. Susan said, "I think we're getting close. Why don't we move you to your side." I lay on my left side. Rich pulled up my knee, and somebody else helped push my knee up from the front. Susan said, "Oh, I can see the top of the head. Would you like to see the head?" She got the mirror. I looked down and remember thinking, *That looks like a wrinkled prune. That's not the head. That's lots of folds of skin.* It was a little disturbing to me, "Oh, that's got a long way to go. I'm not seeing much."

She said, "No, you're almost done."

I didn't want to see any more after that, so they took away the mirror. We had to work a little bit at that point because the baby had his hand up by his ear. I pushed for thirty minutes and tore a bit to get his head through.

Our newborn came out and I felt a wave of relief wash over me. Our baby boy was born at 12:40 and he made it out safely. I only needed four stitches.

We knew he was to be named Ryan, but I had these dreams that a girl came out. We asked in the dream, "Where's Ryan?" I was glad it was Ryan because I already felt bonded to him.

The midwife brought him right up to my chest and I nursed him immediately. Rich was at my side. He took beautiful pictures. When I look at them, I think, *Wow, that's the most beautiful I've ever looked.*

I didn't know my body could do this. What a joy to see our baby. He cried for a minute and he looked up. He looked at me and looked at Rich. It was as if he was like so *that's* who you guys are. A knowing look. He was so calm.

My husband is a pastoral counselor therapist, and when Ryan immediately put his hand up to his face, everyone jokingly said, "Oh no! He looks like a little therapist."

The most sacred experience to me was to be fully participating. I don't think I could do that if I were medicated or "out of it." I felt excited to fully participate in *spite* of the pain, to feel what your body can do and is made to do naturally. That whole sense of being co-creator with God in that creative experience was a highlight of my life.

Release of Fear
Sherri's Story

In the hallway of the hospital, I'm pregnant and confined to a wheelchair, unable to run away. The nurse comes toward me with an extra long, sharp needle. She keeps jabbing and jabbing the epidural into me. I jolt awake at night to find my heart racing in my throat. Again. That nightmare haunted me. I used to be terrified of giving birth.

I prefer a natural lifestyle because of my mom. My mom started working at a health food store. I worked there, too. Before that, we grew up eating Ding Dongs, Twinkies, and Doritos. When I went to college, I majored in nutrition. I found that God gave us food and herbs to heal our bodies. Since 1987, I haven't taken an antibiotic. I use diet and natural ways to balance whatever is imbalanced.

Ted and I were married for eight years when I had nightmares about being pregnant. A friend who was working with a psychologist believed that everything we perceive was imprinted on us while we were still in the womb. He helped me process Prenatal Imprinting: taking me back to the womb by closing my eyes and reverting. This was simple; I went back. What happened is that I felt my mom's fear as she was giving birth.

A baby, growing from conception, picks up energy. *Molecules of Emotions* by Dr. Candace Pert and Deepak Chopra states that the baby's nervous system develops at seven weeks. They experience everything emotionally, spiritually, mentally and physically.

After working through that process, my nightmares stopped. I told Ted, "I'm okay to have a baby now."

That December, we visited a friend's house for a beautiful Christmas dinner. We all shared stories of that year...which was life-changing for me. I realized the most important thing is family and not my career.

Dave, our friend and Ted's coach, said, "I'm glad that you shared that." He described a dream in which my mom came to him in an angelic form and said, "It's time for Ted and Sherri to start having a baby. The time is now; that window of opportunity is open."

"Ted, that's a major sign that it's time to start trying," he said.

In January, during my next ovulation, we went to Kauai. The next day, I woke up and realized it was my birthday. Turns out that our daughter,

Jasmine, was conceived on that day. I know this because that day was magical. We took a helicopter ride off the Napali Coast of Kauai. It's 400 feet of cliffs up the mountains. We saw a full circle rainbow. The pilot who had been there for thirteen years and flies out almost daily, said that was only the second time he'd ever seen one. This rainbow encased us. I got teary. We saw a whale that afternoon and went to a little exclusive glass beach.

The next day we went to a small outside art gallery and fell in love with an artist's paintings. She paints mermaids in the sea and little fairies. We went to a vegetarian cafe for our lunch. After ordering, all of a sudden it hit me: I felt pregnant. I felt nauseated, yet, I felt hungry like I needed to eat right away. I felt someone else's presence with us at the table.

I started crying. "Ted, I'm pregnant." I knew it. There was artwork all over the wall. I knew it was a girl. I felt her presence. She said to me, "I love that fairy painting." I told Ted. We went back and bought the artwork. It was a timeless moment.

The first birth book I was attracted to was *Gentle Birth Choices* by Barbara Harper. That confirmed why I wanted to give birth naturally, in a peaceful setting. Another book was, *Magical Child* by Joseph Chilton Pearce. I read in that book that intelligence is moving from the unknown to the known. At the point of birth, we experience the most drastic change of intelligence from the known to the unknown. All of a sudden we breathe and we hear clearer than in the womb.

My favorite book, *Ideal Birth* by Sondra Ray, concepted rebirthing. During a rebirth, someone went back to their own birth experience. Their mom had an epidural. She as a baby being birthed felt her mother's body go dead, cold, lifeless. She thought that she had hurt her mom. Reading that was powerful for me. Babies feel they are conscious of what's going on emotionally and spiritually. That was a big reason why I wanted to do it naturally, which was a huge step for me, since I was scared about having a baby before.

When I read about waterbirth, I found it intriguing. It talked about the baby staying attached so she could get as much oxygen as possible through her breath and the umbilical cord.

I prayed that God would put people in my path to help me create a good birth experience. My goal was to be safe, have the least amount of pain as possible, in a safe environment, with the right people, and the best way, in the perfect moment with the least effort. That's what I prayed about. Every day I went on a meditative walk with nature.

I read an article in *Redbook* about Cindy Crawford's home birth experience. She started taking prenatal yoga classes from Gurmukh Kaur Khalsa, in California. The other women in the class had midwives and Cindy wanted to learn more about it. Her favorite book was *Active Birth* by Janet Balaskas. What I took from the story was not to care what other people think because it's up to you. It's what's best for you and your baby.

After reading that article, I searched for two months for a prenatal yoga class because they weren't doing them at the Yoga Institute yet. I finally found one at the Birth Center on Lovers Lane. I felt great and was in the best shape I could be. I even wore a bikini during pregnancy. I did not hide myself.

I faced fear again, this time from others. At a party, four people gathered around me and said, "Oh, why are you doing it naturally? I couldn't do it naturally." One of them, an aerobics instructor, who is strong physically, said, "You are too tiny to do it naturally. I had to have a C-section."

I held up my shield. *Let them get their emotions out...it all goes back to them,* I thought. I felt as if I were being attacked, but they didn't realize that. I stayed focused. I went in the bathroom right afterwards. I breathed and released all the negative energy that had come flying at me.

A couple of people I met had recommended the Birth and Women's Center, so we walked in and went for a tour. It was breathtaking, all antiques, plush velvet pillows, a four poster bed with the lace canopy, the hardwood floors and the bathroom.

I read an article in their packet about a lady who created a sacred circle with all the ribbons that were on her presents from her baby shower. She put that around her during birth. I read her poem and was touched. I cried, "This is the place, Ted, this is it." We felt comfortable with the midwife and the place and we started going there.

One midwife at the birth center taught a childbirth class based on *Birthing From Within*. It was perfect for us. The other midwife promoted the *Bradley* method. I signed up for both, to learn the medical information and to empower myself by connecting to the more creative-emotional side of the birth, too. But going twice a week was too much. We did the first one only.

I enjoyed connecting with the people who chose midwives. What I learned that helped during my actual birth experience was the pain techniques they teach you. You actually experience those during the class. You hold your hands in ice water, an example of "nonfocused awareness." That's what I used during my actual labor.

We wanted a waterbirth, but we weren't stuck on having one if it did not feel right. I didn't have to go buy another book on waterbirth. I knew the benefits already. The water felt good, as if it were a midwife's epidural. They've scientifically proven: sitting in a tub of hot water is like being given Demerol.

One idea from the childbirth class was to put your prayer and notes in a little binder so your partner can refer to them. We used it in labor. Ted read poems to me. I love these: "Childbirth is safe. I'm safe in God."

Ted grew up on small farm eating natural food. He enjoys the natural living way, too. He and his family were all cool about our natural birth.

During pregnancy, I took black seed currant oil and ate only olive oil. I took spirulina, red raspberry tea, and I took the PN-6 supplements from Nature's Way. I eat a lot of raw foods—gourmet raw vegetarian food. I craved chicken and salmon, too.

My mom didn't tell my dad for about seven months where we chose to give birth. When he found out, dad said, "You've got to have it in a hospital. What if something happens?" You deal with that a lot; *what if something happens?*

"Baylor Hospital is three minutes away," I said. "I have total faith that my body is intelligent enough to know what to do."

My sister is pregnant right now, and I gave her all my books. I think one leads by example. If people are interested, they'll follow.

The *Birthing From Within* class encourages expressing oneself through art. It's easier getting connected; even Ted drew some art. This is what helped me spiritually. I did a drawing in class with all these little lighted beings, little angels around me. I saw a golden door illuminated.

An example of a great question from the book: What do I need to know about giving birth or being a mother? What I needed to know is that Ted felt the same and knows what I need when I'm giving birth. How do I know he will be connected to my needs? He was drawing and asked, "How can I comfort Sherri?" It was a transformational moment.

Everybody has fears and concerns. My fear was pain. I'm not good with pain. The thought of a needle going in my arm is scary for me. But I focused when I was pregnant. I was determined to manifest the type of birth experience that I desired.

How did I deal with the pain? I researched it, like studying for a Master's degree. This is the most important time for my baby's life. I put her first. It's not about *me* dealing with pain. It's about *her* coming out safe and drug-free.

Someone who knew I was into natural ways asked me, "Do you have a hypnotherapist?" I thought, *maybe there is a reason I need to check out hypnotherapy.* A friend referred me to this lady who was connected to a liaison of the government about hypnotherapy. She was on his board of directors. We had three sessions. I listened to her audio tape everyday. I learned how to monitor pain, turn it on, turn it off, and how it tells one when something needs to be changed in labor.

I talked to my baby a lot during pregnancy. I focused on having my own quiet time. I would lie on the couch, breathe and talk to her:

- About breastfeeding—I told her that she would like my milk.
- About birth—I told her that she would enter this world when the time was perfect and we would all be here for her. I said my manifestation prayers. This is what I desire to manifest—an easy, pain-free, quick birth. I felt in-tune with her when I was pregnant. I've never felt that focused.
- Choosing a name—I asked her what she wanted her name to be. I always wanted "Jasmine." I registered for a girl without even having a sonogram. *Should I do this or not?* Gary Bukoff's *Soul Story*, says when you are multi-sensory, you have a sixth sense. You're in touch beyond the physical. That was my confirmation. Okay, I'm registering for a girl because I *know* it's a girl. I don't need a sonogram to confirm it.

When we traveled to San Jose, my friend cut fresh Jasmine flowers and put them by our bedside. When I came home, some ivy outside had not bloomed in four years and I didn't know what it was. The blooms that appeared were Star Jasmine. The vine Carolina Jasmine that we planted six years ago bloomed. That was my last sign.

"Jasmine" is a Persian name that means "eternal bloom." Her middle name is Hyana—"beautiful flower."

I wore my blessing bracelet made of crystals with prayers from all of my friends, a spiritual experience. Around the tub, we made a sacred circle of ribbons from the baby shower and my wedding ribbons. We had a water purifier for the bathtub spout. Jasmine was born to Sarah Brightman's music. We brought gifts for our baby: my grandma's baby ring, gold coins to symbolize abundance, flowers, my grandma's silk booties.

Heirlooms that she inherited. The whole atmosphere she was born in was important to us.

Labor lasted only seven hours. I labored at home, outside by the pool. I used peppermint oil. It helped lower my pain. I listened to music. At the birth center, we walked a lot during labor. Three hours of walking. Walking in awareness. It's all about being aware of what's going on around you. Ted would say, "I hear the birds. I hear the leaves blowing in the wind. I see the children's playground over there."

Instead of contractions, I called them "expansions." I had less pain during childbirth. Besides the back labor, I didn't feel much discomfort. Ted massaged my back and I used an herbal heat pack. The midwife's assistant massaged my back. The midwife wished she had videotaped it to show other husbands and inspire them to be supportive. Husbands sometimes don't know how to show support.

I squatted at the bedpost. That helped accelerate my dilation. I was stuck at 4 centimeters which is what most people do in a hospital because they are on their back. After squatting for an hour, I did the "Haa" breath with every single expansion that I had. "Haaaaaah" helped me when I squatted. I went from 4 to 10 centimeters from squatting.

One thing that I wish someone had told me beforehand is how to push. I was pushing up in my throat. Ted was behind me in the jacuzzi. We moved in three different positions. Ted was right there, my *rock*. I told him how to hold me. I wasn't in pain, but I went inside myself.

The midwife, Cheri, is a strong woman. I held on to her.

I made noise. That's important. I closed my eyes the whole time. We talked to the baby saying, "Jasmine push yourself out." She came out into the water and into my arms. Jasmine was born weighing 6 pounds, 2 ounces. I felt relieved because I didn't think I could push anymore.

I got emotional and started crying. Ted talked to her and to me. They put Jasmine on my chest to breastfeed. I love that photo of Ted after the birth. He's so *bright*. Here he is, a professional soccer player, giving our tiny newborn daughter her first bath. His face is lit up. He said it was the most incredible moment of his life.

Afterwards, I was exhausted, worn out, yet I felt relieved. I felt empowered. I'm not giving power to someone else delivering my baby. Ted and I delivered our baby with the assistance of a midwife. When you deliver your baby, you are responsible for it coming into the world. I rate it a ten plus, a magical birth. We went home eight hours later.

What I realized is natural birth is not for those who fear. Have faith in

God and the universe. You have to be mentally focused, emotionally and spiritually. You need to be in good physical shape to do it naturally. Your body is working to create a life inside of you. Your body knows how to give birth. It's creating life. Look—(she touches her daughter)—this grew inside of me, little toes, a little brain. It's amazing.

About 300,000 women give birth every day. Our bodies own an innate intelligence to birth naturally. Our bodies were designed to do it. If we give our bodies and minds the power and work *with* it instead of *against* it, we can empower ourselves as women and take ownership. This is the gateway through which babies come into this world. They deserve to come in without anything that's going to inhibit them, their nervous system, their bodies, emotionally or spiritually.

If something happened, I gave up the need for control. I knew that all experiences in our lives benefit us. They are a chance for us to grow and develop spiritually. I released that fear. I chose faith because fear and faith don't go together.

Envision Your Birth Day Worksheet

The process of turning scared into sacred is done by recognizing the need for emotional and spiritual preparation. List all your fears, every single one, on a sheet of paper. Talk with your caregiver about any you need to get off your chest. Now burn it. Those fears are gone because you got rid of them. Breathe. You are more powerful than you know.

From now on, only listen to positive stories. Avoid telling anyone that you want to go natural because it invites unwanted criticism. Keep natural birth close to your heart.

Keep a positive relationship with your provider. They will partner with you and help provide as close to what you want as possible.

Envision your day of creating new life as important and even more memorable than your *wedding* day. However, let your baby pick the date. A whole hormonal orchestration naturally happens when your baby signals the right time. It's a day of transforming from maiden to mother and a reason for celebration. If you think about it in this light, you transform birth from a medical procedure to the sacred event that it truly is.

1. Where do you want to birth? Do you envision a hospital room, a birth center or at home? In your mind's eye, what does the room look like ideally? Dim lighting? Fresh flowers?

_____

_____

_____

_____

_____

2. Who do you want officiating? An obstetrician? A midwife? Do you want to have a doula? (see Chapter 2)

_____

_____

_____

3. What kind of music would be the most relaxing for you?

_____

_____

_____

4. Do you want an altar? If so, what is on your altar? The element of sacred can be simple, yet meaningful. Include a mantel—a grandmother's scarf or your favorite colored fabric. Other items could be a symbol of faith, elements of nature, photos of loved ones and a symbol of new life, like a rosebud.

_____

_____

_____

_____

5. What would you like to wear? A hospital gown is optional but can save your own clothes from getting soiled.

_____

_____

6. Attract what you want through meditation, prayer, through faith, and any mantra that keeps your mind positive. (Example: "I feel a fast easy labor.")

_____

_____

_____

7. Listen to your intuition—keep a dream journal close to your bed and draw or paint art for this new time.

_____

_____

8. Food—you should be allowed to drink and eat for energy during labor.

_____

_____

9. Mentally teach your baby—send visual pictures to your fetus of head down, front facing your spine to avoid spine-to-spine back labor, known as posterior labor, and images of the cord away from the baby's neck.

10. Who will be invited? At what time? During labor? After the birth?
Keeping it to those special people you love and keeping it intimate
helps you feel like you're not performing for a crowd.

_____

_____

_____

_____

_____

The more you envision and proactively plan for your birth, the more
special and satisfied you will feel. If anything isn't going as you thought,
speak up. You have the right to tell others what you need, diplomatically,
of course. There's a time for *letting go* of fear and control and allowing
yourself to enjoy the power of birth. Seeing your beautiful baby is a
blessing.

Other notes:

_____

_____

_____

_____

_____

_____

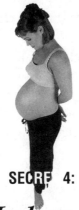

Don't Take Labor Lying Down

Gravity Is Your Friend

Did you know that the most painful position in childbirth is lying on your back? Women in labor pain aren't aware that lying supine restricts blood flow and makes contractions intolerable. Yet this is the position used in most U.S. labor and delivery hospitals.

Outside of pregnancy, women find themselves on their back with their feet in stirrups (known as the lithotomy position) only for their vaginal exams and pap smears. The main reason women are instructed to lie supine is because that position provides visibility for the caregiver during labor and for cutting an episiotomy. It provides hospital staff convenience for hooking the patient to a monitoring belt and an IV. Yet birthing supine hurts because the baby is actually born uphill. No wonder women want an epidural!

Before the advent of hospital births around 1900, women gave birth upright. The reason? Gravity is your friend. Ancient sculpture and art drawings depict women being upright for their labor and delivery.

In other cultures, women squat to birth their babies. These women *instinctively* birthed in the way that felt most natural. Squatting opens the pelvis more than any other position—up to *30 percent* more. Practicing squatting during pregnancy can strengthen the legs, making birthing easier. In her book, *Rediscovering Birth*, Sheila Kitzinger cites a study revealing that women who squatted experienced shorter second stages, tore less, and were less likely to need oxytocin or assistance with forceps. Upright labor and birth lessens the pain, and allows movement. Pushing becomes easier, also.

A Guide to Effective Care in Pregnancy and Childbirth, by Murray Enkin et al., provides thorough medical evidence-based information. The

Cochrane database and controlled studies condense what is beneficial or harmful in obstetric care. The evidence makes a strong case for:

1. Freedom of movement and choice of position in labor.
2. Respecting women's choice of position for the second stage of labor and birth.
3. Maternal movement and position changes to relieve pain in labor.

Upright during labor could entail walking, swinging, rocking, pulling, leaning, dangling, dancing, sitting on a birth ball, sitting on a birthing stool or toilet, getting on all fours, lying sideways with one leg elevated and squatting. Some new studies are underway to determine the most effective position for delivery. If history is any guide, what the statisticians will find is that labor is *less mechanical and more intuitive*. Women know what feels right in the moment. A good caregiver who supports movement in labor may suggest: "Let's try this...would you like to sit on the birth ball?"

The one exception to birthing upright is the *rare* instance of prolapsed cord, where the cord is coming out first. For example, ambulance paramedics once brought a woman with a prolapsed cord to a Dallas hospital while she was sitting up on the stretcher. Wrong. The cord supplies oxygen to the baby. That's why, in this instance, the laboring mother should have been in a position with her pelvis elevated.

Who are these women who birth upright? Amazons? No, they are like you and me. One woman describes herself as a "wus." Another admits she has a low pain threshold. And another curvaceous woman, says she wanted to see what her body could do. In this chapter, you'll read about birth positions in action with stories from two moms—a physical therapist and a childbirth educator.

You'll find a list of other comfort measures that will help you achieve the best labor you could ever wish for. Freedom of movement is the key.

Hospital Cynic

Most women seem more focused in the negative realm of pain, or
what could go wrong. They're not educated in what harm the inter-
ventions can do. They say, "Oh, the baby's heart rate dropped." Did they
know that's a common side effect of the epidural?—Jennifer

For trauma and high risk, abnormal pregnancies or any health reason,
I'm all for the medicine and interventional care. I'm not against it, but I
think it's overdone and over prescribed. Women aren't educated or given
enough choices and encouragement for how our bodies are supposed to
work. Ninety-nine percent of the time our body works in the right way.

It's not a doctor's fault; that's the way that they're educated. They're
taught and focused about the human body not working well. That's what
they're geared for.

Some of my friends ask, "Why in the world would you want *no* anesthesia?" I tell them:

- I'm a little bit cynical, I don't trust hospitals and doctors as much as
  most people.
- I question the reasons behind what they do.
- I've *worked* in a hospital before, have seen how many staff people
  were in the charts and how easily the charts get messed up.
- They tell you things are safe, but they may not be.

My mom was asleep during childbirth with me. My dad was in a chiropractic college. My parents grew stronger in their faith that chiropractic helped a lot of people, and they influenced me growing up. As they got
more independent and confident, they stood up to pressures of outsiders
to do things a certain way, saying, "We don't have to do it that way."

I have a Bachelor's in Business and a Masters in Physical Therapy. If I
had to do it all over again, I would go to chiropractic college like my dad,
become a naturopath, or go into alternative healthcare. Physical therapy
ended up intertwined with the medical-hospital system, but it wasn't
quite as "alternative" as I was hoping.

My husband, Art, and I met in high school and we married after college. Ten years later, we weren't sure that we could conceive. I said, "We
can't get our hearts set on this right now because we've been married a
long time and haven't had any pregnancies. A lot of our friends had infer-

tility. It may not happen for us, either." But the first month after we started trying, I popped up pregnant. It was meant to be.

Later, when we went to Bradley childbirth class, Art said, "You mean
they stick a needle in your spine? I don't want you to have an epidural,
either." In the beginning, he was supportive, but he had his concerns. He's
your typical man; he doesn't quite get it. For our first baby, I considered a
home birth, but that's where he drew the line. He's more mainstream.

When he started telling his friends and people at the office, he came
home and said, "Jen, maybe we should talk about this. Maybe this isn't the
best thing for us. Everybody keeps telling me we're *crazy*, asking 'Why in
the world are you doing this?' They say that home birth is unsafe." They
were questioning him about my decisions.

"Art, don't let people scare you like that. It's because they don't know.
They're not educated about it. Or, it's their whole philosophy, their way of
life. You're not going to change their mind overnight. You almost have to
grow up with the natural philosophy like I did."

We compromised. "Okay, I won't birth at home," I said. "Okay," he said,
relieved. Although Dinah's birth center feels like a home, it wasn't *our*
home for him.

Even though I chose a natural way of having a baby, I was still scared.
I had my concerns. I used a midwife, whom I liked. Even though there
were midwives affiliated close to hospitals, I wanted *distance*. I wanted
control. I wanted to call as many shots as I could within reason. Dinah provided that. She had backup if she needed it, but not too close.

In pregnancy, the concerns were the health-related "what ifs," not so
much the pain. I knew that women have been giving birth for years. If
they can live through the pain, I can too. I'm no different than another
woman who's had natural birth. Yes, it's going to hurt. You expect that, but
you're not going to die from the pain. You *think* you are. The rational side
of my brain says my child is not going to die from the pain, either.

In the midst of birth, I wanted someone to know when to comfort
me, like get some hot cloths. My husband tries and pretends he's with me;
he's not a real nurturer. He would do anything that I asked him to do, but
I would much rather have a woman or doula help. I felt that I had enough
experience and care in the room with my midwife, her assistant and Art.

Labor was longer, more intense and harder than I expected. I educated myself and had faith in myself, but I think I still had some fear of the
unknown. I started fearing whether or not I could actually do it. Part of it
was the fear of becoming a parent and having a child, not giving birth. *Am*

I going to do this? Can I do this? Hours later you get to the point where you think, *I can't do it.* I'm not in a situation where I can get the drugs. When they're checking the baby's heart rate and checking you, you think, *Oh my gosh, is everything okay?*

But deep in my heart, I believed that my baby and I were okay. I had good care. I felt that they knew what they were doing. I trusted Dinah to tell me if a time came that it wasn't going to happen the way I expected.

I told Dinah my preferences. "This is the way I want to do it, but if I can't, I'm okay with that, too. I'll be disappointed, but I'm not going to risk my life or the baby's life to say 'this is the way I did it' to show everybody else." I wasn't going to be obstinate. I trusted her to know when to draw the line. I actually think she let me push longer than she does most of her clients at their first birth.

Contractions started at home about midnight and I labored until about 3:30 a.m. It got to the point that Art couldn't stand it anymore. He said, "We need to go." We went, even though I knew it was too early. At the birth center, Dinah checked me and I was only about 3 1/2 centimeters. She said, "You can either stay here and relax or you can go home. It's up to you." I chose to go home, which threw my husband for a loop.

"If I don't hear from you, I'll call you in the morning," Dinah said. She called at 7:30 a.m. After we talked, she said, "Okay, I think you should come back in." Ten minutes after we got off the phone, my water broke.

We got to the birth center at 8:15 a.m. Dinah thought it was going to happen faster, but my son wasn't born until 12:40 p.m. I pushed for a little over two hours.

The midwife said to her assistant, "Her vital signs are fine, the baby's heartbeat is fine, it's going to take longer." Counter pressure on my back helped. They all took turns pushing back on my sacrum. Dinah was with me every second, massaging my perineum with olive oil and telling me with every contraction if I had enough elasticity to push: if this is a good time to push where I wouldn't tear.

During pushing I didn't think I was going to do it. Didn't want to do it. Lost all motivation. Didn't care about anything. Didn't care what happened to me. Didn't care what happened to the baby. I wanted it over. I thought, *I don't want to do this. Can't do it.* I lost it.

My husband is weak. I know that if I had gone that long and if I had been in the hospital, he would have let me say, "Give me the epidural."

Dinah and her assistant convinced me that I could do it. They kept talking to me, changing my position all the time. "Let's try this." They worked with me using their experience, convincing me that I was close, I had gone through all of this, I was fine and the baby was fine. That was one of the reasons I chose this way. It prepared me for the fact that I knew that if everything is going okay, the drugs are not an option.

I was all over the place during pushing. I was on my side, next on all fours. I went from squatting to standing. When our baby son was born, I was standing up, leaning forward over the bed.

Dinah said, "Oh my gosh, I can't believe how strong her legs are." I felt I had more *push* that way. Dinah caught our baby. We had a son, Brady.

Ah, afterwards I felt relieved. Overwhelmed. Happy. I felt great.

Now, I try not to "sugarcoat" it for people. I do tell them that a lot of the horrible stories you hear about natural childbirth are because they take place in an atmosphere where people aren't trained for it and aren't geared for it. That's not their goal. They have too many people to take care of. They aren't trained on how to massage the perineum. They don't have the time to watch your every single contraction. They use machines.

It seems a prescription exists for hospital birth and it's harder to do it naturally. Even if you're lucky enough to find a doctor willing to work with you, the staff and nurses in the hospital may not know you want to go natural or may not be as willing to help.

I've talked to women whose doctor didn't deliver their baby. Someone else on call from the practice did. The nurses that they knew weren't the nurses on the shift at the time. Nobody knew anybody. They didn't know you. They all bring their own different ideas and philosophies to work. I've heard great stories about nurses who will give options, and I've heard stories about the ones that are just doing their job, getting moms in and out. They don't stay.

Women asked me later, "Did you have an episiotomy?" When I tell them no, they are amazed. I had a first-degree tear with Brady. I tried to do my Kegel exercises (using the muscle that cuts off urinating). I did sitz baths with cypress and lavender essential oils. I tried to drink a lot of fluid, prune juice and other common sense things. I healed up great.

With a ten-month-old baby to take care of, we got pregnant with our second child. I had finished breastfeeding Brady. I hadn't even had a period yet. Brady was sleeping well. I was still in baby mode and I felt excited that my children would be close together in age.

It was an easy pregnancy yet, the closer I got, the bigger I got, and with taking care of a toddler, the more overwhelmed and anxious I became. I was a bit scared of taking care of two. I told Dinah, "I know I've done the natural birth, and it was wonderful. I know I can do it, but a part of me asked *why* am I going to do it, even though I'm not scared of it."

I think the biggest issue was pain. Why do I want to put myself through this again? My body hurt more because I was huge and picking up a toddler. Yes, I had to acknowledge my doubts, get them out, and had to tell my midwife about them. Dinah calls it "realistic anxiety."

My friend and I talked about how that last month of pregnancy is almost overwhelming. You are afraid of how you are going to mother a new baby, having to take care of such a young person. She said *worrying* about it was actually worse than *doing* it. She was right. Yeah, you're tired, but you do it automatically.

With the second one, I have to admit that I was looking less forward to the natural childbirth than I was with the first. However, it was great. My second labor took half the time. He was due on May 15th and he came on the 7th. As before, labor started at 1:00 a.m. and I labored at home until 5:30 a.m. We weren't even packed.

I told Art, "It's *time*."

"Are you serious?" he asked. We got up, called Dinah at 6:30 and got to the birth center by 7:15.

Dinah said, "Oh my gosh, you're fully dilated to 10 centimeters, you can push anytime you want." I pushed thirty-five minutes. I was leaning over on all fours with my head down on the bed.

That's the beautiful thing about working with a midwife. You can move however you want and you're supported. It's not an inconvenience.

Our son, Shane, was born at 8:01 a.m. and we were home by 11:00.

I liked everything about natural birth and all of its benefits:

- Individual care.
- Making a lot of your own decisions, where and how you want to give birth.
- Knowing that those decisions will be respected when you feel out of control and vulnerable. It's easy for some caregivers to say, "Let's go back to the way *I* want to do it."
- No drugs, no catheter.
- I didn't have to stay in the hospital and came home when I wanted.
- My baby never left my sight. We even napped together an hour after he was born.

I can't imagine doing it another way. Oh, it was the most *empowering* feeling. I felt like, *bring it on!*

Labor and Birth Positions

You will instinctively know what position feels comfortable during labor. Or, someone on your team may suggest a position. These are some of the ways women labored or gave birth in this book.

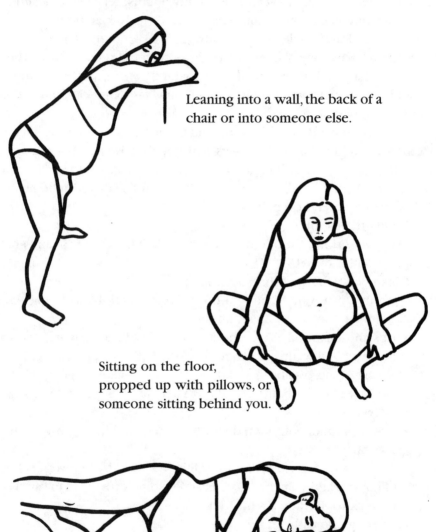

Leaning into a wall, the back of a chair or into someone else.

Sitting on the floor, propped up with pillows, or someone sitting behind you.

Lying on your left side with your right leg supported by pillows or someone holding your leg up.

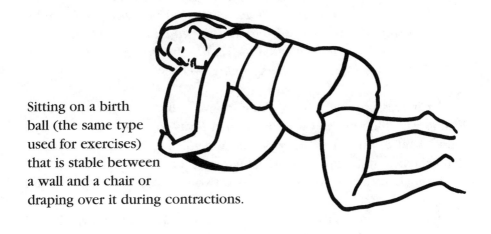

Sitting on a birth ball (the same type used for exercises) that is stable between a wall and a chair or draping over it during contractions.

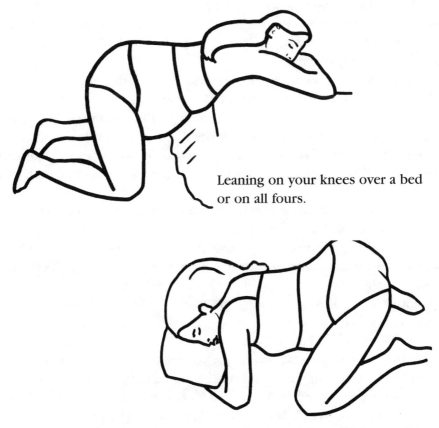

Leaning on your knees over a bed or on all fours.

Lying in a the yoga position called the "child's pose" or raising your hips up while resting your head on a pillow.

The Intimacy of Home Birth

*"My bathroom felt cocoon-like. It was dark and my husband brought
in candles. Through the window, the dawn lightened the
sky and with it came the reality that this birth
is happening today."*—Gwen

I felt pressure that other women in my family didn't have pain medication with their births. I wasn't sure that I was going to do it naturally. I didn't want to project to other people, I'm going to have a natural birth, that's the best thing, and y'all are all wrong.

I confided to one woman who had two children, "Yeah, I feel like I should at least try."

"Oh, you're going to *try*," she said cynically. Like that's all you'll do. I realize this mom had two induced labors, but why would she say that?

Before I got pregnant with Elana, I'd trained for running a 10K. I'm a *poor* athlete, but I possess the drive. After the 10K, I realized I could run a half marathon; I'm ready. I did and it helped me to build my confidence in what my body could do.

With the first pregnancy, I focused on the birth to the point of *obsessiveness*. I grew concerned about being able to handle the pain. From what other women told me, I knew it was painful, but I wouldn't understand what that meant until I was in the thick of it. It's true. I decided to change providers and switched from a female obstetrician/gynecologist who seemed too rushed to a certified nurse-midwife who practiced at a hospital.

"I'm concerned that if something doesn't happen the way you want, you may be devastated," said my husband, Dave.

"I know that the possibility exists that it won't work out. Something might happen and I may need medication or even a cesarean. Perhaps I won't be able to breastfeed for some reason. But from this point forward, I want us to go forth as if we're *going* to do this, like planning to run in a race," I countered.

At the hospital, I labored in the tub to relax. I felt like I had an out-of-body experience, like I was *watching* myself. Out of the tub, I ended up lying on my side in the bed, but I was unwilling to try the birth ball or listen to music. Self-doubt surfaced like, *If I had the epidural, all this pain would go away.* Visualizing my cervix opening and the baby coming down helped me overcome it. During the crowning, the staff asked if I wanted to watch. I did, but when I saw the mirror, I said, "No, I don't want to see that. The baby's not going to make it. The head is not getting out of me without some serious damage." Dave looked down with curiosity, saying, "Wow."

Oh God, I don't want to tear. It burns, I freaked out. Finally, I resolved, *Push. Get it over with. It's not going to happen unless you do it.*

The baby shot out. I looked at our newborn thinking, *My God, this baby is huge.* I couldn't believe this person traveled through my birth canal. Amazing. Elana weighed 6 pounds, 11 ounces.

No one announced the sex. A couple of minutes ticked by. "Is it a boy or a girl?" asked the midwife. It was exciting to find out ourselves.

Afterwards, though, the nurse scared us. "The baby's breathing is a little irregular and her temperature is not stable," she said. Now that I teach childbirth classes, I know that's normal. But the nurse took our baby away to the nursery. My husband followed her. All of a sudden, by myself in the room, I felt a lot of bleeding. I paged the nurse, "I want someone to come in here because I'm bleeding a lot." That's normal, too.

I yearned for my baby. I wanted to nurse her, but the hospital staff was not cooperative. One nurse told me Elana got a little bit of formula.

"I do not want the baby to have *any* bottles and I want her in my room to breastfeed her right now," I said, visibly upset.

Later, the nurse came back. "Oh, I had your baby confused with another baby. She did not get any formula." However, it was five hours before my newborn got back in our room.

At night, I didn't get any sleep, either. With every shift change, a nurse came in and looked at my butt. I found that annoying. "What are you looking for?"

"If you have any stitches, we want to make sure that you're not getting an infection," the nurse said.

"I *didn't* have any stitches, you don't need to see me." On a scale of one to ten, I'd rate the birth a seven or eight, but my hospital experience was a four.

My main motivation for home birth with our second child, Camille, was the experience of separation at the hospital after the birth of Elana. I feel that home birth is something that should be more widely available to women. We have to talk about it and be willing to do it if people are ever going to make this *shift* in thinking about birth.

Most people were supportive. But a few people said, "Oh my God, you're crazy."

Dave was hesitant, but trusted my instincts. I centered myself with prenatal yoga which gave me the time to focus on this pregnancy and on this baby.

I taught childbirth classes at Lovers Lane Birth Center one night a week, where Dinah was the midwife. A few students had switched from their doctor to her birth center. I was fortunate enough to attend one of the births. I liked her style and personality. I met other midwives, but Dinah could give me more individual attention.

Dinah came to my house at thirty-six weeks. Her guidelines are such that if you give birth before thirty-seven weeks or after forty-two weeks, the hospital provides the neonatal care if needed. I didn't choose a midwife for the birth, I chose a midwife for the kind of *care* I was going to get. One of the things that was most important is that Elana, our first daughter, was welcomed at my appointments. I could bring her with me and she could hear the baby's heartbeat which helped her make the transition to welcoming a sibling.

I didn't have a lot of concern about something happening during the labor or my health being jeopardized. I didn't worry about the baby's health, either. I know that the unexpected can happen, but a hospital was five minutes away. Most transfers are not done for emergency reasons, but because labor is taking too long. I know that the possibility exists that I might transfer to have a cesarean, but I felt like if something like that were to happen, it would be unusual.

A famous study by the researcher Marjorie Tew, who expected to prove outcomes are better for babies born in the hospital, found quite the opposite. Through statistics, she discovered birth is *safer* the less it is interfered with. She wrote, *Safer Childbirth? A Critical History of Maternity Care.*

Like my first birth, I felt frequent contractions over a weekend. Sunday was my due date. I thought, this is *it*; I'm going into labor. After a bad cold the week before, I felt tired and coughed a lot. Sunday I wanted to rest. I woke up late that night and knew I was in labor, but the contractions weren't bothering me yet.

I went to the bathroom and saw the big laundry basket ready and filled with supplies for our home birth. A friend was coming to take care of Elana. I gathered items for the cake they were going to bake to celebrate the baby's birthday.

By 4 a.m., contractions were seven minutes apart. I put more air into the birth ball. It was nice that my husband had moved earlier to help Elana transition to her own bed because I didn't wake him up. I think he did that consciously knowing I needed to get sleep. I'm open-minded to a pain-free birth. But as the labor got more intense, I thought, *this is not pain-free.* A friend of mine almost had a pain-free labor, with only a few contractions at the end before pushing, which is when the pain came. What worked for me was focusing through it.

A vision came in my mind: a gray cloudy figure pushing open a door. During a contraction I would imagine that figure pushing with a lot of resistance, like trying to push it open. That image helped me.

At 6 a.m., I called Dinah and said, "I'm in labor and giving you notice before you started getting your kids off to school."

Dave woke up and came stumbling in, groggily asking, "Why are all the lights on? What's going on?"

"I'm in labor. Go take your shower and hurry because I want the bathroom." After he finished, I got in the bathtub.

I didn't want a waterbirth, but I did want water to labor in. Our bathroom and tub are small, but I was comfortable. I filled it slightly with water, had a water pillow against the back and ended up lying on my side in the tub. I went back and forth to each side using hot water. I told him to turn up the hot water heater so I didn't run out. Elana woke up shortly and she couldn't believe I was in labor. She saw me in the bathtub and I smiled at her saying, "The baby's coming today."

Dave and Elana set about making the bed and getting all the supplies out. My friend, Sherry, arrived. Elana became preoccupied with her. I expected her around us more during labor. But she stayed with Sherry, baking the cake. I could hear them doing the dishes, left undone from the night before. *Oh, thank you.* Elana came back to the bedroom only a few times while I was in labor.

I vocalized through contractions and found it helpful. Elana came in saying, "That's funny." We had practiced making noises before, even pretending to give birth. One night, for example, we were in the bathtub together. Elana said, "Why don't you pretend to have the baby." I went, "oooohhhh," and Dave rushed in, "I'm checking to make sure that you're not actually giving birth in here." The role-playing helped. People told me that's what usually frightens children, the sounds their mom makes, more than anything else.

My bathroom felt cocoon-like. It was dark and my husband brought in candles. Through the window, the dawn light peeked across the sky.

I had a few contractions at the end that lasted two minutes. I told Dave, "It's not stopping. It should have stopped by now." He kept timing and telling me how far apart the contractions were. "I don't want to know. Quit telling me that," I said. He hit his watch and I could hear the beep. "Stop that beeping."

"What time is it?" I asked, trying to figure out where Dinah would be, at the birth center or on her cell phone.

"I don't know." Dave was trying to make sure I wasn't trying to keep track of time.

"Oh, you need to call Dinah." *Why do I try to talk women into doing this? This sucks. I am never doing this again. I'm glad this is the last baby I'm having. This is hard.* I didn't feel the out-of-body experience like I did before. Maybe it was because the contractions were further apart and I had more time to think.

In the tub, I had the slightest urge to push, "It's coming." I felt like, oh good. I know I'm getting closer to birth. I tried to get on all fours in the tub but that wasn't comfortable. After a few more contractions, I got out and I sat on the toilet.

"There's quite a bit of morning rush hour traffic," Dinah reported by phone.

"Gwen's pushing, but everything's okay," my husband said, trying to be calm. I learned later that when I had the urge to push, he bolted out and told Sherry, "She told me she had to *push* and I don't know why I'm out here and not with her." He ran away, temporarily. Luckily he came back. He sat on the bathtub and I could lean on him. My legs started to go numb so I had to move.

I did my own vaginal exam to see where the baby's head was and I could tell it was still far up. I wasn't terribly worried, but my husband was. It seemed that I sat on the toilet only a few minutes when Dinah arrived and came running in.

Dinah helped me to our bedroom. She went and got the rest of her supplies. At first, I knelt by our bed and leaned on it. I didn't feel comfortable in that position, I got my birth ball, put it on the bed, and was on my knees leaning over the ball, hugging it. That was comfortable, but my legs were crampy and shaky.

"This baby feels *big* to me." Whereas Elana felt like she was sliding down, Camille felt like a bowling ball. I felt a lot of stretching up in the birth canal. I was on all fours.

I pushed for thirty minutes, the same amount of time as before. Dinah suggested that I squat because my legs were cramping. "No, I don't want to squat. I want the baby to come."

Instead of being an observer, Dave rubbed my back. I told him that I wanted more touch this time, but he was talking to me. I felt annoyed by his talking and wanted touch only.

I vocalized during the contractions. When I pushed with Elana, I felt like everything was under control, deliberate. It felt good to push, but if I didn't want to push, I didn't have to. With Camille, though, I said, "WOOOOWWW." I was bellowing like a cow.

"Oh, it burns." I said. The midwife put some olive oil on me.

"That's good, you're stretching," she reassured. "Do you want to feel the baby?"

"Ewe, it's wrinkly," I said. Her head came out nice and slow. I tried to stay under control. I heard one author compare it to a little angel on one shoulder and a little devil on the other.

"Come on, push. Get it over with. Get that baby out," the devil says.

"No, take it easy. Take a deep breath. Don't push too hard." Listen to that angel. You may not tear as badly or better, not at all.

The baby's head came out and she stayed for a moment. I felt stretched with her head out and her shoulders still in. It lasted only 30 seconds, but I felt a definite pause.

"Push gently," Dinah instructed.

"Okay." I didn't have a contraction. We waited for the next one. I was still on all fours. It's a good position to prevent tears, the reason that I chose it.

When she finally came out it felt like she *spilled* out. Dinah caught her and waited for the cord to stop pulsating before cutting it.

Sherry announced, "It's a girl." We named her Camille.

When I turned around and saw her, she was "roly" compared to Elana. I picked her up and she felt different. I brought her to me and felt ecstatic. She cried immediately.

I love the photo of my husband after the baby's birth. He's *beaming*. I'm exhausted.

Elana sat close by like, *what do I do now?*

"Come over and see her," I encouraged. Elana came over hesitantly. She looked at her. We let her hold her new baby sister. When Elana was a baby, she would suck on my finger and didn't take a pacifier. She offered Camille her finger.

I felt good, exhilarated. The fatigue set in and I felt wiped out. I asked for ice on my perineum to prevent swelling. But I became cold and shaky. When they took the ice off, I was fine. I ate a snack and drank juice.

Dinah weighed and measured Camille. Everyone guessed her weight. Because I had been measuring small, I was thinking maybe 7 1/2 pounds. She weighed 8 pounds, 8 ounces.

"Ah-haaa, *this* is why it took a while for her chest to come out." Dinah said as she measured her chest. Her chest measured as big as her head. "Chunky girl," Dinah quipped in her British accent.

It felt much more relaxing. Your own home and bed is ideal. Home birth was wonderful for Dave, too. There are options in the hospital that are more natural, but I think if you birth at home, the likelihood of interventions decreases. You're much more likely to have a natural birth, if that's what you want.

You wouldn't think anything of spending $1,700 to go on a vacation and that's what our out-of-pocket cost was for the birth. The midwife charged about $2,500 at that time. A birth center costs more.

I haven't started teaching Bradley classes again, although I'll be interested to see how I incorporate what I've learned from my home birth.

Comfort Measures

Mind
- Talk to your baby about a good, safe birth prior to going into labor
- Envision positive images of hold in your baby—your end reward
- Use hypnosis
- Let go, get out of the way mentally, allowing your body to work
- Obtain support from your husband, partner or from a doula
- Visualize opening like a flower
- Imagine your cervix expanding like raindrop rings in water
- Take childbirth classes to know the stages of childbirth, to meet other expectant couples and to ask questions
- Communicate with your provider ahead of time and ask them to select staff such as their favorite supportive nurses

Body
- Tone for birth endurance: Kegels, swim, walk, or yoga
- Enter a hospital or birth center in active labor—unable to talk through a contraction, which comes less than 5 minutes apart, lasting for 1 minute
- Breathe deeply
- Stay hydrated, sipping on water or juice for energy
- Don't take birth lying down: gravity is your friend
- Use varied positions—
    on a birth ball,
    sit on toilet,
    on all fours,
    squatting opens the pelvis 30 percent more,
    lying on your side with leg lifted,
    recline with pillows or recline into your husband,
    lean into your partner standing,
    rocking,
    dancing
- Touch: massage, counter pressure, and accupressure
- Accupuncture
- Apply heat compresses—wet towels or rice socks microwaved
- Use cool cloths on your forehead

Body (continued)
- Hydrotherapy: using water to relax—a bath, shower, or birthing pool
- Make low-pitched sounds, loosen your jaw
- Summon deep strength to push
- Ease up when the baby is crowning to keep from tearing
- Ask for the availability of Nitrous Oxide, N2O (50% nitrous and 50% oxygen blend, "laughing gas" used in dentistry) which wears off immediately when one stops breathing it (Used in Canada and Europe)
- TENS machine with electric currents works for some (Used in Europe)
- Continuous support of a doula to encourage you and run interference

Spirit
- Trust in your body and your intuition
- Believe in helping the birth process
- Make a birth altar in your room
- Focus on a favorite photo
- Use faith
- Walk outside in scenic areas of nature
- Feng shui: have pretty, fresh flowers, dim lights, play soothing music, lighted candles (except in a hospital)
- Aromatherapy—lavender relaxes
- Invite only those you want at the birth with positive energy.

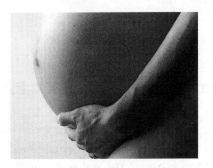

SECRET 5:

Know There's a Reason for the Squeezin'

Why do the majority of women in this country now choose to give birth under an epidural? The reasons are complex. We live in a culture of instant gratification where pain isn't tolerated for many reasons. We have been taught from the time we are little girls to distrust our bodies, and to view its many functions with disdain and dread. There is also a certain cultural taboo against women complaining about their pain and physical issues. Fear of loss of control and anxiety about the unknown, as well as the need for "civilized" ladylike behavior make it difficult in our society for women to surrender to the physical and emotional feelings of labor.

Dr. Christensen explains the historical and religious influences of pain management. Epidural information and the alternatives—the midwife's epidural or waterbirth, and the use of Nitrous Oxide gas—blend this chapter with two waterbirth stories.

Agony and Ecstacy:
Understanding the Paradox of Pain

Underlying these cultural attitudes is a Judeo-Christian belief system, handed down through thousands of years of church patriarchy, that claimed the pain of childbirth was retribution for Eve's sin, and it was visited on all women. Current theological interpretations debunked this as myth, but the age-old belief remains lodged in the minds of many women.[1]

The paradox is that facing pain with consciousness and courage, instead of fear of punishment, can be one of the most powerful ways to realize deep spiritual transformation—an understanding lost in our medicalized approach to pain management in labor.

A Brief Historical Overview of the Management of Labor Pain

Throughout history in all cultures, there exist medicinal plants and potions used to treat pain. Midwives and female healers used the medicinal plant cornucopia to help ease the pains of childbirth. Birth took place in the context of a community of women and family support. Pregnancy and childbirth were considered miraculous events, though fraught with the possibility of danger and death. Spiritual forces were invoked for help. In ancient times, women and midwife-healers were honored for their role in and contribution to the health and continuity of the community.[2]

But, the rise of Western "civilization" did not lead to a corresponding elevation in the status of women. With the spread of male religious institutions, women and female healers became increasingly disdained in society and were even linked to demonic forces. During the "burning times" from the 1300-1700s, these twisted attitudes culminated in a sanctioned assault against women. The Church's obsession with original sin, extreme fear of and disgust with the functions of the human body and women's sexuality, led religious leaders to consider the use of pain medications in childbirth a sin punishable by death for both the midwife and the mother.[3] Most people today are unaware that over 80 percent of the 6–9 million women tortured and killed as "witches" during this 400-year period were healers and midwives.

Social Suffering

When the first use of obstetric anesthesia in the form of spinal and caudal blocks was attempted in the late 1800s, physicians had to receive special dispensation from the church authorities. Queen Victoria was one of the first to deliver her seventh and eighth children with pain medication.[4]

The use of these anesthetics was at first objected to by early obstetricians who were concerned with the unknown effects of these techniques on the mother and fetus.

However it was the women, particularly the well-educated middle and upper-class associated with the suffragette movement, that demanded that all women have the right to pain relief, and challenged the Church's dogma.[5] At the turn of the century, the cultural belief that pain and suffering of women was necessary for the building of moral character gave way to new thinking: By preventing pain, hunger and curing disease, it was thought that many social problems could be alleviated. Along with their social and political rights, women demanded the right of relief from their suffering. At the same time obstetrics and gynecology became recognized as a subspecialty of medicine, particularly with the advancement of surgical techniques and the increasing use of forceps for difficult deliveries.

Knock 'Em Out and Pull 'Em Out

As the use of forceps became routine, there was an increased need for stronger and more effective anesthesia, leading to the proliferation of different methods. By the 1940s and 1950s, the majority of births had moved from the home setting to the hospital and were attended by physicians. The standard for state-of-the-art birth was forceps delivery of a patient isolated from her family, basically unconscious from inhaled nitrous oxide and narcotics, and tied down flat on her back to control her wild thrashing from the ketamine, given to create amnesia.

During this era, babies were born "floppy," were routinely resuscitated, immediately circumcised, and sent off to the factory efficiency of the nursery. Separated from their infants, mothers were only allowed to visit their babies to feed them formula on a strict schedule, and sometimes not until days later. Most women thought this was the way to give birth, and the predominately male medical profession was happy to oblige with advances in medications and technology. Dominion over the forces of Mother Nature was manifested as the Almighty of Science and Technology.

Birth Consciousness Awakens

Over the past forty years, a more humane and family-centered approach to childbirth developed including the development of epidurals, which have allowed women to consciously experience their births without pain, with their families and partners present. These changes originated as grassroots activism by women beginning in the 1960s.

As epidural technique was refined over the next twenty years, a counter-culture developed: more and more women became interested in returning to the safety, wisdom and strength of their bodies in an unmedicated state. *Birth Without Fear*, written and published in the 1930s by a maverick English obstetrician, Grantly Dick Read, extolled the value and safety of the natural birth process. Once again, interest in natural childbirth and breastfeeding paralleled the activism of the feminist movement. Many women felt they might be sacrificing something powerful and spiritually transforming in handing over control and responsibility of their bodies and babies to the medical establishment. They began questioning the dogma of the medicalized, fear-based model of obstetrics, and the safety and long term outcomes of the many routine interventions imposed on their bodies and their babies.[6]

The home birth movement and midwifery were reborn after its death under church-ordered prohibitions of the mid-century. First published in early 1977, *Spiritual Midwifery*, a how-to book of inspiring stories by Ina May Gaskin, head midwife at The Farm commune, explored the powerful spiritual elements of the birth process. The move toward allowing vaginal births after previous cesareans was inspired by a few brave women who chose to have their babies at home, a decision that demonstrated to the medical establishment that contrary to their conviction, it was possible to have a safe vaginal delivery after a Cesarean.

In the 1990s, however, some health insurance companies refused to pay for epidurals claiming they were unnecessary. That decision forced women to undergo a trial of labor rather than be able to choose a repeat cesarean section. A public outcry ensued over forcing women to suffer or depriving them of the *choice* over what would happen with their bodies.

Feminine Spirituality

Along with rising feminine activism, the past forty years has witnessed a dramatic change in the attitudes of women, theologians, anthropologists, and historians engaged in evaluating and interpreting age-old cultural doctrines. Their findings have converged with advances in scientific thoughts about the nature of reality stemming from revelations of quantum physics and the cross-cultural dialogue over Eastern forms of medicine—with its emphasis on the presence of "Chi" or "Prana"(different names for the spiritual life force felt to be directly involved in disease and healing).

Today men and women increasingly recognize the value and sacredness of the human body. The Earth is ultimately the Mother of us all and the vessel through which all Life manifests itself. Many women who have chosen natural childbirth believe a Sacred presence will guide, protect and direct them through the unknown.

Evidenced-Based Medicine

Over the past ten years there has been a major emphasis within the medical community on "evidence-based medicine." Yet, 70 to 80 percent of current medical practice is not based on documented evidence of the efficacy of whatever procedure or treatment is being used. Much of current medical practice has been based on outdated research handed down through the medical establishment without question, or on presumed benefits of a technology or procedure which has not been thoroughly tested.

An example of this in obstetrics is in the use of continuous electronic fetal monitoring (EFM) in low-risk women. This technology, widely adopted in the 1970s, became routine before its benefits were assessed. It was presumed that by continuously monitoring a fetus in-utero during labor EFM could improve outcomes and decrease fetal deaths and the incidence of cerebral palsy. Yet, none of these benefits has been proven. Many major studies have shown *no benefit* over intermittent monitoring with old-fashioned fetoscopes.[7]

EFM has only served to dramatically increase the rate of cesarean sections for low-risk women, with no improvement in fetal outcomes. Ironically, electronic fetal monitoring became the ammunition to fuel the spread of medical malpractice suits against obstetricians, further entrenching the fear-based model of medicine. Other examples of interventions used without scientific evidence are the routine restriction of food and water intake, and the routine use of enemas and pubic shaving. The first has now been shown to be detrimental to a woman's normal body physiology and the second serves no purpose at all.

A landmark change in the application of research-based findings came about in 1989 with the publishing of *Guide to Effective Care in Pregnancy and Childbirth,* by Ian Chalmers and his colleagues at Oxford. This compiled and analyzed all of the quality research from around the world regarding the effectiveness and outcomes of obstetric practices. The findings documented the safety and efficacy of midwifery care in uncomplicated pregnancies and challenged many of the long-held beliefs regarding appropriate obstetrical management. It also revolutionized the way medical practice is evaluated for efficacy and outcomes in *all* fields.

In May of 2001, the Maternity Center Association (now called Childbirth Connection), an advocacy group for family-centered maternity care, convened a national symposium on pain management practices involving experts from all fields of childbirth. Their findings included extensive reviews of high quality studies and in depth analyses from the fields of obstetrics, pediatrics, nursing, midwifery, anesthesiology, medical education, public health, consumer advocacy, childbirth education and medical anthropology. The multidisciplinary studies and conclusions were published as a major supplement to the *American Journal of Obstetrics and Gynecology* in May, 2002, and represent the most comprehensive information available regarding the safety and effectiveness of epidurals. Non-medical approaches to pain management were evaluated. Most of the studies quoted on epidurals are referenced from this milestone publication.

Variables in the Experience of Pain

Expectations

What is not addressed by medical caregivers is the psychological, social, physical and cultural environment in which pain is experienced. The interpretation of labor pain as negative or positive has more to do with a woman's *expectations* and *understanding* of the process involved, along with the emotional and physical support that she receives, than the *intensity* of the sensations themselves. What to one person may be the experience of unwanted fear and immense suffering over which she has no control, may to another be the exhilarating challenge of facing a difficult task with courage and fortitude. Why else would anyone want to climb Mt. Everest or undergo the painful training to be an Olympic athlete? Even though both have pain, the ultimate experience or interpretation of the pain is different.

Satisfaction in Birth

Despite our cultural and medical assumption that a woman's satisfaction with her birth experience is related to the degree of pain prevention, study after study has found this assumption to be utterly false. In an extensive review of the childbirth and medical literature involving over 40,000 births, Elizabeth Hodnett, R.N., Ph.D. concluded that the four most important factors relating to a woman's positive birth experience are: personal expectations, the amount of support from caregivers, the quality of the caregiver-patient relationship, and involvement in decision making—*not* the duration or intensity of pain.[8]

Pain Management Options

Research has shown that U.S. women have far fewer options, particularly with regard to pain management in the hospital setting, than women in other developed countries around the world.[9] Advocates for natural childbirth say women need more access to nurse midwives, doulas, and free-standing birth centers; they need less-restrictive, outdated hospital policies. Such changes can happen only if women educate themselves and demand the right to these choices from their insurance companies, hospitals, doctors, and legislators. At the same time, women need to take responsibility for their choices by helping to advocate for tort reform of medical malpractice environment. Our litigious and fault-finding legal culture has only perpetuated and strengthened the fear and rigidity of the current medical model, thwarting the best intentions of those physicians and practitioners who would like to see change made.

Perpetuating the Mind-Body Split

Epidurals are effective in relieving the pain of labor, while at the same time allowing a woman to be conscious and awake during the birth. However, an epidural is also the ultimate metaphor for the separation of mind and body perpetuated by our culture and Western medicine. Fearing pain, women are programmed to want immediate relief without ever considering how this decision disconnects them from the birth of their child.

American women learn at an early age to tune out, turn off, medicate, or use drugs to escape from the wisdom of our bodies' intelligence. For example, if, as children, our bodies tried to warn us about something potentially harmful—such as inappropriate physical advances from a relative—we might have been told that what we felt or perceived wasn't real, that there was nothing wrong. We learned early on not to trust ourselves, to dissociate our body's feelings from reality. Yet many experts say this unconscious separation of mind from body and the desire to escape from pain is at the root of all addictive behaviors from drug abuse, to alcohol, carbohydrates, sex, work, relationships, gambling and other addictions.

Access to Transformative States

During labor, a woman goes through a powerful and ancient process which is by nature designed to take her into deeper levels of expanded consciousness—accessing inner wisdom and connecting to a force greater than herself. When a woman enters into this state, consciously choosing to be present, to face the pain and fear, to surrender to it, there is access to powerful spiritual states of transformation which may serve her throughout her life. Fear, pain, loss and suffering are part of the human experience, no matter how idyllic a person's life circumstances. To go through intense pain, whether it be emotional, psychological, physical or spiritual and to come out on the other side with a deep sense of serenity and joy, is transformative. This truth is at the core of every religious tradition, including Christianity, Judaism, Buddhism, Islam, Hinduism, and Native American Spirituality. Many women often vocalize "I'm going to die" while in labor. This rarely has to do with physical death but with the spiritual equivalent of dying to one's ego, of recognizing that our physical and psychological concept of who we think we are "dies" and we sense the presence of Spirit in our bodies. The process is the same as those who have serious illnesses or accidents and undergo "near death experiences."

Labor Power

Most women associate significant pain with something being drastically wrong. But, I would remind my patients that the pain of labor means that something is *right*! The paradox of labor pain is that these powerful sensations happen because the uterus and body function exactly how they were *designed* to work. The uterus, one of the body's most powerful muscles, contracts and does the work of firmly massaging the baby down through the birth canal to bring a miracle into your arms. Simply being aware and reassured that your body is capable and ecstacy is possible even in the midst of pain, can help women gain confidence in their body and see the purpose of labor in a whole new light. If one chooses to have an epidural because of special circumstances, she may be able to cope with contractions with far less fear. Consequently she might delay the use of pain medications or an epidural until advanced labor, when there is less likelihood of interference with a normal vaginal birth, as described below.

Choosing What Works Best For Us

The question is not whether epidurals and the use of pain medications are good or bad, or whether women who choose them do so because they are weak. There is a role for this technology when used appropriately. It comes down to the difference of being forced to deliver without pain medications when needed, or consciously or unconsciously pushed into using pain medications without considering other options. It is ultimately about loss of choice and loss of freedom.

It is one thing to consciously choose to have an unmedicated birth because you have educated yourself as to the risks and benefits. It is another thing to have no choice because you are a single, unwed mother, delivering in a county facility where routine epidurals are not available. Or even being a middle class, educated woman forced to endure severe pain by a "well meaning" spouse who believes he controls your body, or believes you shouldn't have pain meds and won't allow anyone to give them to you even though you are begging for it. (Several of my patients experienced this ordeal.)

My belief is that it is a woman's choice. Often, educating her that she has the capability, strength, and courage to labor on her own, is all the encouragement she needs. Being told that her body is designed to give birth—that given lots of positive emotional, physical, and environmental support, she can do it—is inspiring. Armed with knowledge of the possible risks of pain medications enables women to make an informed choice.

Unfortunately, most women in our culture don't have any idea what epidurals entail and what the risks and benefits are. They harbor erroneous assumptions about the quality and safety of midwifery and therefore aren't able to make informed choices concerning what's best for the health, safety, and emotional well-being of their pregnancy and their baby's birth.

Understanding Epidurals: Informing Your Choice

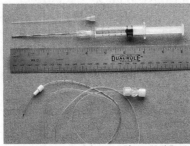

Photo: Neil Farris

Over the past 30 years, epidurals have become the most commonly used form of obstetric anesthesia in America. Approximately 80 percent of all American women receive them during labor. Epidurals work by numbing a woman from just below her breasts down to her toes. Medication is injected in the epidural space (epi- outside of, dura- the membrane covering the spinal cord) and bathes the spinal cord and the nerves coming in and out of the spinal cord in an anesthetic (numbing) solution. This solution blocks transmission of pain, and blocks impulses through the "motor" pathways which innervate the pelvic musculature and legs, preventing movement of these muscles.

Epidural Benefits and Drawbacks

The benefits of an epidural are that they provide for an almost painless birth, which is the goal for many women in our culture. In addition, they are extremely useful for emergency complications involving surgery, as well as for providing a positive, awake experience for mothers undergoing cesarean sections—planned or otherwise. However, there are downsides:

- Epidurals do increase the length of labor.
- They often lead to a cascade of unwanted interventions including the use of Pitocin.
- They often cause a non-infectious fever in the mother, which may lead to an unnecessary workup of the infant for infections.
- They are associated with increased operative deliveries including cesarean sections and the use of forceps and vacuums.
- All of these interactions can lead to difficulty establishing early mother-infant bonding and a less than satisfactory overall experience.

That is not to say that epidurals are bad. They can be very helpful for a woman who has extremely high levels of anxiety, poor pain tolerance, and no support. In these cases, there can be a beneficial effect of lowering the abnormally high levels of cortisone and adrenaline, the maternal stress hormones. The problem is that most women get an epidural with little or no understanding of the risks and benefits involved, nor with the knowledge of other effective tools for pain management.

Understanding Labor Pain

In early labor, pain sensations are primarily due to contraction of the uterus and stretching or dilation of the cervix. This pain is generally more easily controlled with narcotics, given either intravenously or epidurally, because of the type of pain fiber and the location of the nerve roots carrying this pain into the spinal cord. As labor progresses into late first stage and second stage with the baby moving down in the pelvis, stretching of and pressure on the pelvic musculature, vagina, and perineum occurs. This pain is much more intense and is transmitted by different nerve roots entering the spinal cord at a lower level. These involve not only the uterine and cervical pain fibers (called visceral nerves), but also the pain fibers innervating all of the muscles, skin, and bones involved (called somatic nerves). At this point stronger anesthetic agents are required epidurally, which not only numb the pain fibers, but also numb the nerves controlling movement of all the muscles.[1]

Remember, however, that these are the mechanical and physiological aspects of labor pain and don't mean that something is wrong. Your body is working exactly as it was designed. Your experience of and ability to cope with the intensity of the pain has far more to do with:

- your expectations,
- having a positive, supportive environment,
- access to movement, baths and other non-pharmacologic methods of pain relief,
- a trusting relationship with comforting caregivers, and
- your ability to participate in and make decisions regarding what is happening.

Epidural Drugs

Epidurals involve the use of two main categories of drugs: anesthetics and narcotics. The most frequently used drugs are the anesthetic agents lidocaine and bupivicaine which work by numbing the actual nerves entering and leaving the spinal cord, thus preventing the transmission of pain along the nerve fibers. In addition, they block the transmission of impulses along the "motor" pathways which prevents movement of all the muscles below the diaphragm. (The uterus is made up of a different type of muscle cell, called smooth muscle, whose contraction mechanism is independent of the nervous system.) Depending on the dose and concentration of the drug, women may or may not be able to move their legs or feel any sensation of pressure or contractions.

Along with anesthetic drugs, many anesthesiologists will also use a narcotic such as morphine or, most commonly, fentanyl. Narcotics work by decreasing the sensation of pain, especially at the level of the brain, but do not affect the motor pathways as much. They are often used in combination with anesthetics, particularly in early labor so that a decreased dosage of anesthetic can be used, allowing for greater mobility. However, they do not work as well in advanced labor because the baby moves deeper into the pelvis causing pressure and stretching of the pelvic musculature. Narcotic epidurals are often referred to as "walking" epidurals because of the theoretical increased mobility. However, the reality of being hooked up to all kinds of tubes, catheters and fetal monitors, the possibility of being sleepy from the narcotic, combined with most hospital policies, dictate that a woman remain in bed.

Epidural Procedure

A woman getting an epidural can usually expect the following sequence of events:

1. First, an IV is placed and she is hydrated with at least one liter of intravenous fluids to help maintain her blood pressure once the epidural is in place. This may take 20-30 minutes.

2. Then she either sits on the edge of the bed with her back facing the anesthesiologist or nurse anesthetist, or lies down on her left side. Her lower back is then cleansed with an antiseptic solution which usually feels cold.

3. The anesthetist feels along the spine for the appropriate space in between the lower lumbar vertebrae, usually between the third and fourth lumbar vertebrae. A local anesthetic such as lidocaine is given with a small gauge needle in the skin to numb where the larger epidural needle will be placed. This feels like a bit of a bee sting.

4. The patient is asked to hunch over, hold still, and press her back out like a cat (not an easy task when you've got a big pregnant belly and painful contractions), so as to open up the spaces between the vertebrae.

5. The larger epidural needle is then placed and advanced through the ligaments between the vertebrae until the epidural space is identified. This feels like a lot of pressure rather than pain.

6. A small test dose of the anesthetic agent is given to make sure that the needle has not inadvertently been placed in a blood vessel or into the subarachnoid (spinal cord) space.

7. A small, flexible plastic catheter is then threaded through the large needle into the epidural space.

8. The rest of the anesthetic dose is given and the large needle is removed, leaving the thin plastic catheter in place. This is then taped to the back so it won't dislodge. (A spray adhesive is often used to hold the tape in place.)

9. The catheter is hooked up to a pump which can continuously infuse small amounts of the anesthetic agent to maintain good pain control. Some smaller hospitals may use the intermittent technique where no catheter is used. In this case, as the epidural dose of medicines wears off, the epidural injection procedure is repeated a second or third time.

10. Once the epidural is complete, a pillow or wedge is then placed under one hip so that the woman is tilted. If she remains flat on her back, the weight of the uterus can compress the large blood vessels in her abdomen, dropping her blood pressure, making her feel nauseated and can cause fetal bradycardia (slowing of the baby's heart rate—see side effects).

11. When the delivery has been completed, the epidural catheter is simply pulled out. This causes no discomfort. However, sometimes removing the large quantity of surgical tape used to hold the catheter in place can cause discomfort and burning as well as painful skin irritation in those with sensitivity to the adhesives.

Techniques

Different techniques may be utilized including: continuous, intermittent or combined spinal-epidural.

A continuous epidural is when a tiny, soft, flexible catheter is left in place, hooked up to a special pump which continuously infuses small quantities of medications to maintain an even level of pain control. It can be turned up or down or "topped off" as needed. The intermittent technique involves injecting larger quantities of pain medications at intervals, then reinjecting when the effectiveness wears off. This method tends to be used where there is not access to the staff and equipment necessary for monitoring and managing a continuous epidural. The disadvantages are that pain control can fluctuate a great deal, as well as there being a greater risk for low blood pressure episodes with each injection.

The combined spinal-epidural technique involves introducing a tinier needle through the epidural needle into the space directly around the spinal cord (the subarachnoid space) and first injecting a small quantity of anesthetic before withdrawing the tiny needle, then injecting the usual quantity of anesthetic into the epidural space. The theoretical advantage to this technique is the immediate onset of relief, whereas a routine epidural may take up to 20 minutes to provide complete relief. However, it is technically more difficult and may be associated with higher rates of abrupt drop in blood pressure and spinal headaches.

Monitoring After the Epidural

Blood Pressure

After the epidural is in place, the mother and her fetus will be continuously monitored. The mother will have a blood pressure (BP) cuff on her arm that will usually be set to monitor the blood pressure every 5–10 minutes for the first 30–60 minutes. Thereafter it will be checked every hour. For convenience sake, this BP cuff is usually kept on the mother's arm and will automatically take the maternal blood pressure. However, if the cuff is uncomfortable, request removal after the blood pressure is taken.

Fetal Monitors

The baby will be continuously monitored either externally or internally at this point with an electronic fetal monitor. External monitors involve placing two elastic belts around the belly. One picks up the frequency and pattern of the contractions, and the other belt picks up the heart rate of the baby by listening through the belly.

Internal monitors are introduced through the vagina into the cervix. An intrauterine pressure catheter (IUPC) not only gives information regarding the frequency and pattern of the contraction, but also directly monitors the amount of pressure and force generated by each contraction. An internal fetal monitor (IFM) is an electrode that is directly hooked to the baby's scalp via a tiny, screw-like needle. Both require the bag of water to be broken.

Theoretically, internal monitors should only be used when it is truly necessary to have additional information about the efficacy of the contraction pattern, or because of questions concerning the fetal heart rate pattern in cases of distress. In reality, they are often used for the convenience of the medical staff and because of medico-legal concerns about documentation, despite the fact that they carry a higher risk of causing maternal and fetal infections during labor.

Committed to Bed

Once wired up to an IV, an epidural catheter, a blood pressure cuff and fetal monitors, the mom finds it hard to move, even with a light or "walking" epidural. I do encourage women to remain at least in a semi-sitting position to allow gravity to help as much as possible. The nursing staff will usually help the patient to rotate positions from side to side every hour. But, lying flat and being immobilized during labor can be one of the causes of poor progress and of abnormal heart rate patterns, as the weight of the uterus on the mother's large blood vessels can compromise blood flow to the placenta.

Relief Begins

Pain relief begins within a few minutes after placement of the medications and usually reaches its maximum effect within 20 minutes. A combined spinal-epidural will provide immediate pain relief because of the spinal component. A good epidural provides maximum pain relief while at the same time allowing some mobility of the legs and the sensation of some pressure which markedly facilitates pushing. Occasionally, women may have "windows" in their pain relief and be able to feel pain in certain areas while the surrounding areas are numb. Why this happens is unclear. It may be due to anatomic "pockets" within the epidural space where the anesthetic does not reach, or due to inadequate placement of the catheter.[2] It can usually be remedied by changing positions from one side to another or by re-injecting or replacing the epidural if needed. At this point the mom is usually feeling great in terms of pain relief.

General Risks

The downside to epidurals can be their effect on the normal progress of labor, the unintended effects on the fetus, as well as the inherent side effects and major risks of any anesthetic procedure. Having an epidural often leads to a "cascade" of interventions which may have adverse effects on both mother and baby.

Satisfaction with Birth

In some cases the benefit of no pain may be outweighed by the unexpected consequences of getting the epidural. Several studies compare birth experiences of women interviewed after having epidurals versus those who chose to have unmedicated births. The women having unmedicated births were happier with their birth experiences and focused more on the joy of the birth and the baby, despite experiencing greater degrees of pain.[3] Those women who received epidurals tended to be less satisfied with the experience itself and focused more on their fear and experience of pain—even though it was less severe—rather than the baby's birth. Some women complained of an empty feeling afterward and a sense that they had missed something or were totally detached from their experience. I learned that a woman needed to have an incomplete or unsatisfactory experience of birth first in order to start educating herself about what was possible and what her choices were.

Common Side Effects
Hypotension (Low Blood Pressure)

Epidurals cause relaxation and dilation of the maternal blood vessels which, in about 30 percent of patients, may lead to a sudden drop in blood pressure, called hypotension.[4] Low blood pressure may cause nausea and vomiting as well as uncontrollable shivering. Maternal hypotension will decrease blood flow to the placenta and can often lead to episodes of fetal bradycardia (slow heart rate), a form of fetal distress. This is usually transient and can be remedied by giving the mother additional IV fluids, rolling her to the far left side to get the weight of the uterus off the major blood vessels, and by giving an IV injection of ephedrine, a type of synthetic adrenaline which will raise the maternal blood pressure. But, ephedrine also causes an increase in her heart rate and the baby's and makes the mom feel jittery. It also can cause recurrent, abrupt, dramatic swings in blood pressure and heart rate on placental function which can lead to decreased oxygen to the fetus and additional stress, potentially leading to a greater likelihood of resuscitative procedures after the infant is born. The long term effects on the fetus when this happens are unknown. These episodes create anxiety for the mother, who is often unprepared and doesn't understand what is happening to her.

Prolonged Labor and Pitocin Use

Studies have shown an overall increase in the length of the labor, especially of the second, or pushing stage.[5] For reasons that are unclear, epidurals often will slow down uterine contractions, requiring the addition of Pitocin, a synthetic form of the maternal hormone oxytocin, which causes contractions. The use of Pitocin can be associated with longer, harder contractions which can lead to episodes of low heart rate in the fetus. Continued episodes may result in a cesarean delivery. Pitocin itself has been associated with fetal hyperbilirubinemia, or jaundice, which may require additional blood work and treatment of the fetus as well as interfering with normal bonding and breastfeeding behaviors.[6] Prolonged Pitocin causes maternal water retention which, combined with the IV fluids, may cause markedly uncomfortable maternal edema of the hands and feet. It also may cause strong, frequent contractions, known as tetanic contractions, which can cause fetal distress.

Pitocin use in general, and epidurals in particular, require the use of continuous electronic fetal monitoring (an independent risk factor for cesareans), which may be either externally (EFM) placed on the abdomen or internally (IFM) introduced into the uterus through the vagina and clipped to the baby's scalp. Because of the concern for stronger contractions, the force and frequency of the contractions will then often be monitored with an IUPC. The use of IUPC and IFM is associated with an increased risk for maternal infection called chorioamnionitis, which can affect the fetus. Used judiciously and appropriately, Pitocin can be especially helpful in allowing a vaginal delivery in someone who has been laboring for hours without making much progress. Yet it is often just added routinely as part of the epidural regimen.

Abnormal Fetal Position

Along with numbing the pain nerves, epidural anesthetic agents cause relaxation of all of the pelvic and abdominal musculature. The normal tone of these muscles, along with the upright effects of gravity, are involved with the progress and rotation of the baby through the birth canal. The anesthetics make it more likely that the infant may fail to rotate into correct position, or may have more difficulty descending through the vagina. These are the most frequent causes of instrumental deliveries and cesareans. Common medical terminology used to describe these conditions are: failure to progress, dystocia, persistent occiput posterior, and cephalo-pelvic disproportion (CPD).

Operative Deliveries

Epidurals have been shown to prolong the second "pushing" stage of labor and to increase the incidence of forceps and vacuum extractor use.[7] It certainly is more difficult to push when a woman can't feel her contractions or the normal urge to push and can't move her legs without help. With instrumentation there is a higher risk of a deep episiotomy and vaginal lacerations as well as fetal bruising. There is well-documented evidence for a higher incidence of third and fourth degree lacerations (involving the rectal sphincter and tissues).[8] Again, "failure to progress" in labor and "dystocia" (baby being stuck) due to mal-presentation or malrotation are the most common indications for the use of episiotomy, forceps, and vacuums.[9]

These interventions may lead to increased blood loss for the mother as well as more pain and later urinary and fecal incontinence (diminished control of bladder/bowel function). In competent hands and used judiciously, forceps and vacuum can be lifesaving for an infant in severe fetal distress or may prevent a cesarean in a mother who has been laboring and/or pushing for a long time and can't get the baby out. But these tools often become just a routine time-saving device whose use may not have been necessary. In addition, depending on the skill and experience of the practitioner, the physician will go straight to cesarean rather than even attempting vaginal delivery.

Controversy exists over whether epidurals have a direct effect on increasing the rate of cesareans. Several large studies have shown no effect, whereas others have shown a definite increase compared to no medication or intravenous narcotics.[10] Multiple factors influence the magnitude of this increased rate, which may be as low as 5 percent to as high as a 50 percent increase in the likelihood of a C-section, depending on the practitioner, the institution and the area of the country.[11] Studies reveal that primary cesarean rates are higher in private hospital populations than public teaching institutions, independent of epidural use. In those studies which have shown a higher rate with epidural use, "failure to progress" and dystocia are the most common indications for first time cesarean sections, not fetal distress.[12] Further quality research needs to be done before any firm conclusions can be reached. A cesarean is considered major surgery and is associated with increased blood loss, infection, prolonged hospital stay and increased pain and discomfort for the mother along with a prolonged recovery period post-partum.

Bladder Catheterization

Once an epidural is in place, the mother loses the ability to urinate on her own. The nursing staff will check the bladder intermittently to see if it is full and will empty it with a catheter that may or may not be left in place. Although this is not painful when the epidural is working, it does increase the incidence of bladder infections and of urethral irritation once the epidural has worn off. In addition, return of normal bladder function may be delayed, requiring prolonged catheter insertion or intermittent catheterizations after the epidural has worn off.

Fever

Another common side effect of epidurals is maternal hyperthermia, or elevated temperature. Although this is considered a "benign" fever because it is not due to infection, it often times leads to unnecessary blood work, as well as the unnecessary use of antibiotics and additional interventions for both mother and baby after birth. This may include multiple blood draws for both mom and baby and separation of the mother and baby for prolonged periods, even though all the tests come back later as negative for any infection.

Antibiotics themselves can then lead to side effects including oral thrush in the infants, and vaginal, breast, and intestinal yeast infections in the mother. Once again, used appropriately, antibiotics can be life saving, especially in conditions such as group B strep infection. However, their overuse because of "benign" conditions is what leads to the problems with bacterial resistance that the medical community is constantly wrestling with, and compounds the discomforts and anxieties that a new mother already faces.

Spinal Headaches

The epidural needle may inadvertently "nick" the dura surrounding the spinal cord, leaving a small hole through which the spinal fluid can leak out. This can lead to a severe headache in the days following delivery which is exacerbated by movement of the head and makes sitting or standing excruciating. It is treated with supine bed rest—lying completely flat—IV hydration and caffeine. If it is particularly bad, the leak can be treated with a "blood patch," in which blood drawn from the patient is injected into the epidural space to seal the small puncture. It is very difficult to care for or breastfeed a baby in this situation.

Back Pain

The issue of whether or not epidurals lead to an increased risk for chronic low back pain has been debated for the past several years. The latest studies which have looked at this question can find no direct link.[13]

Itching and Shivering

More annoying than anything else, uncontrollable shivering can be present in 10 percent of patients. While it tends to diminish over time, it can be treated with epidural narcotics if persistent. One of the downsides of epidural narcotics, however, is the side effect of intense itching in up to 50 percent of cases, as well as the possibility of women feeling lethargic or sleepy because of the narcotics.

Major Complications

Serious, albeit rare, complications of epidurals include seizures, cardiovascular collapse, and respiratory arrest. Because the spinal cord is surrounded by veins and arteries, the needle may inadvertently puncture a vessel and inject the medication directly into the blood stream. Should the entire dose be injected this could lead to maternal seizures and cardiac arrhythmias (irregular heartbeat), including complete cardiovascular collapse where the heart stops. Obviously, either condition is extremely detrimental to both the mother and the fetus and requires immediate delivery.

Another rare but very serious complication is inadvertent injection of the entire anesthetic dose into the spinal space rather than the epidural space. This leads to a "high" spinal block involving the entire spinal cord, causing paralysis from the neck down, which includes control of the diaphragm making it impossible to breathe on your own. Should this happen the woman would be intubated (a plastic breathing tube placed into the windpipe) immediately and placed on a respirator until the spinal has worn off. To prevent these complications, ensuring that the medication is being injected into the appropriate space, the anesthesiologist will give a small test dose at the time of initial placement of the epidural. They will ask questions such as: "Do you hear ringing in your ears, is your heart racing or do you have a funny taste in your mouth?" The answers to all these questions should be "no."

Effects on the Fetus

Neonatal Behaviors and Neurological Outcomes

All of the anesthetic agents which enter the maternal bloodstream, even those given in the epidural space, are transported across the placenta and into the fetus. We know that the fetal brain and neurological system are extremely sensitive to any type of insults and chemicals both in utero and in the early days and months of life. There is literally an explosion of growth and interconnections made as the brain cells multiply, myelinate (develop an insulating coating), and link up with one another. How are these nerve cells being affected by powerful narcotics and anesthetics? Certainly the common use of IV pain killers such as morphine and Demerol are known to have immediate adverse effects on the infant which may include respiratory depression (breathing difficulties), decreased muscle tone, lethargy, and interference with mother-infant bonding and breastfeeding behaviors.[14]

Subtle Effects

The blood level of narcotics and "caine" drugs given epidurally are much lower than in women who have received IV narcotics, so the level the fetus is exposed to is much lower. Although there are not the same major visible effects on the infant from the type and dose of drugs commonly used in epidurals, more *subtle* changes have been documented. Some studies have shown no effect on the fetus from the use of epidurals. But, when more sensitive testing mechanisms are utilized, significant differences have been found compared to infants of mothers who received no pain medication. These include differences in the baby's motor movements (such as opening and closing the hand, a kneading movement that aids a baby in breastfeeding), response to stress, and less response to the human voice.[15] Another study of epidural-exposed infants compared to non-medicated ones showed less alertness and decreased ability to orient during the first month of life.[16] More studies need to be done to know whether or not there are any long term adverse effects from these potent nervous system drugs.

A Natural High

Part of the evolutionary mechanism of preparing an infant to adapt to life outside of the uterus is the beneficial mechanical and hormonal effects of the labor and delivery in stimulating the baby's nervous system.

We also know that labor stimulates the production of maternal endorphins and opioids, nature's natural pain killers, as well as the production of dopamine, serotonin, and prolactin (the bonding hormone) which helps to make the mother feel "high," joyful, and responsive to her baby. These natural endorphins are markedly diminished in mothers receiving epidurals. Another study comparing epidural versus no-drug infants at one month of age showed that the mothers of epidural-exposed babies viewed their infants less favorably in general and found them more difficult to care for.[17] On the flip side, a mother who is extremely anxious can produce excess amounts of epinephrine (adrenaline) and stress hormones which can have a detrimental effect on the baby's outcome. Although the baseline level of adrenaline and cortisol is elevated in all laboring women, prolonged high levels of these stress hormones can cause fetal distress by constricting the blood flow to the placenta. And babies born to extremely anxious mothers are more likely to be jittery, irritable, and have a harder time latching on for breastfeeding. Epidurals can be helpful in these cases, but so can the presence of a doula or labor support person. A doula is trained to nurture, comfort and reassure a woman, thus decreasing her anxiety and helping her cope with the pain of labor, as well as in helping her bond with and breastfeed her infant once she is delivered.

Long-term Questions

How the babies' delicate neurochemistry may be affected in the long term by exposure to such strong narcotic and anesthetic drugs is unknown. There is currently research being conducted in this area. The teens and twenty-something Americans of the 1960s, the first to widely and openly experiment with and abuse mind altering drugs as an entire generation, were born to the first generation of American women who were routinely given powerful IV narcotics, "twilight sleep," and nitrous oxide in hospital births. A recent retrospective Swedish study has confirmed this link.[18] We already know from twin and adoption studies that infants of women who smoked during pregnancy are much more likely to become smokers as adults even when raised in non-smoking families. The same is true for alcohol exposure during pregnancy. Those babies born to alcoholic mothers and raised in non-alcohol consuming families have a higher incidence of alcoholism themselves. The roots of addiction may be deeper and more insidious than we think. That doesn't mean that just because a woman used IV pain relievers and an epidural during one day of labor that her baby will grow up to be a drug addict. The disease of addiction is far more complex than that and has many stronger links to environment, genetics and cultural messages and values, but these associations do give pause. Clearly, much more research needs to be done.

Neonatal Interventions and Procedures

As noted, epidurals are often associated with maternal fevers which in most U.S. hospitals lead to the infant being evaluated after birth for infection. This evaluation may include several blood draws and a spinal tap, as well as placement of IV lines for antibiotics. All these procedures involve separation of the mother and baby even though all the tests may come back negative after one or two days. In addition the effects of maternal fever, unrelated to infection, on the neurologic system of the infant are unknown. Several studies have shown a possible link of unexplained neonatal seizures with non-infectious fever in the mothers. Much more research is needed in this area.[19]

Respiratory Difficulties

We know that babies exposed to IV narcotics such as Demerol, Stadol and Nubain during labor are more likely to have respiratory depression at birth requiring extra stimulation and oxygen and injection of an anti-narcotic antidote.[20] But, studies have not shown the same direct effects on infants' respiratory function from the epidural medications used. However, indirect effects may be present which can compromise the infants' respiratory integrity. Those babies born to mothers with fevers, instrumental deliveries, recurrent fetal bradycardia and prolonged labors, as well as prolonged rupture of membranes, are more likely to experience transient tachypnea (a too-fast breathing rate). This often requires placement in the nursery with additional oxygen and interferes with a baby's ability to breastfeed in the first hours of life. C-section is a risk factor for this condition because the infants do not receive the beneficial mechanical effects of amniotic fluid being squeezed out of their lungs by passage through the vagina. All of these risk factors for transient tachypnea are indirectly increased by epidural use.

Jaundice (Hyperbilirubinemia)

Several studies have shown a one-and-a-half to two-fold increased incidence of hyperbilirubinemia (or jaundice) in epidural-exposed infants compared to no drugs.[21] Jaundice is a condition in which the infant's immature liver is unable to process the breakdown products of blood cells (bilirubin), leading to high levels in the blood stream which then cause the skin to turn yellow and may have a detrimental effect on the developing brain if very elevated and left untreated. It is unclear whether the elevated bilirubin is a direct effect of the epidural or because of the increased use of oxytocin (Pitocin) and instrumental vaginal deliveries, known risk factors for jaundice, both of which are more likely with epidural analgesia.[22] Neonatal jaundice evaluation and treatment requires several blood sticks of the baby as well as treatment under special lights if severe enough, again leading to separation of the mother-infant pair.

Breastfeeding

There has been very little quality research on the effects of epidural on establishing and maintaining breastfeeding. Some studies have suggested a decrease in breastfeeding at six weeks and six months, whereas others have found no difference. We know that the ease of initiation and the likelihood of prolonged breastfeeding is directly facilitated by early, supportive, and sustained contact of the infant with his mother. Obviously, any situation which interferes with this bonding may make the process more difficult than it needs to be. Intuitively, babies (as well as moms) suffering from any of the aforementioned unintended epidural side effects may have more difficulty. Compared to the side effects of IV narcotics used for pain, however, epidural babies do better with initiating and maintaining breastfeeding. Further research needs to be done in this area.[23]

Optimizing Birth Outcomes

The most important thing a woman needs in labor is a feeling of security, comforting, nurturing, and support. Unmedicated women in labor require a lot of physical and emotional support. They need the constant presence of companions, touch, reassurance, privacy, and a safe-feeling environment. They need the ability to move about in labor, to walk, sit, stand, squat, rock, take a bath or shower, and to be able to freely make noise. The hospital environment in most places in the U.S. is not equipped to do this. There is a chronic shortage of nurses who have too many patients to take care of and too much paperwork to fill out (for legalities, if they arise). Many L&D nurses are trained only in the medical disease model of birth, as are obstetricians, so that they have never gotten any training on how to support women who do not want medical interventions. Add the cultural discomfort we have toward women vocalizing their pain and psychosexual experiences, especially in as public a setting as a hospital, and it is no wonder that it is much easier for patient, family, and staff, to keep the mother quiet and immobilized in bed.

Using epidurals is neither good nor bad. They have a life saving role to play. The issue is that women generally aren't educated about the risks of having one and the benefits of not having one for both mom and baby.

If a woman has to have an epidural because of unexpected events, fetal distress requiring immediate delivery or other complications, or for an extremely long or painful labor that she is no longer able to tolerate, or if that is her choice to begin with, then she can feel good about her decision. If she can, it's best to wait until she's at least 5-6 centimeters dilated before she gets one. Studies have shown that placement late in labor is less likely to interfere with a normal vaginal delivery.[24] I urge women to let go of any guilt, shame or sense of failure and know that they have done their best. They can still have a meaningful experience. Do what you can to help create a calm and sacred environment around yourself. You have the right to choose.

Waterbirths:
The Midwife's Epidural

Most women enjoy their bath, a time for washing away stress as well as cleansing away the grit from mind and body—a pause for oneself, fluid reflection with a fresh floral scent.

The same response comes for women in active labor. Slipping into water is called the "Aaaahhh" effect, the liquid epidural or the midwives' epidural. A bath during strong contractions soothes, relaxes, and opens the cervix while helping to keep the perineum intact.

The baby's transition from womb to clean water provides a familiar environment. Bringing the newborn gently to surface for its first breath, many new parents marvel at the baby's quiet awareness.

With the introduction of birthing pools in the 1970s in France, there was an alternative to offer laboring moms relief other than Demerol (a pain killer). Michel Odent, M.D., from France, says, "We could introduce the mother-to-be into the aquatic birthing room so that she could watch the beautiful blue water and hear the noise of the water filling the pool. The room had been painted blue, with dolphins on the walls. From that time on the question was not, 'When will you give me a painkiller?' It was more often, 'How long does it take to fill the pool?' The dilation of the cervix can already progress dramatically before water immersion...if the environment is private. We learned that the birthing pool can replace drugs."

Not all hospitals support waterbirths, but some LDR units have tubs, jacuzzis or birthing pools specifically for laboring. Typically, birth centers get more requests for waterbirths. In a bathtub, one is in a sitting position alone versus a Jacuzzi where there's also room for the husband. Specially designed birthing tubs, which can be rented, allow for the most movement.

Waterbirths

"It's impossible for babies to gasp for breath until they come into air," says Barbara Harper, founder of Waterbirth International. A waterbirth checklist includes:

• Use filtered water from a faucet with a carbon filter attachment.

• Women with hypertension (high blood pressure) experience a drop in blood pressure about 10–15 minutes after entering a warm bath.

• Heat water warm enough so mom doesn't chill, yet not too hot for baby, 98.6 degrees, similar to the womb. The temperature should not exceed 101 degrees.

• The emerging baby first entering the water will not drown while the cord is still attached.

• Bring the baby to surface to feel air and to take its first breath, keep its face above water, and do not resubmerge.

• Hypothermia of the baby is prevented by skin-to-skin contact with the mother along with a hat for the newborn's head and a warmed towel after birth.

Study Confirms Safety of Waterbirths[25]

Using more than 2,000 waterbirths, a study in Switzerland showed that an episiotomy was performed in only 12.8 percent of the births in water compared to 35.4 percent of bed births. Mother's blood loss was lowest in waterbirths. Fewer painkillers were used and mothers reported the experience of birth itself was more satisfying after a waterbirth. The average arterial blood pH of the umbilical cord as well as the baby's Apgar score at 5 and 10 minutes were significantly higher after waterbirths.

Conclusion: Waterbirths do not demonstrate higher birth risks for mother or child.

During transition from laboring to pushing, most women feel that they need something. If a midwife asks you, "What do you need?" a bath may be the answer.

Birth of a Midwife

Former High-Risk LDR Nurse, Rebecca Burpo, CNM

I didn't sleep well for a week after witnessing my first home birth as a midwife's apprentice. Everything I ever knew before as a high-risk labor and delivery nurse in a busy hospital was of no use. It went right out the window. I was used to women coming into the hospital, putting on their gown and getting into bed. I would walk them around the room and get them up, but they were still patients.

This woman remained fully clothed. She was 5 centimeters dilated when we arrived. She and her husband said, "We're going to walk around the neighborhood." I thought, *Oh, you don't let a woman who's 5 centimeters go walk around the neighborhood. You can't do that!*

"Okay," said the midwife. Everyone was calm except for me. *The midwife told me I had to be quiet. I must keep silent.*

The mom came back in. "I'm starting to get uncomfortable. I think I'm going to get into the swimming pool." She came in later and said, "I want to go upstairs and go to bed." Cheri checked: she was at 8 centimeters.

"I think she's going to go shortly," the midwife told me. *How can she? She's calm. How could she give birth shortly?* This was nothing I'd ever seen before.

"I can't get comfortable. I want to get in the tub."

"Do you want a waterbirth?" the midwife asked.

"I just want to get in the tub right now because I'm having trouble relaxing."

She got in the tub and in two minutes, Cheri called me, "Becky..."

I looked into the bathroom as the woman proceeded to birth in the tub. When the baby came out, he swam. I mean he literally did a breast-stroke in the water before she brought him up. I was mesmerized. I started crying. It was the most beautiful thing I had ever seen.

The energy in the room filled with incredible joy. Everyone was happy, excited and welling up with tears.

In the maternity ward, I was used to women who were barely conscious or who were out of it altogether. They had to sleep. Someone else took care of the baby. But this woman was alert.

We stayed through her recovery, leaving her ready to rest in bed after nursing her baby. When I went home, I questioned, *how could I have made a career in childbirth my whole adult life and missed this?*

That summer I went to more home births as well as birth center births, and knew this was where childbirth truly happened.

In nursing school, I always wanted to be in Labor and Delivery, taking care of women having babies. I wasn't into illness. I became enthralled with all of the technology. *This is cool. I can learn all these skills that nurses like to do.* I felt I was a *total* nurse because I could still provide emotional support. "High-risk obstetrics" came into being, and I started doing cardiovascular monitoring, as well.

In 1990, I interviewed in Dallas to set up a high-risk unit at a local hospital. After the interview, I visited Parkland Hospital because I had done my obstetrics rotation there as a student, twenty years ago. Walking down the hall, I stopped at the nurse recruiter's office to look at job postings. The recruiter walked out, "What do you do?" When I told her about the interview, she asked, "Have you ever thought about being a midwife?"

"Oh yeah, I've always wanted to be a midwife, but I've never been in a place where they had it."

"We're starting a midwifery program here in September," she said. That struck a responsive chord, but I took the hospital job because I needed the money. I didn't have the luxury of going back to school at that point. I worked for three years. Every year though, when things started getting to me, I thought about calling Parkland's program.

We had come to depend more and more on technology, and as a result, I witnessed a 40 percent C-section rate. I couldn't believe it. Inductions, too...everyone was induced. At that point in my career, I questioned, *what has happened that women can't birth on their own anymore? This is not why I became a nurse.*

One night I went with several people from the hospital to hear Bill Moyers, the author of *Healing and the Mind.* He talked about people who were at the forefront of healing in our community. "You have them right here, people who are into the whole person. This is Ron Anderson, the President of Parkland," he said. Moyers had written a chapter about him in his book.

Ron stood up and spoke powerfully about the midwives at Parkland and how they had changed health care for the indigent population. His positive speech inspired me that night. I called the next day to request an application for the midwifery program.

I envisioned practicing midwifery in a hospital. Several people said, "Oh, Parkland is not *real* midwifery because it's not real touchy-feely. It's a medical model, like being a mini-doc." That wasn't going to hurt me because I wanted to know all of the medical information. I started training and enjoyed it, but it was the hardest thing I've ever done. The training was intense. There was only one break. I went seven days a week for one year. (Most programs are two to three years long.) I had one week off halfway through for the annual meeting. It was incredibly strenuous with so much information to learn. I would finish one module, take the test, and get the next module presented an hour later. Then I needed to read another thousand pages. It never let up for a semester break or holidays. The program is a little more student-friendly now.

I started learning about midwifery as a profession when I wrote book reports. I read *Spiritual Midwifery*, by Ina May Gaskin, which changed me more than anything. I developed a *thirst* for midwifery.

The convention was held in Tennessee and Ina May Gaskin attended. I had written to her before to see if I could tour The Farm's Birth Center, but I hadn't heard back. At the meeting, she said lots of people wanted a tour. If we could get out to the rural area, she would spend the afternoon with us. While most of our colleagues went shopping, I went with a carload of people out to The Farm, a vegetarian commune. The young women there birthed their babies naturally: another mind-changing experience. I *really* wanted to go to an out-of-hospital birth and see what this was all about because it was different. It felt as if it was my destiny.

Summer came, time to work as a midwife's apprentice, doing the full scope of care. I had to find my own clinical site to finish the program. By that time a midwife had opened a birth center in town and I worked there.

At 6 a.m. on my first day the midwife called and said, "Would you like to go to a home birth?" That was the first home birth and waterbirth that forever changed my path of becoming a midwife.

Women who come to me as a midwife are exploring their options. They are looking for something *else* beyond the hospital. Two right now are first time moms. Yet for most of my clientele, it's their second or third babies. Most went to the hospital and had an epidural the first time. It left them with a feeling of dissatisfaction or they had a poor experience. That's what they all have in common. They didn't necessarily have a *bad* experience, but it's not what they had anticipated.

They say, "You know, I had a good birth. I had no complaints, but..." Something was missing and they couldn't put their finger on it.

The epidural gives a detached feeling. Some women say they feel removed from their bodies, not experiencing labor. They're in a passive state watching birth with no sensation.

A percent of my clients deliver at home. Sometimes they want to because they have become anti-hospital. They don't want any institutions.

I have some clients who start out saying they want a birth center birth. On the disclosure statement that I give them, I compare home, hospital and birth center births. After they've come for check-ups, they read and start to think. "Oh, *home*, that would be the most comfortable. That would be the best for me."

Once clients make the leap to leave the hospital, the move from birth center to home is easy.

My husband and I have three children, all born naturally, in a military hospital. I didn't know there was a choice. I knew I would have natural childbirth. I would not even consider putting drugs into my body during labor. Intuitively, it didn't seem right for me.

I like to have the husbands come in for the consultation. I find it easier to talk to the guys because I have sons. I know where they are coming from. They have that strong sense of being the protector of the wife. It's their responsibility. They have to do what's safe for their wife, and I acknowledge that when I'm talking to them.

Here are some of the most frequently asked questions by parents:

1. *Is natural birth safe?* I tell them, "Yes, natural birth is safe." I try to individualize it. I believe each woman should choose what's right for her. I give an evidence-based brochure that summarizes studies of home births and birth center births as well as my personal statistics of over 4,000 patients since 1994.

2. *What about pain?* Pain is a major factor in birth. I think women have always been concerned with it, but it seems to be growing. There's a real fear of discomfort in our society right now, a feeling of not being able to make it, of not being strong enough to get through it.

3. *If I can't do it, do you have something for me?* It's always a choice. If that's what you want, I have arrangements to take you to a hospital so you'll be in a safe location to receive an epidural. Once you receive it, you move into a "high risk" category because of the potential for side effects. I don't think people think of it that way because it's so common.

For comfort in labor, water is like Mother Nature's "epidural." I do have some drugs here that can relax the moms, but only one person has ever used them. Most women find that they don't need them.

A lot of the pain is engendered when they go to the hospital with strangers in a strange environment. When they're in a familiar environment with people who are supportive, it makes the difference in how they perceive pain.

I don't intervene. I don't break the mother's bag of water unless it's at the last minute. I don't do things that are going to intensify the pain. I don't induce them.

The benefits of natural childbirth are many. First is a sense of empowerment for the woman. It makes you feel strong and confident in your abilities for the rest of your life. Second, it is best for the baby. You give your baby the gift of a drug-free labor. They come into the world without having been exposed to narcotics.

The birth experience depends on the woman. What is good for one woman is not necessarily appropriate for another.

The southern mentality is that women like to be taken care of. Being a Texan, I can buy that to a degree. A majority of the women who birth with me are not from here, though. We do know that more epidurals and more inductions are done in the southern states than any place else in the country.

A study in Sweden, where they have nationalized healthcare, spanned twenty years and covered thousands of births. With accurate records, they follow their citizens looking at drug abuse in young people in relation to their births. Those who received any kind of drugs at birth were more likely to have drug problems later in life than those who were born drug-free. It's published in their medical journal, but it's been quiet in this country.

Birth is a normal physiological process that's simply *as safe as life gets*. It is a manifestation of love and a time for rejoicing.

Becky Burpo interviewed for this book prior to opening the Allen Birthing Center, in Allen, Texas, a lovely Victorian style two-story historic home that includes birthing tubs in every bedroom. www.allenbirthingcenter.com

Dolphin Spirit

"Rima's ability to birth two babies under water, when her first child died by drowning at age four, is a testimony to the incredible adaptability of human beings and our capacity to receive guidance and be healed."—from Elizabeth Noble's foreword in
The Healing Power of Birth by Rima Star

For my pregnancy with Shay in 1968, I had no special nutrition or childbirth classes. The birth became frightening to me because I was given no information by the hospital staff. They shaved my pubic area, strapped me down, knocked me out with gas, cut an episiotomy (without consent), and the doctor used forceps to pull the baby out. The hospital even gave me drugs to dry up my breast milk. I bottle fed. Now, I want to encourage women to take responsibility for their bodies and to realize they do *know* how to give birth.

At age four, Shay accidentally drowned in a swimming pool. After the hospital told me that he had died despite their efforts, I cried and cried. I remember a friend, Dave, who drove me in his car while I pounded on the dashboard in utter despair and disbelief. He kept me from losing my mind or possibly from even losing my own life.

I eventually learned from this after all the grieving and worked to not only heal my heart but heal my own birth as a baby.

When the doctor gave my mother a cesarean, he accidently cut behind my ear. Until five, I had recurring nightmares of getting cut by knives. Through the rebirthing process, though, I empowered my next births of my own children and helped others, too. Rebirthing is processing your birth through breathwork while under water using a snorkel.

I dreamed of dolphins during my second pregnancy which led to water therapy and home waterbirths for our next three children. I've been swimming with dolphins since 1988 and think in images when I'm around them. During one of my first dolphin swims in a lagoon, I was taken in a circular path in the water by hanging onto a dolphin's dorsal fin. The dolphin is trained to return back to the dock after. With only mental images, I suggested how I wished to go around one more time. The dolphin was about to take me back to the dock. Suddenly, she swam around one more time! I was hanging onto her dorsal fin, thrilled.

I notice the shapes that dolphins swim in—figure eights and hearts—plus their synchronicity. With each dolphin trip, I receive tons of information. It all unfolds in time. My vision is for a healing birth center near dolphins.

For my second pregnancy, I didn't take prenatal vitamins or extra iron, but I did eat Spirulina and took extra vitamin C and calcium. My doctor was delighted at my health and thought I could have a home birth.

Being delivered cesarean myself, I wanted to visualize my baby being born vaginally. I got books and we studied the anatomy of the female reproductive system.

My husband, Steven, and I would tell the baby how she would move her head and body.

The last two weeks of my pregnancy I felt absolutely gorgeous. A friend gave me a chant from *The Course in Miracles* by Dr. Helen Schucman. I did this chant with my highest thoughts about labor and birth in mind.

"My mind is God's mind,
  my body is God's body,
  my spirit is God's spirit."

I chanted this many times during the last two weeks; it was a fine gift.

Another friend asked me about pain right before I was to give birth. "My body is made to give birth, and the pain is not going to last forever. I won't die," I said.

When a woman is nearing 10 centimeters dilation, the labor may be at its most intense. This is called transition, and it is when you feel like, *I may not make it through this kind of pain.* This is when some suggest you should breathe fast and leave your body. What I did was to go *deeper* into my body and the sensation. My whole training in rebirthing taught me to go into it by taking a deep breath, letting go, and relaxing.

Those who have not been taught the Western medical model deliver their babies naturally from an upright position so that gravity is used to its fullest benefit. I learned that the main ingredient in having an ideal birth experience is not being controlled by fear. Fear causes tension; love inspires relaxation.

I birthed our daughter, Mela, in a tub at home and love the photo taken of me holding her with the look of pure joy on my face.

Weeks later, when I needed to clean house, but Mela wouldn't take a nap, I would breathe, relax, and let go. The more I surrendered to her, the more I was able to do other things I wanted. The more I resisted her, the less she cooperated with me.

I enjoyed nursing Mela. Physically it felt wonderful to nurse, and it helped my body complete my mothering cycle. I enjoyed the skin-to-skin contact, and we spent many hours gazing at one another. Never again would I trade the bonding and closeness that nursing creates. And, of course, nursing was a lot more convenient than the bottle: her milk was always ready.

For the waterbirth of our next daughter, Orien, the most encouraging words for me was when the midwife said, "Your body knows how to give birth to this baby. You can trust your body."

A friend said, "Rima, push past that point where it hurts."

Steven later wrote, "God designed a woman to give birth. It is fear, not the size of the baby's head, that almost always complicates the birth. Rima was beautiful—the epitome of a goddess giving birth. Women show their strength and courage during this experience, and it is inspiring for a man to see this in his wife."

Hank, our son, was also born through waterbirthing.

Joseph Chilton Pierce, author of *Magical Child*, claims that the first rapid brain growth spurt occurs during the twenty-four hours after a baby's birth. He says that stillness is the greatest enemy of the newborn; clothing and blankets wrapped around the baby inhibits its freedom of movement. We used his ideas with our babies.

However, a cotton cap immediately after birth for the newborn's head helps the baby to conserve body heat, prevent heat from escaping through the head, and prevents hypothermia (a decrease in body temperature) even if it's a summer day. The newborn needs time to regulate its own body temperature once outside the womb.

All of these births led me to the work I now do through The Star Institute in Austin, Texas. I've attended over 200 waterbirths and assist others using integrative work and healing.

Nitrous Oxide for Comforting Childbirth

Is there an option besides birthing drug-free or with an epidural? Yes. It's nitrous oxide* or "laughing gas," used in dentistry since 1844. For laboring moms in many countries in the world, it provides a sigh of relief.

Although most U.S. hospitals offer epidurals for pain, nitrous oxide (N_2O) may soon be an option as it is in the U.K., Scandinavian countries, Canada, and Australia. And it's safer. Without obliterating pain, the gas used for obstetrics contains a balanced mixture of 50 percent nitrous oxide with 50 percent oxygen. When it is inhaled, a laboring mom feel relaxed, even euphoric. She can feel her contraction but may think, *who cares?*

N_2O works by increasing the release of endorphins, corticotropins, and dopamine in the brain. It helps the mom manage labor by taking the *edge* off pain and anxiety during contractions, during delivery, or for suturing. The mom administers the gas herself by inhaling it through a mask. If she decides she doesn't want it, the effect of N_2O dissipates upon exhalation within minutes without any residual effects.

The beauty of N_2O is the lack of adverse reactions that epidurals have. There is no drop in blood pressure, and it doesn't negatively impact the natural forces of labor. The newborn doesn't need to be resuscitated. The baby's alert state and ability to breastfeed remain intact. The gas is eliminated quickly by the lungs, not slowly by the liver.

Why hasn't N_2O been widely offered? Although once used in the U.S., it became less available as hospitals began to offer epidurals. N_2O is inexpensive and easy to administer by obstetricians, family physicians, midwives, and nurses, but it doesn't have the lucrative potential for pharmaceutical companies, nor the marketing.

Nitrous oxide is currently provided at the University of California at San Francisco Medical Center by physcians and midwives and at the hospital at the University of Washington in Seattle. The American College of Nurse Midwives supports the use of nitrous oxide analgesia for labor.

The growing group of natural birth moms, midwives, birth centers, and hospitals stand poised for N_2O to make a comeback. For women who want to avoid an epidural or those who can't have one, N_2O should be available in all hospital OB units. Although it's not actually "laughing your baby out," it can help in a safe way.

---

* Mild side effects include nausea which is present in labor anyway and a sense of disorientation, which some women like and others do not.

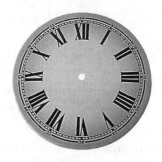

Learn Hospital Strategies

Buy Time and Let Go

I advised Lisa to stay at home until she couldn't talk through a contraction, because once you go to the hospital, your arrival time is documented. "It's like punching in on a clock," I told her. "Your progress becomes measured by the hour. Even with your husband at your side, bring a female doula or a friend to support you because the nurses will be in and out. Keep upright as much as possible during active labor—don't take labor lying down. You can do it."

As Lisa sat on my patio sipping her iced tea that sunny day, I shared with her the benefits of natural childbirth. She didn't think her doctor would support it. At thirty weeks into her pregnancy, she switched to another doctor who was known for delivering natural births. Lisa shares her successful birth of Jacob.

Stretching Time

Lisa's Story

After Erika brought me over to talk with Kalena (the author), I switched to a new doctor who supported natural birth in a hospital. I saw my new doctor for my first two visits and had one visit with each of her female partners so I would know whoever would be on-call. Each doctor answered my questions and was nice. My doctor gave me the impression that if I needed an hour of her time to answer questions, she'd give it. I did not feel rushed at all with her. She was laid back and thorough.

My doctor's partner was on call when I went into labor. When we called her at 1:00 a.m., she suggested we head down to the hospital. I told her I felt fine and wanted to *wait it out*. When we called her at 6:00 a.m., she said we should go in to avoid heavy traffic, but she agreed to let us come in at 9:00 a.m. We arrived at 10:00. I knew stretching time enabled me to go into active labor and avoid interventions at the hospital.

"If you don't significantly progress by 1:00 p.m., we'll have to use Pitocin," the doctor told me. I didn't want any of that, so we began moving and walking around. She checked on me a few times and was in and out pretty quickly, which I imagine is typical.

She almost didn't make it back by the time I started to push. When she came in the room, the resident, who had been helping me, stepped aside. The doctor was calm and encouraging. My husband and I both liked her.

My labor nurse, who was thirty weeks pregnant, supported my natural birth. I asked whether she was having drugs for her labor. She said she planned to have an epidural. Despite her own preference, she guided us by suggesting different positions and gently saying that I was doing well. So well, that before I knew it, I held our newborn son in my arms. I did it!

We had a friend with us (thanks to Kalena's recommendation). After I delivered baby Jacob, my friend asked the nurse if she might reconsider going without an epidural based on my positive experience. "I might." she said. I sent her a card later letting her know how helpful she was to me. She was wonderful and I hope she'll give natural childbirth a try.

I felt supported during my labor, but the hospital part definitely felt like a do-it-yourself deal. A different postpartum nurse gave me foam for an episiotomy (that I didn't have), handed out some Ibuprofen, and pointed to a stack of maxi pads with a cold compress on the counter. She reviewed a chart for me to mark when I used the medications and another for when Jacob nursed, pooped, and peed. I wanted him to room in, but I didn't sleep much.

Early the next morning, the nurse took Jacob to the nursery to be seen by the pediatrician, and I fell back to sleep. I woke up to the doctor standing over my bed. "Are you ready to go home?" she asked.

With the doctor's question I thought, *I can do all this in the comfort of my own home and sleep much better.* So home I went.

Now that the baby is here, natural childbirth is nothing compared to six weeks of sleep deprivation. I'm still feeling a bit like I'm walking around in a fog. It'll be great to shake that off. Oh, how I miss sleep.

I'm glad I switched to another doctor. Something was signaling inside me that I needed to follow my instincts. Our son, Jacob, benefitted from natural birth and his birth has made me a better parent, even if I'm a groggy one right now.

Choosing a Midwife in a Hospital

Susan Akins, CNM
Member, American College of Nurse Midwifery (ACNM)

I deal with *well women*—no high-risk with hypertension or diabetes. I cannot perform breech or multiple births, either. I don't use forceps nor do surgery.

I'll share two examples of women who switched from an M.D., and chose me as their midwife during their pregnancy. One patient first went to a practice close to her home.

"I want an unmedicated birth," she said.

"*We* know when you need pain medication," the doctor replied.

She switched and drove an hour to my office. Another mom told her doctor that she thought she could go natural.

"My mom and my sister have had good births. I think I can, too."

He said, "If you want to try something hard, go climb Mt. Everest."

The most important time during labor is *transition*—between the first stage of contractions and the second stage of pushing. A midwife encourages you: "You are strong. You are powerful. You are almost done."

The midwife stays with you, but the doctor may not be in the room until at the end to catch the baby.

Most women who choose a midwife do go natural. These women have learned how to *trust* their own body.

A small percentage of women want the care of a midwife, with medication. For whatever reason, they may not be sure that they can birth naturally. Perhaps the intensity of birth is more than they can handle because it reminds them of something else painful that happened in their life. But *they* are making the choice and *that* is what is important.

The best thing about natural birth is the *power* women feel. It changes their lives. They're stronger than they thought. Pain is a normal part of life, and birth is a normal process.

Because hospital nurses see many more high-risk births, they sometimes fear natural birth.

These are my "Top Five Reminders" about natural birth:

1. **Get informed.** Ask questions. The only stupid question is the one you don't ask. It will eat away at you. I promise I won't laugh *at* you, only *with* you.

2. **Participate in decisions.** *Choose* the kind of birth you want as opposed to allowing a doctor to choose for you.

3. **Surrender to the process.** This is hard to express to expectant women. You can read, study, take birth classes and prepare for pain management with techniques. However, during labor, a time comes for you to *get out of the way*. Let your body do what it is designed to do.

4. **Let nature keep going.**

5. **Trust.** Trust that your body knows how to birth. Trust your intuition. And trust your partner and your caregiver.

The hospital environment is impersonal, so personalize it. Bring your own T-shirt, music, and photos. *Who* is with you is more important than *where* you are.

One time during a birth, the baby crowned, but the mom did not push. Together, we spent forty-five minutes talking and negotiating her baby out. The mom wanted drugs. It was too late, but I said, "Okay." The nurse glanced at me skeptically, as she left to get the medication. As soon as she walked out the door, the baby was born. It was like the mom needed permission, wanted it granted, felt okay and pushed.

A doctor I knew had a woman in labor who wanted an epidural. She was making great birth noises. Most women who get loud during labor have the most outstanding births.

We told her after she delivered, "Great job!"

At the postpartum visit she was sooo upset. "It was the worst experience of my life...I felt out of control. Didn't know what I was doing," she said.

I realized that the perception, from a health provider's view, is not always the same as the woman's. The birth was too much for her even though she was a powerful attorney in her career. She needed to learn how to let go and accept the birth process.

I remember a mom who looked *peaceful* during her baby's birth. She focused within. Her husband was a great supporter, too. I remember a soft light shining on her face making her glow. She looked surreal.

Last Chance
Amy's Story

"**W**e might have to induce you," said the midwife.

Amy, a thirty-three-year-old Microsoft employee in Washington State, blinked back tears. She had walked around dilated at 3 centimeters for three weeks. She was one-and-a-half-weeks overdue and losing a little amniotic fluid.

Amy's mom, Barb, a registered nurse, influenced her towards natural childbirth. Barb saw many hospital births and she recommended no IVs and no numb legs. She had read *Childbirth Without Fear* by Grantly Dick-Read and the Bradley books. She found a physician who did hypnosis and gave birth to Amy naturally in the early 60's. She joined La Leche League and breastfed knowing it was healthier than formula for her babies.

"You can do this," she encouraged Amy.

"If Mom can do it, I can too," Amy says. "I wanted a female caregiver, a woman who viewed childbirth as a *process,* not as a pathology. My next door neighbor was a midwife. My best friend in high school became an obstetrician in her early twenties. Birth is managed from the doctor's view. You push uphill, on a bed. It's all for the doctor's benefit, not yours."

At six weeks into pregnancy, Amy explored water birth. She collected information over two weeks. Reading *Spiritual Midwifery* by Ina May Gaskin showed statistics of 1,500 drug-free births with zero maternal deaths. Amy read another book, *Complete Pregnancy and Childbirth* by Sheila Kitzinger. She rented videos, toured birth centers and interviewed eight midwives. "I asked the midwife questions that I found like, 'Has a baby ever died in your care? What's your C-section rate? What's your episiotomy rate?'"

As a first time mom, she was scared that the pain would be overwhelming. "I used prenatal yoga to relax during pregnancy and used breathing techniques for labor." She also worried about her husband, Larry, who faints at the sight of blood.

"I preferred home birth because I felt that my own choices would be taken away in a hospital." Yet, she chose Evergreen Hospital, which is rated as one of the Top Ten "baby friendly" hospitals in the U.S. "I was concerned about leaving too fast, and at some birth centers you leave three hours after delivery. In a hospital, I could stay longer. I bonded with the midwives, who were the first to listen to our baby's heartbeat. These midwives were integrated as a team into the hospital, not as an afterthought."

Evergreen's services include classes* for childbirth preparation. They presume a woman wants to birth naturally. It's one of the most progressive hospitals in the country. Yet only 15 percent of births end up drug-free. They offer breastfeeding classes, a postpartum counselor, and mom and baby support groups.

"During pregnancy, I worked out at the club but my blood pressure went too high. I walked and did yoga. I used two prenatal massage gift certificates that I saved for the last two months of pregnancy when I was uncomfortable."

Amy got home from the check-up with the midwife, who talked about inducing her birth. She cried and called her physician friend.

"Don't get hooked up with Pitocin. Walk around for twelve hours, not twelve minutes, not two hours, but *twelve* hours. A little pill called the 'magic bullet' can be inserted in the vagina by your caregiver to get labor going, if needed. Wait until you are dilated 5 centimeters, after that you can do it," the doctor said. After the phone call, Amy felt relieved. She had a game plan.

"I looked at the bottle of Castor Oil that I bought for labor if needed. On the label was written 'Last Chance' because the store had put it on sale. It was my last chance to get labor going. It cleaned me out."

At midnight, Amy said to her husband, "Either I have food poisoning or I'm in labor."

They had packed five bags of special birth items: special pillows, a birth ball, scones, a neck pillow, and more. "I had a birth plan which I slaved over, but didn't even look at it."

They went to the hospital about 2 a.m. It took twenty-five minutes to get there. Amy didn't want a bumpy ride. Her mom, in the role as her doula, came with her.

After arriving and checking in, Amy found out she was 8 centimeters dilated. "I can do this!" she cheered. The delivery and post-labor room looked like an apartment with a Jacuzzi tub in the room. A two-to-one nurse-to-patient ratio exists at this hospital.

"Another worry I had was: what if I get a labor nurse who is not sympathetic?"

"We can get you another one," the midwife reassured. The nurse they got was skeptical at first.

Amy got undressed. They didn't make her wear the belt for checking the fetal heartbeat. She wanted the freedom of motion and used the birth ball. Amy got in the Jacuzzi tub for about forty-five minutes. She held Larry's hand and then her mom's. "I asked for stories of places I loved, like a day in Hawaii. We had gone to the islands during pregnancy and I could be transported mentally away from labor to recall the relaxing feeling, and envision the swaying palm trees, gentle sea and the sweet breeze of the island."

She wanted a change from the tub, distractions, and new things to try. "Our baby girl, Stella, was tilted 30 degrees from a perfect launch position. She spiraled down to where I felt back labor. My husband held my hips together. Standing up felt better, and leaning forward with weight on my hands took pressure off my tailbone. I was lying down to sleep in between contractions. The bean bag to lie over, stomach down, felt good."

"Where's the birth bar?"

"I'm getting it," said the labor nurse, who now took her seriously. The midwife stayed the whole time. "I was in transition when they draped the sheet over the bar. I climbed up the bar using my upper body with each contraction."

"Come on Stella," the midwife coaxed the baby.

"I pushed for one and a half hours and was exhausted."

"Focus on pushing, don't waste your energy screaming or yelling," said the nurse.

Amy learned how to vocalize labor in prenatal yoga, but she did a bit of howling like a dog instead. Larry almost fell over laughing.

People took turns rubbing Amy's back. Amy tightly squeezed Larry's hand. A solo cello CD and Bach music played all through the birth.

"I had women around me that knew how to support me. They knew what I was going through, and kept me active saying, "Try this." After labor, the new parents gave the CD to the labor nurse as a present.

Stella was born with her arm up and elbow by her head. "I screamed when the elbow popped out because I tore." She was born at 6:58 a.m., and weighed seven and a half pounds.

"Yes it's pain, but it's pain with a *purpose*. Every contraction brings you closer to your baby." The nurse later sent a thank you note saying it was such a privilege to witness the birth.

"Other moms that hear my birth story say they might try to do a natural birth the second time. The five centimeter rule helped and the library had books regarding pain and childbirth were helpful, too. For outer pain,

I localized it elsewhere, like hearing stories of other places. Inside, I felt *I can do this*.

"Being older and mature, I had personal and professional successes and failures. If you are younger, you may trust that *others* know best. However, get as educated as possible. I wanted an *active* part of this experience, not have this happening *to* me.

"What I tell friends about natural birth is this: Push. It feels like pushing a basketball out. But I promise your bottom will not explode."

Example of Classes at Evergreen Hospital:

Labor & Birth Basic (five weeknights)
Labor & Birth Basic Weekends (two Saturdays)
Labor & Birth for Teens and Young Adults
Refresher Labor & Birth (two evenings)
Hypnobirthing
Practice Only—Labor Coping Skills (two hours)
Multiples Labor & Birth (two evenings)
Multiples Seminar: More Than One Baby
Pelvic Health Class
Yoga for Pregnancy
A Day About Baby (skills on a Saturday)
Infant Feeding & Pumping
Car-Safe Kids Class
Car Seat Inspection Clinic
Exploring Child Care Options
The Happiest Baby on the Block
Bringing Baby Home—Avoiding "marital meltdown"
Dads Only
Expecting a Grandbaby?
Siblings
Family Maternity Center (FMC) Tour
FMC Tour in Spanish
Parent-Baby Classes
This is Not What I Expected
Starting Solid Foods
Breastfeeding Your Older Baby and Child
Parenting with Love and Logic

Evergreen Hospital
Kirkland, Washington

Located north of Seattle and close to Microsoft, Evergreen Hospital has been voted one of the "Top 10 Places to have a Baby" by *Self* Magazine. They received an award from UNICEF for their breastfeeding support to new mothers. In walking the halls, this hospital doesn't *look* any different. Yet through their Nurse Manager, Linda, and a labor and delivery nurse, Judy, you will discover how they assist natural birth patients with doctors or midwives, and strive to meet the unique needs of the community.

Evergreen handles about 4,400 births a year. The mothers are highly educated. They've done their research on the pros and cons of natural childbirth. The percentage of natural birth is not nearly as high as it once was. In 1997, it was about 65 percent. Now, more women have epidurals. The hospital does support VBACs, but the C-section rate is getting higher—around 33 percent.

"Evergreen's philosophy is to provide what the community needs," says Linda. Most of the classes offered exist because of a community need. (See Class List)

For example, the staff has been partnering with a Muslim community in the area to try to figure out how to get childbirth education to their population. These women won't go to traditional childbirth classes because men are present. Culturally, their classes need to be women only. Evergreen has helped to develop specific plans for these patients.

"If you're not aware of what their cultural needs are, you can't address them. I've learned you can't decide what they need. You go *ask* them what they need. We went to their Mosque's 'Open House' and met the women. They are happy coming here for classes and childbirth, yet we're trying to meet their needs within the parameters of what you can do in a hospital," says Linda. If they need a C-section, Evergreen Hospital can't guarantee that the anesthesiologist is female. However, most of the women in the Muslim community have natural childbirth."

At Evergreen, another kind of collaboration takes place: physicians and midwives. It's a partnership rare in most hospitals in the U.S. The physician needs to trust in a midwife's decision-making 100 percent. Some of the obstetricians don't have midwives. In a hospital, a midwife is surrounded with more people to consult with than working alone at a home birth. The midwives at Evergreen have a collaborative relationship with the physicians and with the nurses. The physicians trust them, and the nurses view midwives as being as capable in meeting the mothers' needs as the physicians. Both are care providers.

Society's expectations are changing. Judy says, "When I had my first child 15 years ago, you couldn't find out the gender of your baby. By the time I had my next two, everybody was finding out. Ten years ago, when a patient came into the hospital, you could ask her, 'What are you having?' She'd tell you. Everybody knew. But now it's going back to people not finding out again. Shifts and trends happen.

"I believe if you want to go natural you should be able to. This hospital is supportive of whatever you want to do. For a while, women who wanted to go natural didn't because they found labor hurt more than they expected. They felt like failures. That whole process has triggered people saying, 'I'm not sure if I'm going to have the epidural or not.'

"At Evergreen, we're supportive and up front if you choose to go natural. I've lived all over and I agree it is harder to go drug-free in some hospitals because of a lack of encouragement by the staff. When my son was born in North Carolina in 1992, most people bottlefed their babies, used disposable diapers and had an epidural.

"When I came to Seattle, people were into cloth diapers. Everyone breastfed. Everyone gave natural childbirth. I had an epidural with our son and people were mortified.

"What you're seeing now in Seattle is people are finding the happy medium."

A huge controversy exists regarding malpractice. "Sometimes midwives in other settings, like a birth center or at home, are the only ones in the room with the mom and think, *the baby's getting ready to come out. If I can give it a few more minutes, we'll have this baby.* A few minutes turn into hours. The patient gets transferred to Evergreen from the birth center," explains Judy.

If a birth center or home birth mom transfers, she goes to the ER. The physicians don't want to accept a transfer because a physician at another hospital tried doing that and lost their license. The physician ended up delivering the transfer patient's baby and the outcome wasn't good. The patient sued the doctor and not the birth center.

Medical malpractice reform is a *huge* topic in Washington State because there are no caps, or limits, on what you can sue somebody for. A $13 million lawsuit settled in Seattle. The obstetricians already pay upwards of $75,000 a year for malpractice insurance.

"It would be wonderful if we could figure out a way to partner with the birth centers so that if the patients came over here, the physician had no liability for what happened prior to the patient arriving. The problem is, how do you know for sure if it happens *prior* to coming to the hospital? The lawyer could argue, 'No it happened *after* they got to the hospital.' That's why all the transfers come through the ER. It's all litigation-based," Judy says.

"I have seen the philosophy of childbirth, anesthesia and even the way they administer it change through the years," Judy recalls. "My mother had me thirty-eight years ago with Scopolamine, which makes you feel like a crazy person. She remembered everything. My mother's a mellow person, but she was out of her mind. When the nurse shaved mom's pubic area, which is what they did back then, she accidently cut her. My mother impulsively *swung* in reaction. She didn't mean to hit the nurse in the face. She broke her nose.

"She didn't want that to happen with her next child. Pregnant with my sister, she said to the doctor, 'Look, I don't care what you have to do to me, but you are NOT giving me those drugs again. I'm not having anything.' My mother even went to Lamaze classes to prepare. Three couples attended the class, but only two finished. My father refused to go. My sister ended up being late, or past the due date, so they induced my mom.

"In 1970, my mother was the first woman at the hospital in North Carolina to have natural childbirth with an induction. Residents and interns came in the room to watch her have her baby because nobody believed she could do it. They put her down on the little stretcher, made her stay in bed, put an IV in her and said, 'If you move your arm, we're giving you those drugs.'

"It was horrible, but she didn't move her arm. She said she was focused on not moving her arm, she didn't care what the labor pain felt like because she didn't want those drugs. Anything was better than that. She birthed my sister naturally. Can you imagine?

"When I had my first child fifteen years ago in California, I thought I wanted natural. But they tried to stop my labor with Magnesium Sulphate, a horrible drug that makes you feel sicker.

"They gave you an epidural if they felt you needed it. It was not something you asked for. That was the norm.

"I probably would have gone natural with my second and third babies, but they were born in North Carolina and the hospital's attitude influenced me. I know some nurses who like for the patients to have epidurals because they don't have to fool with them. It's less management for the nurses.

"With my last child, I had a spinal at 9 centimeters. That's the best thing I ever had with pain management. I knew she would be born quickly. I could still feel her coming out, it took away the contractions, it was short-acting and I could walk around right after.

"With an epidural, it's hours before you can walk and that's not what I wanted. I wasn't a labor nurse when I had my children. Since I am now, I have a better idea what my options are."

"I've been to hospitals that still make you stay in bed because they think, 'What if she prolapses her cord?' The nurses sit at the desk and watch the monitor screens. They don't stay in the room with the patient.

"Some of the Evergreen nurses, who weren't used to that way, would go over to the other hospital and would get grief from their nurses. 'Don't go in the room and monitor the patient. Don't get active.' But I'm concerned about giving hospitals a bad rap. Evergreen is different.

"Natural birth moms are not monitored continuously at Evergreen. It's every thirty minutes during early labor, every fifteen minutes in active labor, every two to five minutes in pushing. Women don't have to stay in the bed. Even Pitocin patients may get in the tub. Whatever they want to do as long as it's safe for them and their baby," Judy says.

After birth, a lactation consultant visits you in to help with breastfeeding. Babies room in unless they need watching. Massage is even available for any patient in the hospital, as well as the family and staff.

Faith in Experience
Kristi's Story

The hospital was sterile, but my mom helped me through a real tough part of my labor. Sitting up in bed, I leaned into her as she held me. Gently squeezing my hand, she whispered prayers in my ears—prayers that we recited when I was a child. My mother helped me in a huge way with my birth. With eyes shut, I focused. When I came around between contractions, I saw my mom and my husband praying the rosary.

I'm the tenth chiropractor in my family. My grandmother, who was the first one, birthed eleven children naturally at home on their farm. Instead of a doctor or midwife, neighbors helped her through labor. However, she gave birth to her twelfth child in a hospital. "That was my worst labor, delivery and birth ever," she said. Because of my grandmother, my mother's philosophy growing up was childbirth should be *natural*.

When my parents married, my mother had trouble conceiving. She lost a baby at two months into pregnancy. One of my uncles, who was in chiropractic school, learned applied kinesiology. He completely changed her diet and worked on her, structurally, so her body was functioning better. Spiritually, she turned back to her faith and became pregnant with me.

Our mother was determined to rear the three of us in a healthy physical and spiritual environment. That was the reason for the career I chose. I knew I wanted to work in medicine to help people.

I have vivid memories of spending summers in Ohio where my mother's family lives. My uncle would treat patients brought to his home on stretchers. He'd take them up to the third floor and they would come *walking down* after hours of treatment. I took that for granted and thought everybody knew about that kind of care.

While I was in chiropractic school, I worked in the ER of a hospital for two years. Loved it. I felt that emergency care medicine couldn't be replaced. I gained insight as to how many people seek medical care, but don't need it. Patients came in with headaches, and with sugar and blood disorders, such as diabetes. They needed the type of health care I had growing up—what I took for granted. Not that I believe traditional medicine is unnecessary. I believe that you have to know when to use what.

I went on to complete applied kinesiology training in California over the next three years. It's more of a diagnostic tool, nonspecific and much more clinically based instead of what people seem to think of chiropractors: cracking backs, necks and dealing with car accidents. I had known the practice of chiropractic to be a complete type of care, treating all kinds of ailments. They'd say, "Take this remedy. Or do this." That is the doctor I'd become when I opened my practice here in Dallas.

My husband and I took a natural family planning course before we got married. When I wanted to start our family, natural birth fit my philosophy. My faith maintains that God designed the body perfectly. By working with people, seeing their conditions and watching how their bodies responded, I gained more respect for the body every day.

I had complete confidence that birth is a process that has happened for about 250,000 years. In researching, I saw how it had changed from something natural and normal to women fearing it, considering only the pain and wanting to avoid it.

I chose to ignore the painful aspects of labor which now I see left me unprepared. At the time I thought, *this is something I want to do because that's the way it should be done.*

I looked for a good obstetrician/gynecologist with a lot of experience, which was at the top of my list. I wanted someone who had been in practice for a long time. You can't top experience.

I asked some LDR nurse friends that don't know each other, "Who do you suggest? Who do you *admire*? Who do you like that you work with all the time?" All three of them gave me one doctor's name who has been in practice for more than twenty years. "Why do you like him?" I asked. They all agreed that he does the "right thing," without fail. They don't question his judgment. Their vote of confidence inspired me.

My husband and I met this recommended obstetrician with the idea of interviewing him. He said, "Let me tell you, *I've* never delivered a baby in all my years of practice. *You* are the one that's doing this. I'll be present in case any special circumstance arises. If you have any questions about that, we can certainly talk about it. I'm not going to impede the process. We're going to do it however you want."

The doctor was completely open to natural birth. He even arranged that when I went into labor at the hospital, the nurses who took care of me had a lot of experience with natural deliveries. They were open and positive. They respected our privacy and time.

During pregnancy, I took the Bradley method and Lamaze classes, where I met an excellent doula. She has four sons that she delivered naturally, the smallest weighed 9 1/2 pounds. She knew it could be done. She started working with me and was there for the birth. My sister, who is a massage therapist, came too. I felt I had a good team around me. I believed the pain and labor and delivery are only for a quantifiable amount of time.

I had read about a study where a group of obstetricians went into third world countries. They asked the women if they wanted epidurals. Astonished, the women asked, "Why do we need pain medicine?"

My husband and I watched videos and saw the difference between medicated and unmedicated births—in the baby's response. I knew, but my husband was shocked. "Those babies were drugged," he said. Their Apgar scores were low (see glossary), they weren't as active and they didn't breastfeed. The drugs crossed the placenta. Pitocin, a medication used often in hospitals to bring stronger contractions, contains inherent risks.

I kept active, did yoga, light weight training, and fast walking. I took a good regimen of nutrients, specific to applied kinesiology.

I used an Osteopath, who practiced acupuncture. It was the *only* remedy for my nausea in my first trimester. I saw her every week and after the first three months my nausea disappeared.

When labor started, I actually stayed home a couple of hours by myself. My husband wasn't home yet. My water broke before I had one contraction. Then they came on strong. I called the doula. "No discoloration, you're okay. I'm going to make my way over," she said. She lived 45 minutes away. I called the doctor to let him know what was going on. My contractions quickly came closer and closer together.

We went to the hospital as soon as my husband got home. The doctor came in and checked me. "Gosh, you're already fully effaced and dilated to almost 5," he said. "This baby's going to come fast."

Yet the baby kept turning to the posterior position. The spine of the baby along my spine caused more pain. My labor shifted to the immediate problem of how to deal with the discomfort of back labor. I was not confined to bed, though. Had my water not broken I could have gotten in the jacuzzi tub. That would have been a comfortable choice, but not allowed in the hospital because there's a risk of infection if your water breaks. I was up, in the rocking chair, on the birthing ball, forward on the bed, my husband behind me. I did counter pressure, too. We did all kinds of things to ease my discomfort.

For the first eight hours I was right on the contractions or stayed ahead of them. But as I started to tire and my labor lingered, I lost the resolve to have a natural birth. That's when all my fears crept in, the great unknowns rising to the surface.

The doula took pictures and the expression on my face was strained. I suspect that stalled my labor more than anything—getting tensed up. Fortunately she suggested relaxation techniques—breathing, visualizations, and various positions. "Uterine surges will cause pressure," she said.

At twenty hours of labor, which is the hospital's policy for time limit, I heard a staff person say, "I'm going to go get a team together just in case."

My husband was petrified and prayed the rosary.

I had a quarter of an epidural. "Let her rest for a couple of hours," my doula requested. I could still stand and still feel my legs.

When it came time to push, my husband was the most helpful. In his own way, he gave a football talk. "You've got to hunker down." He centered me and helped me focus. I pushed.

"While most physicians pull the baby, I'm here to guide," our doctor said. I saw what he did. As the baby's one shoulder popped through with the head, he put his index finger into the armpit from the backside. He guided the baby out with leverage. He stopped when the contractions stopped. "Is it a boy or girl?"

Samuel was so cute. He didn't even cry. His eyes were wide open. I said something and he looked right at me and at my husband.

Now that I'm pregnant with our second baby, I'm working on how to deal with pain, especially back labor if it happens again. I envision this birth completely different. If I had more tricks in my hat to rely on, I could speed up the labor or make it more comfortable. We enrolled in a class about hypnobirthing, for deep relaxation. The mind can only hold one thought at a time.

My husband said once, "I don't think I'll ever be able to go back into our home if you have a baby there." He now wants a home birth, saying, "It'll be better." He has made a huge transition.

Samuel is now fourteen months old. Our second child is due in a few months. For this birth, I'll make peace with it. Get centered. It's normal to have those fears from the first time, but now I know better.

I'm going to have even fewer people in the room, less distractions. Fewer things going on. I will stay focused, make a real concerted effort and hopefully it will be a little easier.

"That second labor is easier from start to finish, and *raising* the child is easier, too," my mother-in-law said. I want to believe that's true.

Storms Trigger Labor for Self-Confessed "Wus"
Dawn's Story

The sky becomes ominously dark as flashes of lightning crack to the earth. Sheets of blinding rain pound the ground. Wild clouds spin into funnels. A family in North Texas thinks of where to take cover. The electricity flickers...and the *contractions* begin. Could the drop in the barometric pressure bring on labor?

When a woman is in the midst of having a baby, she can become oblivious to whatever chaos is occurring around her. Getting a baby out takes over as the primary focus. Dawn, a magazine writer, shares how she gave birth in the midst of such intensity.

When I was 29, my husband and I were about to have our first child. I saw The Birth and Women's Center when I was doing research. I walked in....it felt like a home. "If we have a baby, I'd like to birth at this birth center," I told him. But my husband favored the hospital as the best place for birth.

I'm not a fan of hospitals. My dad was dying of cancer, and my family was leery of doctors because my father wasn't getting cured. But they still thought that the hospital was the best place to have a baby. I showed articles to justify my position, but to no avail. My father didn't live to see Noah, our first son.

I called the Birth Center and asked what doctor they recommended. They said to see Dr. Christensen and her practice included a midwife, Susan. I would have loved to have Susan at that birth center or even at my house.

I signed up for natural birth classes that included Bradley. The great thing about Bradley is that the dad-to-be *learns*. My husband learned so much that he now answers questions for pregnant women at work.

My motivation for natural birth was:

1. Never loved doctors
2. Didn't want to give up control
3. Afraid of C-section—how to avoid it during birth
4. Wanted to be "there" for the baby
5. Let nature takes its course

After natural birth, friends asked, "Why?" I'm a researcher by nature; a journalist. It seems these days women know nothing of childbirth. Women plan their own wedding, yet put their baby's birth into a doctor's hands. I could say that birth is incredible. I never talked to a person with a medicated birth that felt that way. Yet, *I'm a wus,* not one to tolerate a lot of pain. Even so, I decided natural was the best way. Plus, I always ask myself, *do doctors always know what is right?*

In preparing for our first birth, I did lots of Bradley exercises. I walked every other day, about one mile, until I felt the baby might fall out. It was a hot summer. I ate healthy and massaged my perineum with oil that smelled like roses.

Our son, Noah, was three days late, even though I had been having Braxton Hicks (mild contractions) for one month. I was tired of being pregnant. One night, Clyde, my husband, made me a root beer float with castor oil.

A storm hit that night. My water broke at 1 a.m. I had Group B Strep infection (GBS) which can be infectious to the baby. At 7 a.m. we went in to the hospital where they administered antibiotics in an IV for strep. By 11 a.m. I was dilated only to 2 centimeters. My contractions weakened, then stopped—like a big interruption. The nurse strapped a heart monitor on me.

Walking picked up my contractions as long as we kept going. Susan worried and she suggested Pitocin. I trusted her judgment, but I couldn't handle the Pitocin and panicked.

Two doses of Stadol through the IV calmed me down, over a four hour stretch.

At 9:08 pm, I pushed for one and-a-half hours. Exhausted, I burst blood vessels in my eyes from the strain of pushing.

"The head is crowning. Do you want to touch it?" Susan asked.

"No."

"The head is coming out. Do you want to see in a mirror?"

"NO!" I felt like saying, "I want to get this baby OUT. Stop interrupting me."

I had picked a friend, a personal trainer, to come with me, a positive cheerleader type of personality. She came to support Clyde, too. One thing Clyde did that helped sustain my energy; he brought fresh squeezed orange juice that he had made at home for me to sip on.

Our healthy boy, Noah, was born and was soon in my arms. He weighed 8 pounds, 4 ounces.

I had practiced with the first birth, but it was harder to practice for the second with a little one around.

I now knew that I could birth naturally. I was no longer scared, knowing it was the best thing. Anything else was *not* an option. Like breastfeeding a newborn; if you don't have formula around, it's not an option.

Sawyer, our second son, was born the night the tornadoes hit Fort Worth. The hospital was losing electricity. Downtown Dallas was under a tornado warning.

I was one day past due. When I saw Susan that day, she said, "Everything's ready to go. You're getting close. I'm working today and tomorrow, and off until Friday."

"We need to go into labor in twenty-four hours." I said. Susan suggested Blue Cohosh, a liquid herb that kicks in labor. It tasted bad, but I took a dropper full every thirty minutes...like drinking shots.

I got Braxton Hicks, which was a happy stage for me. I played Enya, lit candles, stayed by myself, lay on the bed, all afternoon. From 6 p.m. until midnight, I called Susan. We headed in. I went through transition on the way to the hospital, asking my husband to stop at every pothole and drive around them on the way.

I'd describe a contraction as a cramp. It goes through the whole stomach area and around the back like a wave, holds, and goes back like a wave does. It can be tolerated...slow forming, slow moving, reaches a peak, goes down and goes away.

Clyde was wonderful. He knew *everything,* as much as I did. As soon as the pain came, I was focused and couldn't handle anything else. He knew what I was thinking or when I'd say, "Remember that thing we learned?" He did massage or counter pressure on my lower back. We worked as one.

At 12:30 a.m. at the hospital, the midwife cleared my cervical lip. In the beginning, I could take my mind to where we eloped—Greece. But then it got harder to focus.

"I can't relax anymore," I said.

"At this time, you need to get mad. Let it out," Susan directed.

I vocalized through the contractions. Would I get that suggestion from an obstetrician? Even my family was surprised that the midwife arrived before they did. It was a personal experience and a special relationship.

Our sweet baby boy was born at 3:45 a.m., after only three pushes. He weighed 9 pounds, 14 ounces. I felt so wonderful.

Birth compares to how you would choose to climb a beautiful mountain. You can hike on a trail, remembering every place that you stopped to rest, seeing a beautiful stream, and smelling the woods. Or, you can fly up the mountain and the pilot does the work. The different ways you get there depend on your choices. My own experience is that there is instant connection with your baby when you *personally* birth your child into the world the natural way.

A Fender-bender on the Way to Have a Baby
Ally's Story

I vividly remember going to my friend's birthday party when I was pregnant. Thirteen women came. Everybody was pregnant or had children, except two. I was the only one who had a midwife and was planning natural birth.

"I had the pit drip," one woman said.

"I'm not having an episiotomy," I told the group.

"Don't you have to have one?"

"No. Why do you have to have one?" I asked.

"You can't get the baby out. Who is your doctor?"

"She's a midwife with Renaissance."

"Have you read that book, *Midwives,* yet?"

"No. Is it negative?"

They looked at me like I had three heads! Half of them bemoaned their births because it wasn't what they wanted.

But you can have what you want. The doctor isn't in control of you. You are paying him or her. I'm not going to give my power over to somebody else.

I wanted natural birth because my mom had. All three of her births ended up that way. My sister was breech. "We're letting the epidural wear off and then you're going to have to push," the doctor said to mom. With my brother, the epidural never took and she almost gave birth on the gurney. *If my little mom can do it, I can do it.*

For ages, women have done this. There's no reason I can't. I knew I wanted a midwife. I didn't want an episiotomy. That scared me to death. And I didn't want a needle in my back.

We work hard when we are pregnant, avoiding alcohol, stopping the smoking, no harmful prescriptions like antidepressants, eating right, and exercising. If you don't take Sinutab, you don't do any drugs, why would you give your baby a big ol' dose of narcotics? Come on...hello? It doesn't make any sense.

It was hard to get my husband, an international rugby player, to focus. Although he was a little bit reluctant, we attended Bradley classes.

"Okay, I'm your team. I need you to treat me like your team. You go out of your way to plan these rugby trips. You arrange the travel, get the cars, and take care of details. I need you to put that energy on me," I told him.

A light bulb went off in his head. He focused on me, and gave me a massage. I shared my visualization with him. "This is how I want to feel...sitting at the beach, warm sun, not hot, and nothingness, no distractions." I had to let him know that as our baby's father, he had to be at the birth and support me.

Out of the four couples in class, three of us went natural. The instructor, Tracy, helped us to know what to expect. She never discounted pain, but said it was for a purpose.

"Once it gets to where you don't think you can't stand it anymore, it is almost over," she said. That's what I kept thinking during the twelve hours from start to finish. The only time I was concerned was when I was by myself while my husband was at work.

During pregnancy, I walked my dogs. Squatting. I tried to do some Kegels. I found it difficult to keep up a strenuous workout routine.

I gained forty pounds during my pregnancy. I ate well and followed the Bradley method. My midwife said, "Don't eat as much protein. If you eat that much protein and if for some reason I have to burst your sack, it's a lot more difficult to burst. That amniotic sack is thick." I ate yellow and green vegetables. I ate better when I was pregnant than I do now. They told me to cut out the ice cream. I listened to them, but I wasn't going to worry about my weight.

Whenever nature said *sleep,* I took a nap.

I talked to women that had natural childbirth. *I stayed away from women who had bad stories.* Everyone wants to tell you their bad story, but I didn't want to hear it. I surrounded myself with positives. My natural birth friends are all career women, strong and opinionated. I knew some from LaLeche League. They weren't the Breastfeeding Nazis: You have to do it; you're-bad-if-you-don't types.

I had an LDR nurse friend, whose mother is Swedish. She would have natural childbirth without question. Her mother nursed all five children, including twins.

"All you have to tell yourself is 'this too shall pass.' If I can do it you can do it," my mom said. I tried to keep a sense of humor. I kept my options open; I wasn't going to fail if for some reason a complication happened and I had to have an epidural or an alternative birth than what I had planned. The goal is a healthy baby and a healthy mom. I knew that my midwives would be positive. They didn't have a hidden agenda.

Can I do it? I blew it off. *Of course I can, stupid. I can do this.* I thought, *I'm a woman, I have the right to change my mind. I'm going to have natural childbirth, subject-to-change. Okay, if for some reason I could not possibly do it, I could scream for the epidural.* I always left that little door open. That was always in my pocket. In the back of my mind though, I knew I was never going to go through with it.

I felt more female than I had ever felt in my life. I finally figured out what I was supposed to do. I'm supposed to be a mom. That was a big shock to me.

Our baby daughter, Emily, came six days before my due date. I woke up at 7:00 a.m., cramping. "I think I'm in labor," I told my husband.

"Let's go walk around the block and see if it stops or keeps up," he said.

I had an appointment that day with one of the doctors, whom I had never met.

"You may be in labor, but you may not be. This may be false labor. What you need to look for are contractions from here to here..." the physician said. He threw me off from everything I had learned in Bradley, including contractions.

I even called the doctor back, "Look, I *really* think I'm in labor."

Yet I went back to my office and was alone most of the day. On the phone, I couldn't talk through some of the contractions. A friend came with my favorite shrimp salad and a piece of chocolate cake. I couldn't eat.

"I'm taking you home," she said.

We called my husband at work. I called my mom when I got home.

"Do you feel it in your back?" she asked.

"Yeah."

"You're in *labor*. You're going to have a baby today," she confirmed.

My husband got home. I kept telling him, "Call the midwife. Call Elizabeth."

"No, let me time the contractions," he said.

"CALL ELIZABETH!"

I called. But I couldn't talk to her through one of my contractions.

"Why don't you come down to the office and we'll go over to Baylor Hospital? Let me check you," she said.

On the way, we became the fourth car in a rear-end collision. My husband got out of the car, growling. It was the 5:00 p.m. rush hour traffic. I called the midwife's office from the car, "We got rear-ended. Don't know if it's bad. I'm fine."

"Go straight to the hospital," they said.

They put the other midwife, Susan, on the phone. I told her we were fine. It was more stressful for my husband. I was in a loosey-goosey state in "labor land."

"Get back in the car," I said to him, and we headed straight to the hospital.

The staff put me in a room and put a monitor on me, strapped me down, and made me lie on my back. The baby's heart rate was fine. But lying on my back was horrible. So was wearing that gross gown. At that point I was like "whatever."

I said I couldn't lay on my back anymore. The nurse let me lay on my side. And they took the monitor off. At about 6:30 p.m., my water broke.

Elizabeth walked in the room. I told her, "I have to push now."

"You have to do *what*?" She looked astonished.

"I HAVE TO PUSH!"

She checked me and I was at 9 centimeters. That was about 6:45-7:00 p.m. I pushed on my side with one of my legs over the shoulder of a nurse. Elizabeth helped hold my leg. I pushed. I *had* to push. *Nothing* is going to stop it. The head was crowning.

"Do you want to see the head?"

"I don't want to see *anything*."

Primal noises came out of me like a Zena Warrior Princess.

I remember hitting my husband's stomach, like a punching bag.

"I'm sorry," I said, looking up at his stoic face.

"No, no, no. It's okay," he said. "You do whatever you need to do. Don't worry about it."

One of the staff came in to take my blood.

"What are you doing? I have to push. Get away from me."

Emily was born and she was absolutely perfect. When I looked at her face, she looked like an angel. She weighed 7 pounds, 14 ounces and measured twenty inches long. She had a small bruise on her head.

I walked to the bathroom and went. If I had had an epidural I would have had a bedpan or a catheter. I had no major tearing. I needed only one little stitch.

I felt amazed and relieved. I'm not pregnant anymore, she's here. I did what I wanted to do: have a natural birth and a healthy baby. It made me feel powerful. I remember saying, "Oh, we'll do that again."

The nurses took Emily to weigh her. When they gave her back to me, she latched on to nurse immediately. I got a little sore for five days because I was letting her hang down too low. I wasn't getting her to open her mouth wide enough, to get her lips out. I had to work on that.

I thought, *I went to the La Leche meetings. This shouldn't be happening to me.*

When I went upstairs to postpartum, a nurse asked, "Can you feel your legs?"

"Yeah, I didn't have anything."

I didn't find the nursing staff particularly helpful. I liked the labor and delivery staff much better. I didn't find the care afterward to be particularly nice. I don't know if I got the weekend staff or what. I didn't like the room or the bed and felt that those nurses didn't care. Every time I slept, someone would walk in my room, handing me a Bible, a menu, or taking my blood at 4 a.m.. *They didn't let me rest.* How does anyone get any sleep? I was upset.

As soon as the pediatrician checked the baby, we left.

There are a few things I'd like the medical staff to know:

• Women aren't stupid.
• If there's no great risk in our pregnancy, there's no reason to have a baby at a hospital.
• Support our choices of what we want.
• If in a hospital, to make it a more *nurturing* atmosphere. Make the beds more comfortable with decent pillows.
• Encourage rooming-in, with mom and baby staying together.
• Just because you have the equipment doesn't mean you have to use it.
• Listen to us.
• More staff training of what a woman's body *naturally* does in birth.
• More training in breastfeeding. No sugar water. Our baby needs to be with us, the mother.
• I can sleep with my baby and it's *okay.*

If I have another baby, I'm either having one at home or at the birth center. I won't go to the hospital except in an emergency. My baby won't be taken away from me again. A home atmosphere is more nurturing. I want Emily at my side, and Mom to cook meals. And I don't want anybody coming in at 4 a.m. to take my blood.

There are many benefits of natural birth. I had a quicker recovery. I got up and went to the bathroom after I gave birth. I didn't have a bedpan or get catheterized. I could feel my legs. My baby wasn't groggy; she latched on immediately. I didn't have a bunch of stitches for an episiotomy. That cut can be worse than childbirth itself.

You feel like this powerful, *I can do it,* woman. In a hospital, women's power is taken away from them. That's why I sought out a midwife. She was sweet and nurturing. What doctor would have massaged my stomach or feet every time I went for a prenatal visit?

Inductions

The majority of inductions done in private hospitals are done for convenience and not necessarily for medical indications. It's rare for a woman to go more than one week overdue these days without being induced. Up to two weeks overdue, or forty-two weeks, remains okay and safe, but rarely happens.

Penny Simkin best describes the path of elective inductions in one of her articles, "The Seduction of Induction." Elective inductions are presented to women as, "Why not induce?" However, it ignores the fetus' role in labor. Simkin points out that the fetus controls the onset of normal labor.

A positive chain of events happens naturally inside the body, including the stimulation of the hypothalamus, the pituitary gland and the adrenal gland. The placenta converts progesterone to estrogen, which increases oxytocin in the uterine lining by 100–200 times. The uterus increases contractions, causing pressure and stretching. Estrogen instructs the uterus, membranes and placenta to produce prostaglandins, which ripen the cervix. Estrogen improves the mother's clotting ability, protecting against hemorrhage.

Examples of inductions for convenience:

• A lot of women want the obstetrician whom they have been seeing most often to deliver them. And since most obstetricians work in large groups, they're only in labor and delivery certain days of the week. They try to schedule the ladies for the day that they are on, and/or work around weekends and holidays.

• A lot of *women* want convenience, too. They would rather plan and pick a date to fit their own schedule.

• For many physicians in private practice, especially if they're sole practitioners and don't want to get up in the middle of the night, it's just easier.

• A physician can get things started during the office hours of 9 to 5. There's strong motivation for "daylight deliveries" for the medical staff.

Common medical indications for induction include: pregnancy-induced hypertension (PIH), signs that the baby is not growing well (interuterine growth restriction or IGR), a suspected large baby, and other medical complications.

Induction Steps

There are different methods of induction.

1. **Cervical ripening**—A common method starts with the *cervical ripening* first. Often that includes using prostaglandin gel or little prostaglandin tampons put inside a woman's vagina. The prostaglandins help to soften and ripen the cervix and get labor started. One might need a couple of applications of the prostaglandin gel over several days. After the doctor puts the gel on, the woman is monitored for a couple of hours and sent home. Then she comes back. We call that "ripening" rather than induction. A lot of physicians will use that.

The prostaglandins actually affect the tissue on the cervix and help to soften up the fibers. It causes contractions, but they tend to be milder than those given by Pitocin. Prostaglandin F2 Alpha is the one that's used.

2. **Pitocin**—The woman is hooked up to an IV and gets Pitocin (oxytocin) started. Some physicians start with breaking the waters all at the same time. Others wait for a couple of hours' worth of contractions and break the waters, depending on how "favorable" the cervix is.

Occasionally somebody will have what we refer to as a "green" cervix, an unripe cervix. A doctor tries to induce them and gives them Pitocin for eight hours. If nothing happens, it is stopped and the woman comes back in a couple of days.

Natural Ways to Stimulate Labor

• **Nipple stimulation**—this involves the husband suckling on the breast for thirty minutes, five minutes per side.

• **Intercourse**—semen has prostaglandins in it. It is the natural softening and ripening agent. Sex will not make you go into labor unless your body is ready.

• **Orgasm** can cause contractions at term.

If you use those three things in combination at term—the end of pregnancy—you'll go into labor. Now if you're doing that before term, you won't go into labor unless you're at risk for preterm labor.

• **Castor oil** can work, but it has some strong, yucky side effects, like bad diarrhea. The oil stimulates the intestines and the intestines release prostaglandins.

• **Stripping membranes.**

The natural triggers of labor happen through some interaction between mother and fetus. After all these years, nobody knows exactly why labor starts when it does, but there is some sort of neuroendocrine reaction. Substances secreted by the baby or the baby's brain says, *Hey, I'm done.* That interacts with the placenta, which in turn interacts with the mother's hormones that kick-starts the labor.

Water Breaking

Occasionally some women will go into labor on their own because their water breaks first. They're not in labor yet, but their water breaks, and *then* they go into labor. The water breaking on its own has no bearing on when the baby will be delivered. It doesn't necessarily mean the baby is coming immediately. Some women go into labor and their water *never* breaks until delivery.

Breaking the bag of water by the doctor has been shown to speed up labor, but only by thirty minutes total. For the most part, it's best to leave well enough alone. If somebody's labor has stalled out and you're looking for *non-medical interventions*, I would first start with **nipple stimulation**. If that doesn't work, you might want to consider breaking the bag of water if that hasn't happened yet. You have to be careful that the baby's head is well in the pelvis so that you don't have a problem with a prolapsed cord, which is rare. It doesn't happen unless the baby is not engaged in the pelvis. You can feel where the baby's head is. If you are five to six centimeters dilated, I think that's okay. If you are only one to two centimeters, you are going to run into more problems.

Breaking the water can make the contractions *stronger,* and that may be what you need if you have a stalled-out labor. From my own experience of four labors, the pain was not worse one way or the other.

The risk of the bag of water being broken has to do with possible infection. The longer you go with a broken bag of water, the higher the risk of infection, "chorioamnionitis," in which bacteria from the vagina spread up into the uterus and can infect the baby.

The baby can be become septic, which means having a bad infection. Plus the mom can end up running a high fever and end up feeling bad. At that point, she needs antibiotics.

Preventing infection means keeping fingers out of the vagina and decreasing the number of exams. The more exams, the higher the risk for infection. With interuterine fetal monitor and interuterine pressure catheter, the risk of infection goes up.

If your water breaks, you should shower instead of taking a bath. If the waters break and a woman isn't in labor within twelve hours then it's appropriate to come in to your doctor or midwife's office and/or the hospital to be checked.

Important Checks If Your Water Breaks at Home:

- If the fluid is green or brown, you need to come in immediately.
- Monitor your temperature, every three to four hours.
- Make sure the baby is kicking actively.
- If your bag of water breaks and something comes out of your vagina that looks like a cord, lie down immediately, put your hips up as high as you can and call 911. Don't let them sit you up.

Questions to ask before an induction*:

Is there a problem? How serious is it?

How urgent is it that we induce? Describe the procedure.

If it does not succeed, what are the next steps? Are there risks?

Are there alternatives including waiting or not doing it at all?

Ask same questions about alternatives.

I remember one lady who came into the hospital ER with a prolapsed cord (the umbilical cord is coming out first instead of the baby) by ambulance. The paramedics had her sitting up on the stretcher. Wrong way! They needed to have the *pelvis up* and have somebody put a hand in the vagina, pushing the head up. Paramedics should know that. Sadly, her baby didn't make it.

Note: The correct position for a laboring mom with either a prolapsed cord, shoulder dystocia, breech or limb presentation of the baby is a knee-chest position, face down with her bottom in the air, even for ambulance transport. This is now illustrated in the Emergency Technician training book for EMTs.

*A checklist by Penny Simkin

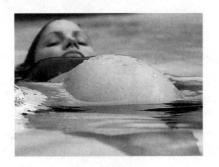

SECRET 7:

Find Out How Birth Centers Bridge the Choice

Free-standing birth centers offer a bridge between home and a hospital. You have the comforts of home—a bedroom, kitchen, bathroom, sitting area—to gather family and friends without tidying up. The environment feels more relaxing than a bustling hospital. But there's oxygen, resuscitation equipment, and a baby warmer tucked discreetly inside an armoire.

In addition to being as safe as a hospital,[1] the main advantage in using a birth center is the personalized, one-on-one care. Your midwife gets to know you—your concerns and preferences. Prenatal visits cover more in-depth information than an obstetrician may have time for. Over a cup of tea, your midwife might review your nutrition regimen, or if you have other children with you, let them listen to their sibling's heartbeat. All of which provides greater relaxation, so important in natural birth.

During your labor, the midwife stays with you to make sure you're *comfortable*. Although epidurals aren't an option, the low-tech approach of a birth center means *lower risks* for you and your baby. Birthing centers offer other soothing options to help you through contractions. They range from scented candles to freedom of movement, the ability to eat and drink to waterbirths in tubs, jacuzzis or other birthing pools. A midwife's confidence along with her encouraging words, dissolves anxiety and empowers you.

In this chapter, you'll find out about three types of training and certification programs for midwives. Each state regulates and licenses midwives. The largest group of licensed midwives is the Certified Nurse Midwives, or CNMs. Direct Entry and Certified Professional Midwives are two others. (Chapter 2 includes a complete description.) Midwives work at more than 200 birth centers in the United States helping deliver about 20,000 births annually.

When a woman in a birth center needs to be transported to a hospital, it's usually because her labor isn't progressing. Only 15 percent of women laboring in birth centers are transferred to hospitals and about 4 percent of those end up with a C-section delivery.[2] Since it takes about 15 minutes from "decision to incision," even in a hospital, it's smart to select a birth center close to a hospital in case transport is needed and the midwife can call enroute.

What comes next are stories of mothers and midwives inside various birth centers across the country.

Family-Centered Maternity Care
Debra DuBois, Midwife

On an active retail street in Oak Cliff, an area south of downtown Dallas, stands an unassuming white wooden house-turned-birth-center.

Debra DuBois, who owned Family-Centered Maternity Care, worked as a high-risk labor and delivery nurse before becoming a midwife. She witnessed women birth naturally unintentionally because their babies were born before doctors arrived. "These women did just fine." she said.

When epidurals were first used, you had to be far along into labor before they were administered.But soon, women got it when they walked in the door. Debra says, "Meet me in the parking lot with my epidural," became a running joke.

In suburbia, many women think an epidural is a standard procedure in childbirth. They ask their pregnant friends, "Are you being induced or having a C-section?"

"Yet, it helps to realize that a routine epidural at 4 centimeters is going to slow labor down," says Debra.

"If you were a nurse, do you want an easy or difficult job?" she asks. The easy way means a woman is medicated in bed, doesn't moan or cry, and doesn't require much attention. That's not pointing fingers or blame, Debra says, because they're not sitting on their duffs all day. It's easier to have ten quiet women than ten needy ones.

"Or you can't be taking care of five other patients at the same time," she says. "What motivates me is: I know the joy that the mother is going to have when the baby comes out and it's over. Everybody is smiling and cheering."

After completing midwifery school, Debra left her nursing job at Parkland, a busy county hospital, to work the next two years at a small birth center. "It was such a foreign concept," Debra says. But before long, she loved it and couldn't imagine even working in a hospital again.

"It's not set up for personalized care," she says. "Where out-of-hospital, with obviously smaller numbers, I can personalize someone's experience for them." About 80 percent of women labor at the center and 20 percent birth at home.

Debra's clientele ranges across cultures. Hispanics represent about 40 percent of her practice. "In little towns in Mexico, you don't go to the hospital. You birth your baby at home. Usually one older woman in the community is the midwife. She birthed all of her children at home. She helps everybody in town, even making house calls. That's the way it is. In big cities, they may go to hospitals, but the hospital C-section rate is high."

In Dallas, outside of the handful of birth centers, only *one* midwife works in *one* hospital in the city. "Because the physicians won't let them in. Plain and simple," says Debra. Susan, the midwife who practiced at Baylor Hospital, and now works in Taos, is excellent. It was a physician that got her in the door. This doctor's power and her belief in midwifery made it happen. But the hospital insisted it would only allow *one* midwife. When Dr. Margaret Christensen wanted to have another one, the hospital authorities said, "If you want a second midwife, you need a ratio of one physician per midwife."

Some physicians see the value of midwives, but aren't willing to fight for them, though their own studies show that patients are more satisfied with midwifery care than conventional medicine. Midwifery care is as safe as with a physician, and outcomes are better than in a physician's care, although midwives don't take care of sick and high-risk women.

"If medicine would adjust to let us take care of low-risk women, our patients would be more satisfied and our outcomes would be better. Plus, we do it for less money. Our whole healthcare system wins."

At the birth center, women are encouraged to walk which helps facilitate labor by allowing gravity to work. A warm bathtub soothes and relaxes, and sitting on the birth ball eases discomfort. Some have waterbirths, but it's not for everyone.

The transfer rate from birth center to hospital is only 6 percent. The main reason is "failure to progress"—not progressing at all or the mom gets to a point and stops. It's usually cleared up with Pitocin. They aren't all emergencies.

Julie, an Asian woman who is married with two children, arrives for her prenatal check-up. Her third baby is due Christmas Eve. Julie always liked to go as drug-free as possible. She didn't know any nurse midwives personally, but she knew that midwifery dates back to the Biblical times, despite its "New Age" reputation.

"My mother had eleven children, and three were born at home. In Japan, most births happen in the hospital. I was born in 1965. That was when everyone went under [was put to sleep during labor]."

Debra laughs, "Yeah, you woke up three days later, hoping the baby in the bed next to you was yours."

Julie's first midwife practiced under an obstetrician. He oversaw his midwives, and he supported them. Julie's first birth was hard because of back labor. "Otherwise, I felt comfortable and was well taken care of."

Misty, a single mom, enters the birth center with her three-week-old baby girl wrapped in a pink blanket. She comes for a postpartum appointment.

While relaxing in a chair, she shares her birth experience. "I knew natural was for me. I'm into holistic health, homeopathy and herbs. Being in a hospital clashed with my lifestyle—getting drugged, getting an IV and being strapped down to a bed. Natural birth is so healthy for the baby and the mom. You heal faster. If women could learn more about how much better it is for the baby, more would be inspired to do it.

"I tell everybody, 'I had a doctor at first, but I switched to a midwife.'" Debra gave Misty materials to read such as *Birthing from Within* by Pam England, articles on waterbirth, and pregnancy magazines like *Mothering*, and *Birth* which helped her prepare for her own natural childbirth.

"My labor was short. Debra checked me at 1 p.m. and I was about 4 1/2 centimeters. She broke my water. I didn't start having contractions until 3:30. The baby was born at 7:30, only 4 hours later. It all seems like a dream now."

"Music helped. I walked around. The birth ball was comfortable. I got in the tub and wanted to have a waterbirth. It seemed like it slowed my labor down, but the warm water felt relieving for my back pain. After getting out, Debra suggested I get on my side to get the baby to turn.

"Debra was busy helping the baby come out. I felt hot and I was sweating. My sister-in-law got a cool wet rag and lightly caressed my forehead, my lips, cooling my arms. Light touch. Cooling me down and relaxing. Really nice. That helped so much.

"Robert, my boyfriend did great. At first, he was nervous about not going to a hospital. He went with me once to the obstetrician. When I switched to this birth center and midwife, he was skeptical at first. All of the what-if's came up? He came to one appointment at the birth center and as we walked out, I looked at him. 'So?'

"I like her. I think it's good," he said.

"Before childbirth class I was worried about how good of a partner my boyfriend would be. I didn't think he was in touch. We watched two natural childbirth videos. The teacher went over things with us that help in labor. After our classes, I felt more secure that he'd be okay.

"When I went into labor, Robert remembered what we learned. He massaged with pressure. He tuned in, 'Do you want me to do massage while contractions are going on? Do you want me to stop when it goes off?' He could tell it was comforting in between but when the pain was intense, I didn't want a massage. I needed him the most when I started pushing. He encouraged me, 'Okay, two more seconds, two more seconds. Bear down, bear down. One more push.'

"Robert didn't see the baby come out. I kept bearing down and my face turned red. He was worried. 'Focus. Think about where you are pushing. Two more seconds, two more seconds.' Hearing that helped me.

"A lot of people were in the room. But I only paid attention to Robert and Debra. Women from his family and mine came and surrounded the bed. My eyes were puffed up from pushing. But I opened them as she was coming out. Our daughter weighed 6 pounds, 12 ounces.

"I felt great. It was just as I wanted it. It wasn't like she was coming out with strangers wearing masks in a sterile room. Instead, it was an intimate setting.

"As I was holding my newborn baby girl, my aunt stood over me just crying. She said, "Misty, I prayed the whole time that she would have a small head.'

"Thank you," I whispered.

A Hispanic mom, Sylvia, sits down on the sofa of the birth center. She gave birth only three days ago to her fourth child.

"My first birth center and first little girl," she says. "I didn't even know the Birth Center was natural...It all happened quickly. I got here at noon. After my water broke on its own, it was only twenty minutes before the baby came."

"You did great," Debra said.

Debra would like to see greater acceptance of midwifery from the medical community. She feels women need to know their options.

"Every single day, I talk to women who say, 'I didn't know about nurse-midwives. I didn't know you could do that. Wow, that's neat.'"

Lovers Lane Birth Center

Waterbirths at the Birth Center and Home Births
— Dinah Waranch, CNM

Dinah, a curly-haired midwife with a British accent, runs Lovers Lane Birth Center out of a cozy brick bungalow house in Dallas, Texas. Dinah's clients want the comforts of home during childbirth. During prenatal visits she makes a cup of tea for the mom and welcomes her young children. The environment feels safer to many women because you can't see monitors and IV's and C-section rooms.

In the book, *Misconceptions*, Naomi Wolf shares her birth experiences in a hospital. She had two C-sections.

"Personally, I got the feeling while she understood you need to have a provider that supports natural birth, that gives labor time to unfold. She didn't understand how incredibly important it is *where* you give birth," Dinah says.

"Women are strong in both mind and body," Dinah says. "Most women can birth naturally without interventions, without drugs. Natural birth unfolds in its own way. It's a powerful expression of each woman's inner self. Birth requires patience and respect. What healthy women need to birth naturally is loving support and the freedom to birth in the way that they choose. But just as your food is more important to a healthy diet than nutritional supplements, your *caregiver and the environment* you choose are much more important than a breathing technique. If natural birth is important to you, choose a caregiver whose expertise is supporting natural birth: a professional midwife. Choose a *birth place* where natural birth is understood and supported, too: your home or a freestanding birth center.

Dinah believes women do have to find the *strength in themselves*. "I can't give it to them," she says.

"For example, a woman who had a previous cesarean and now wants a vaginal [called vaginal birth after cesarean, or VBAC], thought she was in labor called me crying, out of control. She was nervous. I went to her house, checked her and she was only at 2 centimeters. Contractions were frequent but not strong or long. She was scared and tense. That's what intensifies the pain, that kind of fear. I breathed with her and talked about it. The contractions went away. She calmed down and she dozed.

"A couple of days later, she came back for a prenatal visit. I gave her the book *Spiritual Midwifery*. It describes greeting your contractions, or what the author, Ina May Gaskin, calls 'rushes.' It's not that she is avoiding the topic of pain. But birth to her is power and love—not pain. For this one woman, that's what worked for her. She absorbed it.

"When she went into labor, this correct middle-class lady arrived here saying with hands waving up in the air, 'Oooouuu, come on rushes.' She had her baby within an hour and a half of coming to the birth center.

"The key is this: To *greet this powerful force* that's bringing your baby, *letting go*. When people can internalize that message, they can do it."

Seventeen years ago, Dinah was pregnant with her first child in Europe where midwifery care is standard. (That's the case in all developed countries except Canada, the U.S., and countries in South America.) She was studying Urban Planning. "For some reason, I couldn't finish my thesis and got a lot more interested in my pregnancy. I birthed my baby with the help of a staff midwife at a hospital. Natural childbirth was a life-changing experience. I thought, *this city planning is not for me.*"

Dinah became a childbirth educator, a profession that had its limits and frustrations. Women came back to her with depressing experiences, particularly once she moved to the U.S. "You teach everybody all you know, get them excited about their births and then it goes completely different at the hospital because birth is medicalized. I decided to become a midwife to provide natural birth for women, a good fit for me, too, since I had three boys of my own, naturally."

Dinah became a certified nurse-midwife (CNM). It meant going to nursing school, working as a postpartum nurse at a hospital afterward, and working with a midwife. To get into midwifery school, Dinah needed hospital labor and delivery experience.

She enrolled in the Community-Based Nurse-Midwifery Education Program (CNEP). "Look at that old black and white photo on my wall of a lady on a horse and the baby in a saddle bag. That magnificent maverick, Mary Breckenridge, became the first certified midwife in the U.S. She founded the Frontier Nursing Service in Kentucky, to serve poor rural women, where high infant mortality existed," Dinah says.

From her experience as a nurse in WWI, Mary learned that European midwives provided safe care at low cost. She started a midwifery service in Kentucky and brought in midwives from Europe. She single-handedly lowered the infant mortality rate.

Mary started her own school, the Frontier School of Midwifery and Family Nursing. In the 1990s, Kitty Ernst, her successor, made Frontier the first distance-learning CNM program. It became the biggest in the country.

"After becoming a CNM, I started a home birth practice with a friend. When she got another job, I thought, *I need my own office.* If I was going to have an office, I might as well put in a room for births, too. I didn't plan to start a birth center. It just evolved.

"People ask me, 'How many births do you do a year?' I tell them about 40. The point is not high numbers, it's *low* numbers. You have to keep the numbers low in order to provide good quality care."

The front door of Lovers Lane Birth Center opens into the old living room, which is now the waiting room. Prenatal yoga classes are taught there on Saturdays. Dinah measures women's bellies and listens to their babies' heartbeat in her office. In a clean and fully equipped kitchen, clients can bring whatever they want to eat and drink during labor. The bedroom has light walls, natural wood furniture, a queen bed with a blue bedspread and blue curtains. An armoire contains oxygen and supplies.

For nutrition, Dinah instructs pregnant moms to eat plenty of protein. "I'm not as obsessive as Bradley, fifty to sixty grams is fine. Use the food pyramid for variety. Vegetarian clients are no problem: whole grains and organics are best. Drink eight glasses of water a day. Graze all day. Avoid skipping meals."

Dinah explains her relationship with her clients. "We've talked on the phone usually several times beforehand...how things are going, how you're feeling, how you're progressing. I evaluate on the phone, whether you seem pretty hot and heavy, ready to go. By the time you come in, you are or you *think* you are. I check you out. We decide if you need to stay or not. If you stay...obviously, you can do anything you want.

"Some women come and they're already intense, it's clear they're going to have a baby soon. They say, 'I need to get in the tub now.' And they have their baby. For other gals, it's clear that they're in pretty active labor, maybe with their first baby and they still have some time to go. They go for a walk outside. They are going to go in the shower.

"Most of my clients ask, 'Do you do waterbirths?' I explain that waterbirth happens often here. That's what the women want. They get in the water and they don't want to get out.

"In the tub, you're limited to sitting. If they are out of the tub, they are able to squat."

"I have to provide all the care. Some midwives attend all the births, while most doctors will not. An assistant will come here when the woman is in transition to help with the birth itself. I do all the care myself, administrative, supplies, everything. I take care of a mom who is low-risk and remains low-risk.

"Sheila Kitzinger got me into natural childbirth. I *love* Michel Odont. I would marry him tomorrow if we were both single. [Dinah imitates a French accent.] 'Eet's ool about luvvv.' And he's right. You have to read his book, *Birth Reborn*. If everyone birthed naturally the world would be a much better place."

Dinah hopes midwifery will one day become *standard* care. It is not that she wants midwifery to replace medical specialists because they are essential for complicated pregnancies or surgery.

Overcoming Body Image and Family Opposition
Jennifer's Two Birth Stories

What attracted me about natural childbirth was the chance to over-come some of the negative things each of us experience as women— like body image, personal power, and other gender issues. I never felt confi-dent physically. Some would describe my body as "curvy." A friend who runs marathons told me, "Having a baby is like training as an athlete." That metaphor worked for her, but not for me. I never felt coordinated or strong. I needed something else to feel proud of.

One of my good friends—the first one to become a mom—gave birth to her second child at home. She educated me. She assured me it would be such a positive experience that I saw her as my *birth mentor.* That was five years before I had a child.

Even though I come from a family of doctors, I favor natural remedies such as acupuncture for healing allergies and asthma instead of shots or inhalers. When the time came to start our family, I looked into natural birth. My research confirmed it was the best thing for me and the baby.

I read about pre-pregnancy nutrition and prepared myself emotional-ly before conception. I read about 20 books. A friend gave birth naturally and in sharing her extraordinary experience, it affirmed my decision to choose natural birth.

I did prenatal yoga. Walking helped me feel stronger. I squatted, too. It was an *emotional* thing; I needed the confidence that my body was going to hold up through labor and delivery. I don't think you have be athletic; you can just be a woman. That clicked for me.

At the twenty-eighth week of my pregnancy, I switched from a busy birth center to one owned by a midwife named Dinah. The first place had so many clients it felt impersonal. I wanted a more "touchy-feely" midwife, someone who shows she truly cares about me and my baby. Dinah wants to see what you're eating, but she doesn't sit and *highlight* with a yellow marker what you should not have eaten. I was on a pre-pregnancy diet for three months and took prenatal vitamins. But with the food cravings of pregnancy, it's impossible sometimes to deny them.

I felt a chemistry and a spiritual connection with Dinah. She is Jewish, like me. That helped. Her dad is a doctor too, like mine. She under-stands me.

My father is a back surgeon, a neurosurgeon. I did not get *any* support from my father or the rest of my family about my decision to birth naturally. "Oh-my-gosh, that's crazy," they exclaimed.

The main thing my family opposed was giving birth *outside a hospital.* "We've evolved. Women don't have to go through that anymore," they said. One of our closest family friends, a gynecologist told me, "You are absolutely crazy. Why would you do that to yourself? Why?!"

I was doing it because I wanted to for myself and my child. I needed to connect with people who saw natural birth the same way I did.

Bradley childbirth classes, books, and like-minded friends became an important part of my support base, an inspiring circle of hope. If women don't do what I did, I can see why they would be scared. The more natural birth stories I read and the more natural birth people I talked to, the more mentally prepared I was for it.

My husband, Sam, mentally prepared, too. By the time we finished the Bradley classes, he was ready to do it without a midwife. He wanted to deliver the baby. I wasn't quite ready for that.

On a Thursday, I started having contractions that kept me up that night. I had to get on all fours and breathe through them. My husband took the next day off work and we called the midwife. "This is it. It's going to happen." The contractions *never* got regular, though. They went from ten minutes, to seven, to five, back to ten again with no pattern.

The next day, we did some things to encourage labor. We made love. I ate spicy food. I walked and stayed active. The contractions got stronger at night and kept me awake again, but by Saturday morning they stopped. I felt exhausted, discouraged.

Dinah told me to rest. "Don't do anything to stimulate the labor or if you do, don't do it after 12 noon. Relax today since the contractions have stopped." I thought about doing acupuncture, but did not. I rested some. Saturday night they came back again, strong. No sleep for the third straight night.

Sunday morning they disappeared and I became discouraged home birth might not happen. But the contractions came back strong that night.

Monday, Sam went back to work.

On Tuesday, we went in to see Dinah. She checked me and asked if I wanted her to strip my membranes. I declined. Sometimes checking is enough to get things moving. I never focused much on dilation. The exam got labor moving. That night the contractions became regular—five minutes apart—and   strong. Dinah came over at 10:00 p.m. We did a lot of walking outside, squatting.

Once Dinah came, I felt more *reassured*. We decided after a few hours of talking, to break my water. Originally I didn't want to do that. But I was exhausted by this time, ready to do whatever Dinah suggested. She broke my water sac accelerating labor. What I didn't know at the time—but learned later—is that when Dinah checked me, my cervix had actually *shrunk* not widened. That's why she brought up breaking the water. The other midwife, Gail, arrived to assist. She was reassuring and experienced.

Both midwives suggested I try to sleep. But that was hard because of the contractions. I used yoga breathing to rest for 30 minutes, and got some energy. Despite the pain, I craved sleep. By 10 a.m., I began pushing. Dinah moved back a little lip on my cervix to shorten the pushing time, which was incredibly painful.

I started doubting myself, *I can't do this. This isn't going to work.*

I began to cry. "Come on Jen, you can do it," Sam said.

"You can. You're doing great," Dinah and Gail said. They *held m*e and *rocked* with me. I wanted it to work, but I also wanted it to be over.

After hours of pushing, I took black and blue cohosh herbs.* We tried nipple stimulation and every birth position known to woman. I pushed and pushed. They could see part of the baby's head. Dinah kept giving me little goals, "I want to see this much of her head in the next 20 minutes or we're going to have to go to the hospital." She started talking hospital because pushing took a long time. All the signs were fine but the contractions weren't strong enough.

Time was up. "Okay, we're going to the hospital," Dinah decided. Everyone packed as I put on my nightgown. After I got up, though, and walked around, those contractions started *roaring*. I walked onto the porch, held the railing and squatted. I could smell the rain. I actually gained a second wind with more energy. My neighbors could've come out and seen me. Dinah was in her car. We were going to follow her the two minutes to the hospital. I cried out, "The baby's coming. It's here. What if it comes out in the car?" All of a sudden, something felt different.

"We've got to *go* to the hospital." Dinah said. I pushed longer than her protocol allowed.

Sam drove. I pushed in the car. When he approached a stoplight, I hissed in a raspy active-labor-possessed voice, "Go through that red light!" I barely made it through the hospital doors. It was like a movie. I squatted in the lobby, squatted in the elevator. Strangers stared at me in jaw-dropping disbelief. I was having the baby. Right now. *I finally let go of whatever was holding me or this birth back.* I could not control myself. Labor kicked in *big time*.

It's rare to see somebody that far along in their labor enter the hospital. The nurses got me right up on the table, but they were in a flurry, sticking me with needles and making me sign papers. They were nice, though. Dinah's backup doctor hadn't arrived yet and the baby crowned.

"Get a resident!" a nurse shouted.

"Don't worry if the doctor doesn't get here," Dinah reassured her, "I've done this many times. She's going to be okay." It was chaotic, but Dinah stood calmly by me. She confidently knew that the baby was coming and she knew the baby was fine because she had been checking the baby's heartbeat and position.

"Do you want to see with a mirror?" Another nurse asked me. But the only thing I wanted was to have it over.

The resident rushed in. I appreciated Dinah saying to him, "This is a home birth mom. As you can see the baby's *here*. She would like to push the baby out *on her own*. She does *not* want an episiotomy. If you could *please* let her do this." He listened. The baby was coming. He let the baby sit on my perineum and he didn't cut me. Even the nurses said, "Wow, they never let them sit that long." Usually if the baby crowns in between contractions they cut you, especially a first-birth mom. He let me push her out, thanks to Dinah's request.

I'm about to cry retelling this story... I was fine. I had a little tear. The baby was born only 30 minutes after we arrived. I held our newborn and the backup doctor walked in, but it was already over. He stitched me. I felt great. As hard as it was, I'm glad everything was okay. I did it.

The first thing Dinah said was, "You're a hero." I had never felt proud of myself before.

Sam was wonderful. We were both crying, looking at our beautiful little newborn in my arms. I asked him, "What is it?"

He looked. "I'm not a doctor, but I think it's a girl," he said. I laughed.

The only thing I didn't want was her cord cut before it stopped pulsing. Right before they reached for the instruments, Sam said, "Can't you wait?" It had clicked in his head that, we wanted to *wait* to cut the cord.

"She hasn't taken a breath yet, we have to cut it," the resident said. He cut the cord. She took her breath and she was fine. I can't complain. Baby Jacqueline never left my side. They let her lie with me for an hour and let her latch on to nurse. I stayed the night in the hospital.

I felt like I had run a marathon. I had used every single muscle. My throat muscles and my lungs ached. My toes, my cheek muscles, and muscles I never felt before hurt.

Why did my first birth take so long? I was a lot more *scared* than I was willing to admit. Generally, *I am scared to let go.* I tend to have a lot of anxiety and worry which doesn't mesh well with natural birth because you have to *let go.* All of those voices of naysayers scared me. I was scared of having my baby at home.

I realized a personal discovery: I need to let go more in my *life.* A part of me wanted to deliver the baby at home just to prove everybody wrong, which is *not* the right reason. That's part of what my hang-up was: I was doing it partly to show all those doctors in my family.

"See, you had to go to the hospital anyway," they said later.

I still had work to do for our next child.

Three months later, I got another opportunity to practice letting go. I got pregnant, which I was *not* planning. The first birth took me eight weeks to recover from. I bled for seven weeks. Four weeks go by and I'm pregnant. I hadn't had time to even process the *first* birth. I felt overwhelmed. My life had been all birth and pregnancy for the last two years.

I had a baby to take care of and I didn't focus on the second pregnancy. No classes and no books. I wasn't worried about the physical part because I'd done it before. That helped me.

What I *did* do, though, is sign up for a couple of sessions of hypnotherapy. I needed to *process* my first birth some more by imagining it and seeing what lessons I could learn. This step became the most crucial one for our next birth. Hypnosis helped heal me.

I had another chance at birth. I wanted to *feel it* this time. I tried not to worry, think too much, over plan or try to control it. I wondered if I should hire a new midwife. I still wanted to go natural, but my first labor was long and hard. I didn't want to go through all that again. I interviewed other midwives, but came back to Dinah. I'm thankful that I stayed with her.

Five days after my due date, I felt impatient for labor to kick in. On a Tuesday night, I ate some spicy food. I felt antsy. The contractions started in the middle of the night. They continued all the next day off and on. I could not be up for nights with another child now. I worried, *maybe I don't go into labor like everybody else.*

We were in denial thinking it would be days. *I'm not in labor. This is just the way it's going.* I had an appointment planned with Dinah that day. When she checked me, I was moving along, 90 percent effaced and a couple of centimeters dilated. I went on two walks that day—one in the morning and one at 5:00 in the afternoon with three friends who had all birthed naturally.

"Jennifer, you've had five contractions on this forty-five minute walk. That means they're getting on, averaging about every 9 minutes," they said.

I had to stop and breathe, "Yeah?" The contractions sped up. "I guess you're right." I still thought labor was going to be long.

Sam came home from work. My labor got faster and stronger. I breathed through the contractions. I took a bath and drank one small glass of wine, which is what Dinah said to do to slow things down because I had been up the night before. She didn't want this to happen again. The wine didn't help. Sam hadn't packed anything to go to the birth center.

I wanted Jacqueline to stay at home. She had turned one. I didn't want her at the birth center because we would not be able to take care of her. We decided to leave her at home and call our neighbor friends to come over and watch her. I wouldn't be scared to do it at home, but it was nice and clean at the birth center. I didn't have to worry about keeping the house clean beforehand or especially after.

"I think this is it."

"No, it's not *IT*," Sam insisted.

"I think you need to call your boss and tell him you're not going to be at work tomorrow," I warned him.

I felt different. Nothing slowed down. I ate and drank since I was sure it would be 20 hours more. I needed energy. I ate and drank through the whole last birth too, which is the *only* reason I made it for 19 hours. If I had been in the hospital, I would have been *starving*.

I called Dinah at 8:00 p.m.

"I haven't heard a contraction yet. Let's talk until I hear you having one," she said. The contraction came and she said, "Oh yeah, you need to get over here, Jennifer."

"Really?" I asked, amazed.

"I'll meet you at the birth center by 9."

We quickly called my friend again to come watch Jacqueline. The contractions were less than five minutes apart, and strong.

When we got to the Birth Center, I was glad to see Dinah because I was already getting a little down *emotionally.* With all day and the night before, I was thinking, *uuggghh, it's going to be long.* Dinah lit candles and played a CD. "We're having a birth." Her excited mood became contagious and that helped lift my spirits.

We walked. I showered. At midnight, after two hours, I cried and thought, *I want to go to the hospital. This hurts too much. I can't do this for 19 hours again.* I wasn't going to last. I wanted someone else to take over and take care of me.

Dinah kept telling me, "You feel like you're not going to last because *these* are the kind of contractions that bring a baby." I was dilated to seven centimeters.

"Isn't my labor moving slowly?" I asked, with my first birth still fresh in my memory.

"You're moving along fine," she encouraged. "Okay, enough of this, let's get happy again." She put African drumming music on. I got into the rhythms. Maybe an hour later, Dinah asked, "Do you feel like pushing?"

"Could it be time already?" I asked, incredulous.

"You sound like you're pushing."

I had been grunting without realizing it. She didn't have time to check me. They quickly ran the bath water because I was going to try a waterbirth. But I didn't want to get in. I bent over halfway with my hands on the high tub. I started pushing. I didn't even squat.

In less than ten pushes, Dinah said, "Here's his head."

"That can't be his head yet." I said. I couldn't believe it—only eight minutes of pushing.

Sam stood in the doorway, dumbfounded. "Are you going to stand there or do you want to catch your baby?" Dinah asked him. She directed him around to my other side. After the head and shoulders were out, Sam caught our baby which is what he wanted to do the first time.

Our son, Nathan, was born while still in his waters. His sack came out intact—a rarity, that is suppose to be good luck. It makes a birth smoother. The pictures of his sack right after they broke it are unique.

I finally understood the kind of contractions Dinah was talking about. The hour right before transition was terrible, but those pushing contractions felt *good.* I screamed in a releasing kind of way, belting it out. I was not even trying to push. I didn't tear, either, and baby Nathan was even bigger, 8 pounds. Jacqueline was 7 pounds, 11 ounces.

I couldn't believe that it was over even when he was in my arms. Sam and I got on the bed, holding him. I nursed him before I gave birth to the placenta, which came out gently. The whole cord cutting was *delayed* until we were ready. I felt great.

The midwives didn't do anything to Nathan. "Aren't you going to weigh him?" I asked. Dinah showed me the placenta first which I didn't get to see the last time. She never took him away. He was perfectly clean. They didn't need to bathe him right away. They drew an herbal bath for me and we got in together.

In the tub, he floated looking at me as I held his head above the water. So sweet. We slept for a few hours. Nathan was born at 1 a.m. and we went home at 6 a.m. This birth came much easier and faster than I imagined. Nothing held back, nothing to prove. Through bringing my babies into the world, I experienced the miraculous journey and mastered letting go.

Northern New Mexico Women's
Health and Birth Center
Elizabeth Gilmore, Lay Midwife and Founder in Taos, NM

Growing up in Mexico City, I witnessed many types of births. You could get whatever you could pay for in Mexico. You could have your baby in the fanciest hospital that's like a hotel, so fancy that you'll see birds in cages, flowing fountains, servants in your room complete with a hanging cradle. Or you could birth in a regular hospital or a clinic, even. Perhaps you'd like for the doctor to come to your house instead, unless you prefer to hire a midwife. Many ways of birth exist with no rules like here in the U.S. I've seen babies born all my life. In my mind, birth is not complicated. Having a baby is pleasant and nice.

My dad immigrated to the U.S. from Moldavia (a little country near the Black Sea, that used to be part of Russia). At age seven, he and his big Jewish family came through Ellis Island. They were so poor that they gave away their youngest child. When my dad grew up, he joined the merchant marines and ended up in Spain.

My mom, an American, met my dad in Greenwich Village as he was on his way to WWII. "I will come back to marry you and we'll live in Mexico," he told her. When he returned and they married, he went to Mexico looking to start a business for an American textile company. He met up with a Mexican friend, went in business with him, and bought out the company.

In 1969, I graduated from the University of Wisconsin. It was my hippie days. I was twenty years old and pregnant with our first child. I ended up staying at a house my mom owned in Massachusetts. Speaking English rather poorly, like an immigrant, people thought I was nuts. My brother-in-law had graduated from medical school, though, I said to him, "Give me your obstetrics book. Obviously everybody in the U.S. is crazy. I'll do it myself." In hospitals forty years ago, women were put to sleep during labor. I wanted to deliver my baby at home.

After staying home for thirty hours in labor, I thought, *well, nobody can help tell me where I'm going. I can't have this baby at home.* We went to the hospital. However, I arrived too late to use drugs. I refused anything they tried to give me. The nurse came in and I told her, "If you come near me with drugs, I'm leaving." Then the doctor came in ready to deliver and the baby came in half an hour. The doctor was shocked.

Even though we disagreed during labor, the physician said, "Wow, that was a cool birth. Could you teach other ladies how to do that? Why don't you help all these ladies have their babies without all these drugs." He suggested that we could use the basement of the Episcopal Church every Wednesday night to teach.

Four of us taught childbirth classes in that basement. We were invited to a lot of home births and to many hospital births, as guests. The contrast was *startling*. We actually saw babies *die* in the hospital. I saw none die at home.

People thought I was a midwife, asking me to deliver their babies at home. I explained, "I'm not a midwife, just an advocate and educator." I finally told the same doctor at the hospital, who suggested I teach, that people were asking me to deliver their babies at home and I didn't know about that.

"If you keep coming to these hospital births," he said, "I'll show you some stuff in case any of those home births have a problem, you'll know what to do." People were nice. I learned midwifery mostly from the parents, about what worked, what didn't, and from kind doctors. Nurse-midwives from a Boston hospital taught us eight classes, too.

Three and a half years later, my husband and I birthed our second baby at home. A team—a couple of my educator friends—supported me for the childbirth. I knew what to expect. Although it took a long time, 21 hours in all, it was easy. My family came, too. This was much more like my Mexican experiences. We filmed an 8 millimeter movie. My brother-in-law, the doctor, was amazed. It was a great birth.

Our last baby was breech and I knew it would cause a big scandal to deliver at home. It seemed anything outside the norm was considered child abuse. I went home to Mexico to let my mom take care of me. I brought my midwife partner. In labor, I did a lot of swimming. Guess what? The baby turned head down.

In 1977, we moved to Taos, New Mexico. Midwifery was about to be illegal. Local midwives found out "a midwife from back east" had arrived. "Oh, I'm not a midwife," I told them.

"You could at least help us make sure that they don't make midwifery illegal here," they said. We developed local licensing and had a public hearing. We finally got modern regulations, written and oral exams. I got "grannied in" as a midwife (by experience as a lay or direct entry birth provider). I became a midwife sort of sideways.

The birth center that I started got accredited in 1983. I realized we needed to educate midwives and started a college without walls. Our enrollment today consists of lots of individuals and groups in the Philippines, Chili, Alaska, and Idaho. (See www.midwiferycollege.org.) When we needed an accreditation mechanism for the college, I started an accrediting agency.

I found other models, like the one for becoming a certified nurse-midwife (CNM), and borrowed it. Because I had been involved in the accreditation of the birth center, I knew it wasn't absolutely insurmountable.

In New Mexico, only one generation has been in the hospital, so most people believe it's good to give birth at home. For example, when doctors were called away during WWII, midwives all over town were providing home births. The doctors returned from the war thinking, *I can't be running around, the laboring women all have to come to the hospital.* A switch happened.

In the 1970s most grandparents didn't think it was strange to birth at home. Locals considered our birth center no big deal. A huge advantage with Hispanics is their culture *loves* children compared to Anglos. It seems as if our society doesn't want noisy kids around, like in certain restaurants or social events.

Yet Hispanics say, "Please bring your babies, bring your children. We want to see them." They are more family oriented. The entire family comes together to have a baby, bringing lots of support. Even teen pregnancies are supported.

The negative side of that is if birth isn't going well, they all freak out, "What are you midwives doing here?" I call that *Family Dystocia.*

The transfer rate from home or birth center to the hospital is about 15 percent. Some births still work out in the hospital. They may need temporary pain relief.

To me, women's dissatisfaction in birth has a lot more to do with how they are treated. Birth should be *revered.* Yet, hospitals are the last place where abuse of people is still tolerated. Having to take your clothes off. Hospital policies like no food or drink, that's abuse. Being trapped and can't go outside. "This is hospital policy, you must wear the fetal monitor." Taking your baby *away* is the most abusive of all. Newborn babies belong on their mother's tummy. It's different in the hospital. OBEY. If you don't, you're labeled as bad and inconveniencing others. You're the non-compliant, difficult patient.

The group of midwives that I work with always see themselves as facilitators. The mother delivers her own baby. What better way to feel confident.

Ask yourself: What's important in having a child? What's important to you as a parent? To get the best child, how would you go about it? What's your plan? Investigate and find out. Get informed, make choices and *own* your birth. Watch home births and birth center births.

Ask yourself, what would be the best thing for me to do? Not necessarily Pitocin and epidurals because those come with a level of risk. Only one cell layer separates the mom's blood from the baby's at the placenta. However, if you tried and your birth doesn't turn out natural, heal any guilt over your outcome. If you did everything you could to make it be the best, that's all that anyone could ask. With the information that you had, you made the best decision that you could at that time.

Get back to basics and simplicity: Postpartum recovery, breastfeeding, and mothering. We need to value women's work. Should we raise our children only to get a career? What about right now? Have something practical going on. Where is the quality of life? Each day matters.

I've done some wonderful and exciting things. Nothing feels greater than participating in raising a child to make a better world. Giving children a perspective of life has been one of the most important times in my life. Because I lived in Mexico City, I found out when I was young that life is short. Driving a car is dangerous. People die. My mother almost died of tetanus. My friend died of polio. Each moment counts.

One of the things I like most is seeing women and their families feel competent in the job of Mom and Dad, to feel that they can do it. "You are a unique and wonderful human being. You are a talented person who has the capacity to make a difference in the world," I say.

Midwife's Approach Suits
No-nonsense Corporate Mom
Shelley's Story

For the longest time during my pregnancy I thought, *I'm going to have a hospital birth; wake me up when it's over.* At thirty-two weeks of pregnancy, we toured the hospital. My husband, Dave, and I didn't like it at all. I like to know and be in control of what's happening to me.

I started having emotional breakdowns. What was bothering me was the obstetrician. I was diagnosed with gestational diabetes and spent three hours in the doctor's office for the blood work, with no information given to me. I was told to watch a video in a room by myself. Nobody answered questions afterward. As I was leaving, they said, "Come back next Thursday at 2." His whole practice was like a factory: "We do this all the time, trust us, go along, you'll be fine."

As the exit door closed behind me, I knew I didn't want to come back.

A friend had her first birth by cesarean because the doctor wanted to move her labor along. She read *Good Birth Safe Birth,* by Diana Korte and Roberta Scaer, and told me about it.

I found a doula who hooked me up with a birth center. I saw the physican who backed it up because I had a weird pain. My sugar levels were normal, but a tumor in my uterus was causing contractions which made me go into labor. At thirty-six weeks, I had to go on bed rest and I took a drug to stop labor. Later on to prepare for labor, I attended a weekend birth class, not affiliated with a hospital.

I didn't know anyone who had gone naturally, but read that for active labor* the average number of contractions is one hundred. I thought, *I can deal with this.* It gave me peace of mind.

When the midwives asked for my birth plan, I said, "Whatever works. No episiotomy." I understood not to be a martyr. I even asked the midwives, "How far do you let it go?"

"We don't. If you are high risk, you're out of here," they said. The Birth Center talks about how you will go to hospital if a problem develops. If they say it's time to go, I know it is. I didn't want lay midwives because if we needed a physician's help there would already be a good relationship with these certified midwives.

I'm a runner and at a healthy weight. But, I carried our daughter low that after six months I would get Braxton Hicks when walking.

Labor started while I was at a Christmas Party, on December 17th. I was due January 5th. We went home and Dave went to bed. I couldn't sleep and hung out until 2:30 a.m. I called the birth center midwife. "We're finishing a birth right now. Can you hold out until 6 a.m.?" she asked. I said okay. Contractions were about ten to fifteen minutes apart at that point.

While driving to the birth center the next morning, I wanted to focus during each contraction. A moving car was too much. "Stop the car. Stop the car." I said.

"No, we're going to keep going," Dave said, intently looking straight ahead.

At the birth center, the midwives wanted to try the ball. I didn't like the birth ball. It hurt to spread my legs. I wanted a hot bath, but when I got in the hot tub, labor slowed. I got out, dressed and walked around the park next door. By that time it was past noon.

I was at seven centimeters and wanted to push. They broke the water to move labor along. It hurt like hell. I walked some more. Then I needed to push. They stretched the cervix, waiting for a contraction to do it.

Internalizing the pain was the way I dealt with labor. With eyes closed, I didn't want to be touched. During transition, sitting backwards on the toilet, I grabbed the toilet lid so tightly that I was numb in my thumb for several months. I focused there, breathing for a while.

I moved to lie down on the bed. I needed to sit up in a contraction. It worked better. Sitting on my side felt good, too. The baby's head was catching on my cervix.

During transition a weak point came that if someone had offered drugs I would've taken them. But it was not an option. It was intense and some contractions were doubling on top of each other. They were not slowing down.

"It is not fair." I protested about my contractions as the midwife massaged my legs, but her hands were rough. "Can't you use some hand lotion?"

At one point, I wanted quiet. No talking. No music. I pushed a big fourteen inch head out, although it took three hours of pushing. I was on my back with my knees up to my ears. It was a tight squeeze. Sylvie, our baby girl, came out bruised.

Five minutes after birth, all I wanted to do was order dinner from La Madeleine and take a shower. They put a chair in the shower for me. I was surprised that I didn't want to hold the baby. I wanted to shower, to order dinner and needed to regroup myself first. I couldn't think of taking care of a baby yet.

They gave me juice. We stayed until 11 p.m. The baby was fine. I had no tearing and was in good shape.

A lot of women want drugs because of the unknown. They don't know what birth is going to be like. But, I opted for natural birth and I felt good afterwards. My friend's experience was not as good. She had an epidural and got a ruptured bladder from the catheter that was put in her. She had to let the drugs wear off, and it was a longer recovery.

If I had to do anything differently, it would be to have a midwife in the *beginning* of my pregnancy. I was afraid to change to a midwife so late in my first pregnancy, but I was empowered by it. I had a doula, the midwife, a midwife's assistant and my husband. Great support.

With our second child, Shawn, I was more calm. Since I carried him low also, I was always looking out for the handicapped zone to park. If I couldn't find a spot at the grocery, I drove to another store because I would get diarrhea if I had to walk too much.

Shawn was due in the winter and I opted for a home birth. Here in Montana, the closest hospital is in Livingston which is 30 miles over a mountain pass in freezing weather. I found our midwife by word of mouth. Midwives here are busy. If you want them, it needs to be scheduled to see if they are in town and can fit you in.

I went into labor at 1 a.m. and hung out. About 4 a.m., I called the midwife. "They're five minutes apart if I stand." She suggested I sit down and told me that she was on her way. She arrived at 6 a.m. I spent only forty minutes pushing and delivered at 8:30 a.m. I would rate it a nine only because the umbilical cord had to be cut from around his neck and I had to hold off a push. It was a weird feeling for the baby to be out and still inside, too.

I recommend breastfeeding your baby. Have you ever taken a magnet to formula and watched what happens? It has five to ten times the iron that breastmilk does. It smells gross and it tastes gross. It's disgusting. I wouldn't drink it. Why would I give it to my child?

Sylvie breastfed great. She made my toes curl. Two weeks into it, it hurt. Yet, I breastfed for seven months and expressed milk for five more months.

Shawn was a lazy nurser. He was distracted easily, fussy, and cried a lot. "Oh, you must be hungry. Here." He was a fat little thing, and nursed for fifteen months.

I'm not a hippie. I'm not a granola girl. I'm all for Western medicine but I do take herbal supplements. I want control of my delivery, my body and my baby. I wanted to have the support from a midwife who would say, "It's okay, this is what is happening. Keep it up."

A no-nonsense approach. That worked for me.

Note: Active labor is defined as contractions coming less than 5 minutes apart and lasting about a minute.

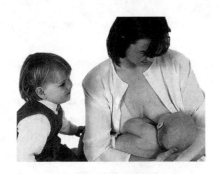

Meet True Stay-at-Home Moms

A Doctor's View of Home Births

Alex Bekker, M.D. and Homeopath* with wife July Bekker, from Peru

Dr. Bekker says his wife gave birth to their first baby at home right before he went to medical school. "I suppose that's why I wasn't against home birth. Going through medical school, I would have been more hesitant and afraid if we didn't already have our first child. I became more aware of all the complications of childbirth. But it didn't stop us from having two more babies at home with a midwife."

"I had been training in Homeopathy for some years, so that's why the idea of natural childbirth was not foreign. A good friend trained to become a midwife around that same time. When my wife, July [pronounced like Julie], became pregnant, we were going to have our child at home without question."

July admits that she never witnessed birth happen before. "My mom gave birth to all of my brothers naturally at home in Peru except for my sister and I," she says. "I was a footling breech [the baby's foot presents first as the baby sits in a bottom down rather than head down position before birth] so she birthed me at a clinic."

"The birth of our daughter, Natasha [meaning Nativity because she was born on December 28th], was a long and difficult birth. I was in labor for two days. She was breech with her back against mine. They would turn her and she'd flip breech again. We treated her with homeopathy, using Pulsatilla (a Homeopathic remedy), which helped her turn and she finally stayed in position.

"I walked a lot, up and down stairs, cooked, went to the movies and walked in the mall.

"Because labor was strenuous and I was up at night, I took a lot of honey for energy. After twelve hours, the midwife suggested going to the hospital, which I didn't want. We danced and sang a song we made up together, an opera spoof for humor. That helped me relax. Alex put a towel around me and we started singing that song. The midwives asked us to walk. Instead we danced. Of Russian descent, Dr. Bekker sung Russian words like *crocaduchi* which means 'little crocodiles.'

"I felt like I was having labor *with* her. I was pushing, like sympathetic labor. My abdominal muscles grew sore.

"The baby started coming and got stuck because she decided to put her left hand on her face. The midwives made a small incision, or episiotomy, and gently pulled her arm out.

"She was only 6 pounds, 11 ounces, small and round. After she came out, they put her on my belly. She didn't cry. Like a little turtle, she raised her head and looked around. Then she smiled, an unusual surprise. She was so cute. I felt excellent, excited."

The next year, Dr. Bekker began his first year of medical school. The birth of their second child was not as difficult as the first birth. Labor did not last as long.

"Our third child was born in my third year of medical school," Dr. Bekker says. "We kept our home birth private because my colleagues might think it was strange. We only told a few close friends.

"All the things that we did at home we would not have been able to do at a hospital. Walking, dancing, singing, eating light, having water, giving Pulsatilla, having friends over with a party afterwards. July might have had a C-section because she's borderline high blood pressure.

"The third baby came too fast." July recalls. "I walked in the room of our house and all of a sudden I heard a scream. A big echo inside 'whoooo.' The baby screamed before coming out. I thought I was crazy; it can't scream inside. I felt strange little butterflies all over the place. I shouted to my husband, 'Alex.' I tried walking towards the bed and felt this urge. He had to catch the baby by sliding under me as I was standing up. I never made it to the bed."

When July went to the restroom, she fainted from fatigue. Her husband gave her some Arnica (a Homeopathic remedy) and she regained consciousness.

July recalls, "I remember the psychiatrist asked me, 'Where did we have the third baby, what hospital?'"

"We didn't have our baby in the hospital."

"Where did you have it?"

"At home." I said matter-of-fact.

"At home?"

Dr. Bekker says he knew from the beginning that he wanted to practice Homeopathy. "My orientation leans towards natural healing. I went through rotations in Obstetrics with the idea of obtaining information. I knew that what I was learning was a small part of the picture, an incomplete part. To put obstetric pathology into perspective, it has to be put into childbirth as a whole.

"If you don't see anything else, your training is such that you don't have any alternative points of view, then what you *see* is what you get. You do what you're trained and you think the way you're trained to think. In medical school, *examining* what you're taught is not something that's encouraged. You're suppose to *accept* what you're taught.

"For example, we were taught at that time that every woman over a certain age must be on hormone replacement therapy (HRT). Studies supported this practice initially. But when the studies were carefully examined, they turned out to be inaccurate."

Dr. Bekker says, "Everything I learned in med school hasn't contradicted what I learned in Homeopathy, which is practiced and respected in many parts of the world. You can go to a Homeopath in England, France and Germany. It's a patient's choice. Health does not come from a bottle. It's innate and natural."

Discussing the safety of home birth, Dr. Bekker compares it to a hospital birth. "Obstetricians have raised the risks of birth with interventions in a hospital, such as not allowing women in labor to walk. Parameters to induce with Pitocin and inductions carries its own risks. The risks of the hospital outweigh the risks of natural childbirth at home."

* Note: Remedy examples are personalized based on individual constitution.
Homeopathic solutions should be discussed with an experienced Homeopath.

From Traumatic First Birth to Divine Deliverance
Michelle's Story

Michelle's mother can sense danger. She'll call Michelle, a strawberry blonde with wavy long hair, to warn her. She told Michelle, "A mother's intuition becomes acute after giving birth."

"Maybe women are built that way to take optimal care of our children. My mother gave birth to me naturally in four hours and to my sister in one hour. She actually caught my sister because the doctor didn't show up in time.

"With the birth of our first baby, Christian, I wanted to go natural, but the nurses discouraged it. When I got in the tub, the nurse told me to get in bed. When I wanted to walk around, I was taken back to the room. I felt trapped. After five hours of labor, the doctor induced me.

"My expectation of a natural childbirth was shattered, and so was my confidence. I gave in to the epidural and felt like crying. The epidural had a terrible side effect on me and my baby. Once it was administered, my heart rate and his heart rate plummeted. I remember feeling my whole body going numb and the room getting dim.

"The doctor cut my perineum with a fourth-degree episiotomy and used forceps. When they handed our newborn to me, his eyes were rolling in the back of his head and he was spastic. I think it was a side effect of the epidural. No one encouraged me to breastfeed.

"Later, a pediatrician told me that our son was two weeks early. I suffered postpartum depression and had serious problems from the episiotomy. My first bowel movement was extremely painful. The cut took over nine months to heal. Sex didn't become comfortable again until my son was a year old. I paid a heavy price for my ignorance."

Afterwards, Michelle read everything she could get her hands on. She talked to moms who birthed naturally. But no one in her family supported her at first. Then one day, her mother-in-law, a nurse, said, "Having your baby at home is safer because you're immune to your own germs."

Michelle searched and found two midwives that worked together, Gail Johnson and Bonnie Kitchen. "The care I received was far beyond what I imagined. I didn't realize how bad my prenatal care was before with the obstetrician until I discovered the kind of treatment I was given with the midwives."

"On March 9th, I felt unusually alert. It was time for our second baby's arrival. I cleaned my house. My nesting instinct to sanitize with safe cleaning products was pleasurable. Around 2 p.m., I noticed that my Braxton Hicks [mild contractions prior to labor] became regular. They weren't painful. In fact, the contractions give me a rush of energy.

"At 4:30 p.m., I noticed a bit more blood than the usual tinge of color normally found with discharge, like a light period. Concerned, I called Gail. She said to meet at her office at 6:00. When she checked me, I was 4 1/2 centimeters. 'Today is a good day to have a baby. Call me at 8 p.m. and tell me your progress.'

"I ate, returned home and put Christian to bed. We read to him, *Welcome With Love,* by Jenni Overend, a picture storybook that explains how a baby enters the world. I called my crew for stand-by and called Gail. I sent my husband, Matt, for food."

Gail arrived at 9:30 p.m. She wore maroon scrubs with a stethoscope which looks familiar to hospital staff if she ever transports a mom to Labor and Delivery. Bonnie Kitchen, another midwife, an apprentice (who monitors fetal heart rate), and Kalena Cook joined her. Gail checked Michelle and found her dilated to six centimeters, 85 percent effaced, at zero station.

"Every time I felt a contraction, I welcomed gravity with bouncing and dancing to Loreena McKennitt's, *The Book of Secrets* music. I drank water from my half-gallon jug. I drank two already and worked on a third one. Water has a tremendous effect on labor. A hydrated laboring woman notices less pain.

"I went to the toilet before lying down to rest. I had to reserve my energy. My husband brought me broccoli, carrots, and pineapples to nibble on and more water to drink. A chest and knee position on the bed felt best. Kalena and Gail joined me and we talked. Gail massaged my back. I enjoyed her cold hands.

"I confided, 'I'm afraid of tearing.' I asked Kalena what it was like for her to push. 'It felt good to push, like I *wanted* to push. That was the surprise for me, that it didn't hurt to push. However, it took a lot of strength. I was winded afterwards,' she said. With their presence I drifted into an *altered state of conscience* as I sensed the contractions becoming stronger. I found both thrill and comfort in each contraction. Though they were intense, they brought me closer to having my baby. I concentrated on each one with slow deep breathing. Every contraction demanded more of my attention.

"At a quarter 'til midnight, everyone left me to rest. I felt alone so I walked into the living room. Matt offered me a massage in his massage chair, but I didn't want to sit on my bottom. I obsessed with the idea that I had to poop. The rectal pressure existed but I didn't feel like pushing. Perhaps with the long healing of my perineum before, I was afraid to push.

"Everyone was hanging out and having a good time. It was a celebration with music and food. I squatted in the chair and asked aloud if this could be transition. 'When you yell out, we will all run to you.' Kalena answered humorously.

"Gail offered to check me. First, I went to the bathroom. The baby was at plus one station, eight to nine centimeters and had a bulging bag that broke upon examination. The water was clear and my contractions dominoed.

"At 1:00 a.m. labor became exhausting. I turned onto my side in bed with Matt supporting my leg. Ten minutes later, Gail noticed I had a small cervical lip that's in the way and it kept me at nine centimeters. I asked her to flip it for me. She did but it felt uncomfortable and she stopped. The lip remained and we waited until it released. I got anxious for this to be over so I asked her to do it again, even though it felt very uncomfortable. She proceeded, I hollered, and she stopped again. She suggested I go to the bathroom instead. I took one more sip of my water and got up quickly before another contraction hit.

"Yes, I needed to poop and pee a lot, too. I heard everyone in the bedroom clapping for me. Leaning into my husband in the bathroom, I started pushing while standing with a lot of power; it felt great. No more pain, just a tremendous amount of power. I reached inside to see if I could feel the head. I felt a wrinkly flesh and it made me worry that it was the umbilical cord. Gail assured me that it is the head. Fully dilated, I continued to push while standing. 'I can't believe this.' Matt said. 'Men couldn't do this even if we were anatomically correct.'

"After drinking more water, I waddled slowly to the bed in the knee and chest down position. I continued to push. The baby's head crowned and I touched him. I got an incredible rush of euphoria. Our baby's heart rate was at 108 which is normal because he's getting squeezed. My heart rate would drop, too. Ten minutes later, his heart-rate returned to 150, a definite sign of the ordinary."

"Gail encouraged me not to push too hard now to avoid tearing. They massaged my perineum with warm olive oil and continuously trade warmed compresses from the crock pot, which felt comforting. 'You are such a star,' Gail said. All of her actions happened in a rhythm that comes from experience and confidence.

"At 2:20 a.m., Matt signaled to our friend, Bari, to get Christian, our son, out of bed. He joined the room wide-eyed in pajamas, fully aware that his brother will soon be here. Our baby's head appeared looking like a gray egg. I opened wider and his bulging of the head appeared. A gush of amniotic fluid sprayed Bonnie and everyone laughed. The midwives patiently waited for the next contraction.

"Gail guided Matt to catch his baby. One more push and our beautiful son, Jaden, was born into his hands. Christian clapped with joy and said, 'Yay! Jaden is here.' It is 2:29 a.m.

"Matt gave Jaden to Gail, and she handed me the biggest trophy I have ever won in my life. Placed on my chest, he smiled and giggled. Words can never describe the moment.

"I latched Jaden on my breast right away and he breastfed.

"Everyone left us alone, our blessed family cherishing the moment of our new arrival.

"Gail poured an herbal bath for Jaden and me, and helped me out of bed. It can be awkward to walk at first. My diaphragm readjusted to the smaller size. I now understand how easy it can be to get the wind knocked out of you while getting up for the first time. The herbal bath felt soothing."

"I was able to breastfeed right away because my milk came in the next day. I was pleased with the way everything worked out.

"Gail knew exactly when to touch me and when not to. I feel fortunate to have her as my midwife. I will treasure the moment in birth when I climaxed to the highest point of womanhood. It was the most amazing event in my life. I hope that God will bless us with more children so that I may once again experience the joy of giving birth.

"In fact, natural childbirth healed me not only emotionally but physically. I was able to have a bowel movement with no problems for the first time in almost three years. I'm regular to a 'T' now. It's wonderful to be able to sit on my bottom without the pain I had the first time I gave birth. It almost feels like I didn't have a baby. I recovered quickly.

"Friends tell me that I've changed overnight. I was no longer depressed. Last night, my friend said, 'You're much more confident now. You are a different person.' I'm not stressed. I'm happy all the time.

Ecstatic. I think one of the reasons postpartum is a big issue is because depression happens after a traumatic birth.

"Matt was happy. He became sentimental when we were all together by ourselves with our sons. He said with watery eyes, 'That was awesome. I love my boys.' He's more emotional than I am. Our neighbors came over and brought flowers. He cried in front of them saying, 'I wish we had done this the first time,' he said."

Shoulder Dystocia

Gail explains Jaden's birth, "The baby's head came out blue and okay. We waited for the next contraction and push.

The anterior shoulder hooks on the front pelvic bone and the posterior shoulder will naturally come out first.

Some doctors yank and pull the baby out, trying to get the anterior shoulder out first, resulting in shoulder dystocia, which causes the newborn's clavicle to break."

Supplies

The midwives brought a crock pot for warmed water with compresses. Some of the supplies included a hanging toiletry bag for small items like aspirin, collapsible trash cans, a heating pad for use afterwards to warm the mom if she is shaking from the adrenaline rush of birth, pads for fluids, gauze to catch any bowel movements, a doppler and a chart to record times in.

Matt provided a spread of food for friends, family and the midwives to enjoy—a fruit tray, a veggie tray, sandwich meat and breads, and spring water.

A Dad's Perspective

Matt's Story of Comparing Hospital and Home Births

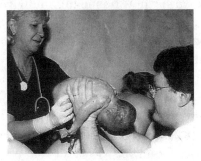

The hospital birth of our first son, Christian, was about what I expected. The doctors and nurses took command over the whole situation and we didn't have a lot of say. Michelle wasn't allowed to walk around or use the jacuzzi tub in the room. The staff wanted to maintain control. Looking back, we *had* more say, we didn't know *how* to say what we wanted. It wasn't a matter of someone saying, "No, you can't do this." They used subtle intimidation that halted us like, "I highly suggest you get back in bed. It's best if you stay in your room. We'll need to come in and check on you, so you need to stay here."

I had mixed feelings. The doctor, who we had some issues with, still allowed me to stand right beside Michelle. When he pulled Christian out, the first thing he did was turn to me and say, "Here daddy, here's your son." He gave him directly to me which was *wonderful*. I was the first person that my son looked at when he opened his eyes. He even peed on me.

The *way* the doctor delivered our baby was another issue, though. He's trained and from his perspective of traditional western medicine, he's excellent. He used a time-sensitive method to protect the mother's health (as he saw it) and to deliver a healthy baby. He used forceps, which he was good at. However, my wife had an extensive episiotomy because he had to make more room for the forceps. To him, I think, he believes that's the cost of doing business.

Never once during that time did I feel this was unhealthy. I thought, *this is the way it works nowadays.* Michelle's physical health was never in jeopardy.

If I compare our first birth of Christian to Jaden's birth at home, the hospital delivery, with all of the equipment was an antiseptic environment. It seemed like Michelle was more of a control subject in an experiment than a mother giving birth to her first child.

When Michelle gave birth at home, the midwives didn't induce her with Pitocin, like when she was in the hospital. She gave birth when her body said it was time. They didn't rush her. They patiently let her labor, allowing her neuromuscular system to relax and stretch the way it was supposed to. When they gave the epidural at the hospital, her dilation immediately stopped.

I watched the midwives, calmly, work as a team. They didn't deliver the baby so much as provide support and reassurance to Michelle as she was giving birth on her own. She was as dilated and relaxed. She had a slight tear, but she recovered quickly. She was even able to sit up the next day.

Gail had delivered 1,500 babies and Bonnie had delivered 1,200. It was reassuring to know they had as much experience as a young doctor in a hospital.

I grew up on a farm and delivered over 100 Angus calves with my dad. In the early '80s, the breeding stock had gotten the calves so large that it was hard for the cows. We attached chains to their hooves and put a great big winch on their behind. When they were trying to give birth, we winched the calf out. Now, the cattle industry has gone back to where they breed smaller calves that can be birthed naturally.

I knew natural birth has been around forever. When my wife brought up the idea that she wanted to go natural for our second child, my mom, a critical care nurse, supported her wanting a home birth. Michelle started researching into it. We compared our hospital experience to what we were learning. Once I understood Michelle *really* wanted to do it, I was behind her.

I'm happy that we made the decision to birth at home, although I wish we had a bigger bed with more room to maneuver. I thought I could help Michelle with the pain. I used some of the techniques I learned doing muscular work as a massage therapist. The theory I read about in books—"You can have a painless birth"—is complete nonsense to me. Michelle felt pain, but she was in a different state of mind. She had forgotten the pain until she watched the video back. Then she said, "Oh yeah, that did hurt, I forgot about that."

It wasn't easy supporting Michelle. When she leaned into me while standing in the bathroom, she was crushing my shoulders. It was if she had robotic hands, but I wouldn't change it at all.

My advice to other men is the same advice whether it's home birth, vaccinations, or circumcision. *Do the research.* Take time away from the job—not one day but a couple of days off. Visit respected midwives in your area, visit birthing centers, visit the hospital. Ask hard questions. That's the only way I know of because it's a change of state of mind. That's only going to happen through a personal conviction—because of a bad experience, or because you take the time to go look.

Don't be afraid of what other people are going to say.

Yoga Helps Mom for Second Birth at Home
Jeannie's Story

After my first birth at the hospital, a friendly attendant came into my room with a wheelchair to take me upstairs to postpartum. She had a gospel singer's hearty voice. As she secured the brakes, I got out of the bed by myself and walked to the bathroom.

She looked up with surprise, "Girrlll. You didn't have drugs did you?"

"No ma'am, I sure didn't," I replied.

"Well, I can tell!"

My husband, Mark, and I had just moved. I thought I had at least a couple of more weeks before my due date. But unexpectedly, I woke up at 3:30 a.m. in labor. Yet I didn't realize I was starting labor since this was my first time. I kept going to the bathroom and checking myself to see what was going on. Thank God I had a bowel movement, I didn't have to go through that with others around. I got up, made my husband coffee, and woke him up about 6:30 a.m.

My doctor had moved during my fifth month of pregnancy. I started seeing her partner, another female obstetrician. I saw the midwife at the same practice quite a few times, too.

One book that I read during that time, *Birth,* by Dr. William Sears, offered an outline of how to do your birth plan. I hadn't made mine yet, so my husband, Mark, busily typed one up as I dealt with contractions. I knew I didn't want any kind of medical intervention. I didn't want an episiotomy, and I didn't want them to take my baby away from me.

Several things helped me to prepare for natural birth. As a hairdresser at a day spa, I enjoyed good support from my co-workers. Everybody was into natural health and nutrition. I received prenatal massage, which felt good. I was determined to give birth naturally.

Every day I talked with people who sat in my chair, mostly husbands. I'd ask, "Did your wife have natural childbirth?"

"Oh yeah, she had the epidural and everything." *Okay, he doesn't understand.*

I was inspired reading *Mothering* magazine.

But, I made the mistake of taking Lamaze classes because I was the only one in the whole room that raised my hand that I wasn't going to take drugs during labor. Everyone turned to look at me like I was some kind of freak. But, at least the classes gave my husband an idea of what was going to happen.

We called the doctor to tell her that my labor had started. "Relax, take a bath," she said. The contractions came fast.

The doula arrived at our house and took one look at me going through a contraction. She said, "We need to go." She was in her early fifties with two children, and has helped deliver four or five other babies, so she *knew*.

Mark and I got to the hospital about 9 a.m.. Everything went smoothly until the nurse put the fetal monitor on me. It felt like a knife cutting into my belly. "Can you please loosen that?" I pleaded.

"No, no. We need to leave this belt on for twenty minutes," the nurse said.

My doctor was preparing to do a scheduled C-section on another woman. But because my baby was ready to go, she had to wait.

During labor, it was funny. I did the Lamaze breathing, but I make a joke out of it, "ha-ha, hee-hee, tooky tooky." The nurses must have thought, *This redhead is weird. She's laughing during labor.*

Mark was scared to death. He was the only male in the delivery room. He held my hand. My massage therapist rubbed certain parts of my back, gave me ice and put a cool cloth on my head. The doula helped Mark relax by massaging his neck. She stood by to run interference in case the staff intervened in away I didn't want."

Labor was painful, but my endorphins kicked in. Knowing what I was going to have—a baby—when it was all over with, helped. I kept telling myself in my head, *I can do this.*

And my group told me, too. "You're doing great." Having other women there was important to me.

I pushed maybe fifteen minutes at most. I wasn't hooked up to IVs or monitor so I was able to move freely. I tried different positions. I labored on the birth ball. At the end of the labor stage, someone put a bar on my bed saying, "Okay, Jeanie pretend you are on your Harley." I grabbed the bar and kept pushing. As the baby was starting to crown, I lay down on my back.

It all happened fast. We got to the hospital at 9 a.m. and our daughter, Zoe, was born at 11:14 a.m.

Mark cried. I've got an incredible picture of him and Zoe. She's on a warming table and she's looking up into his eyes.

Zoe stayed with me for an hour while I nursed her. Mark went up to the nursery with her. The nurses wanted to do all these things saying, "Her body temperature is low."

"You give that baby back to her mother right now. She'll get her temperature up," he said. They brought her to me and she never left again.

When I got up to the postpartum room, the nurse offered me some Tylenol and Motrin for pain. "I gave birth to a baby without medications. It's over. Why would I want that *now*? No thanks," I said.

It's true that every pregnancy feels different. With Zoe I was not sick at all, but with this little boy, ah, I felt sick. I felt bad for a few weeks, but it passed. I worked out doing aerobics, water aerobics and prenatal yoga.

Yoga ended up being the best thing I ever did. It was incredible. I came together with other pregnant women because I wasn't working. We all shared our stories, our fears. The experienced moms would answer questions for the inexperienced women. Kind of like a La Leche meeting. The "child's pose" was the position that I labored in. The yoga breathing and going into my mind and taking my body elsewhere helped.

I had two appointments with the midwife I saw before. She gave me a list of midwives that would do home births. I was going to do three interviews but I liked the second one, Becky, the best. She was sweet and had two boys. What sold me on her is she used to work at Presbyterian Hospital as the head obstetrical nurse. She didn't like what was going in the hospital with the high cesarean rates and intervention. Becky came to my house every month in the first few months and in the last few weeks, she came weekly.

She was calm, nurturing and down to earth. A few times she wanted me to do something medically that I didn't agree with. I told her I wasn't going to do it. For example, I came down with the flu. She said I needed to take some over-the-counter medicine, but I refused.

"Did you ever take that medicine?" she asked.

"No," I said. She was cool with that.

We had company over one night. I was exhausted. My husband and the guests were drinking wine. They were getting on my nerves. I put Zoe to bed, and the guests finally left around 10 p.m.

I lay down for an hour. I didn't know it at that time, but I had been losing a small amount of amniotic fluid. I thought I was losing my bladder a little. I slept for about an hour. Everything was ready in the back room for labor except my music. I got up to go the bathroom and went back to bed. Then I went to the bathroom again. *Okay, this is happening.*

I went into the den and as I sat down to get my CDs, my amniotic fluid flowed out. *Oh great.* I was in total denial because I needed sleep. *Oh no, this isn't happening.* I got my music and took it to the back room. I had several contractions and lay down in the child's pose thinking, *time to call my midwife.*

"Becky we never discussed at what point I should call you, but I'm in labor," I told her on the phone.

"How far apart are your contractions? Call me when they're 15 minutes apart."

I called my friend Karen, the doula. I knew she was closer. She had helped deliver seven babies before. She arrived first, at 1:30 a.m., but she was freaking out because it was happening fast. "Jeannie, please don't have this baby before Becky gets here."

"You need to talk to *him*," I said pointing to my belly. "Don't talk to me."

She called the midwife. "Becky, you need to get over here," she said frantically.

Karen was helping me with contractions. I was on my hands and knees in the child's pose. She had the birth ball. It didn't feel great this time, so I didn't do it. I moved around the guest room. Candles were lit. It was cool. All the supplies were set up, clean sheets with a shower curtain underneath.

Becky arrived at 2:30 a.m. She unpacked her huge bag containing supplies and oxygen. I was taken aback for a second, thinking, *that's the stuff she needs if something goes wrong.* In the unlikely event something were to happen, Becky knew people at Presbyterian and at the fire station. She remained calm, pulling her stuff out. I felt at ease with her serenity. I felt comfortable in my home. I put worry aside.

Next, who was going to go wake up my husband? The gals discussed back and forth as I warned, "Whoever goes back to the bedroom needs to tell him to *put some clothes on* before he gets up out of the bed."

"Okay, Karen, you go wake him up because you've given him a massage before. You've seen most of his body." We heard rustling.

"Mark? Are you dressed?" Karen asked.

He got up about 3:30 a.m. He called our minister because we asked her to come take pictures. As a Methodist minister, she's been on death beds, but this was her first birth experience.

"You need to get over here because this is happening," he said. She lived right around the corner but she barely arrived in time.

I put the music on. I brought an enlarged picture of me at the beach sitting on this huge area of coral. Seeing the waves, listening to the music took me to a different state of mind. Deep Forest, Enya and mystical chants. Music helped me not to think about what was going on. Yoga teaches you how to relax also.

Your natural endorphins take over. It is a mind-body experience.

I progressed quickly. "Karen, tell me to breathe," I said.

"I thought you were doing fine."

"Just tell me." I said emphatically. The labor intensity got to me for a few minutes.

Becky told me that part of my cervix covered the baby's head. She reached down inside and pulled it to the side. I was on my hands and knees. Then I turned over and had him on my back. I pushed maybe three times and our newborn boy arrived. Baby Zach was born by flashlight at 5:07 a.m.

Quick and easy three-and-a-half hours this time. Yoga and breathing is what got me through the second time. Zach weighed eight pounds, one ounce. I didn't even tear. I felt tired, but exhilarated.

I'm glad I had the first hospital experience. Yet the second birth was *much more comfortable* in my own home. My husband cooked up a huge breakfast feast for everybody while I had my sweet little boy wrapped in a towel, asleep on my chest.

Dealing with Posterior Labor
Tracy's Story

I'm doing something wrong. This labor is taking so long.
"You are doing great. You can do this," the midwife told me. You need that kind of encouragement, at least I did, laboring with my first child. The posterior position of my baby in the womb, with his spine against mine, gave me incredible back pain during labor. But, the midwife's support and various pain relief techniques kept me going.

I chose natural birth after reading about a magazine editor's home birth. Then my sister gave birth in a hospital. The obstetrical nurse lay across her belly to push the baby out. It was all about time; the birth needed to happen before 7:30 p.m. I don't know why. I knew right then that a hospital birth was not for me. I attended three births of friends: two in the hospital and one at a birth center.

I didn't want to lose control of my birth to let someone else take over and use interventions against my wishes. Instead, I liked the phrase "the tincture of time" used in *The Thinking Woman's Guide to a Better Birth,* by Henci Goer. Everything I witnessed first-hand and read about alleviated my fear. I wanted to give birth at home and my husband embraced a home birth.

What helped most during pregnancy was the Bradley childbirth exercises which prepared my muscles even more. I was already fit from having walked two-and-a-half miles daily for seven years. I swam. I wore support hose for varicose veins. Bradley provided techniques that deal with emotions, too, in the book, *Natural Childbirth the Bradley Way,* by Susan McCutcheon. I visualized the picture of the sock coming over the baby's head like a turtleneck in my mind. I wrote in a journal, prayed, lit lavender candles, and listened to soothing music.

One pregnancy ritual I did for another friend was to anoint her for birth.

The first sign of labor came when my water broke at home. My back hurt. With the rhythms, my belly button got hard. I used acupuncture to stimulate contractions at pressure points on my little toe and above my ankle.

I felt freer to use several techniques for pain. I vocalized. Touch helped tremendously. Five different women—two friends, two apprentices and the midwife—gave me counter pressure by pushing on my lower back. The tub provided relief. The water gave me thirty minutes of no pain. I took showers, too. Heat helped, as did getting in various positions. When the pain in my lower back spread to my upper thighs, I saw the sensations as a sign of progressing.

Prior to labor, the midwife and I talked about the possibility of going to the hospital. I said, "One of us has to be dying, either the baby or me." During labor, the midwife was generous with her time. I pushed longer than what she usually allowed. The baby crowned for forty-five minutes.

Galen was born at thirty-eight weeks, weighing 9 pounds, 4 ounces, with long black hair. To avoid an IV, I drank one pint of fluid for every pint of blood lost afterwards.

Because of my inspiring birth at home, I trained to teach childbirth classes to other women. I love teaching and making a difference.

What I tell new moms-to-be is, "Nature's designs are rarely wrong. Women were born to have and nurse babies. Somehow, we have come to doubt our ability. Natural birth provides you with confidence and a strong connection to your children that can guide and sustain you for mothering. This confidence comes in part from staying *active* in the process versus a passive observer. You know you are strong after actively birthing your baby. If you did that, you feel like you can do anything."

For the birth of our son, I was in charge. It was a dream come true having our baby at home. After Galen was born with family and friends around us, we had a Blessing Service. It was inspiring.

Tracy's second child, a pretty daughter named Ava, was also born at home.

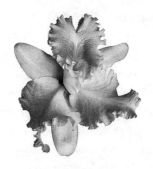

SECRET 9:

Make a Mind-Body-Spirit Commitment

Despite Physical Challenges, Obstetrician Chose a Birth Center

Melissa Crochet, M.D.'s Story

At ten weeks into my second pregnancy, my ovary twisted on itself. I knew something was wrong. I writhed in pain. At first I thought it was appendicitis. It became a nightmare because we had our toddler, Ethan, with us and we needed my husband's mom to help care for him immediately. So my husband, Jay, called her from the Ob/Gyn's office who was going to perform my surgery. Jay's mom was teaching and she had to leave her class immediately. She needs directions when driving in Dallas and Jay stood in the doctor's office looking out from the third floor window directing her on his cell phone turn-by-turn to the building.

With clenched teeth, I said, "Just get her heeere ...." Finally she arrived.

We all went down to the parking lot. The nurse carried our stuff and I walked bent over in pain. It would ease off and then *yaaaaa*. I got in the car and just wished we would go. Jay stopped and turned. His mom wanted directions on how to get from there to our house. I heard him say, "Well, you need to take...well, no...don't go that way. It would be quicker this way." I was in the back seat. I just took my hand, beat on the glass almost breaking it, and yelled at the top of my lungs, "GET IN THE CAR!" I was in so much pain. It was horrible. I couldn't tolerate the scene: just have her follow us to the hospital first and *then* give her directions to our house.

Arriving at the hospital I felt a little better. Still, I was worried.

A laparoscopy showed that I had a huge corpus luteum cyst—not uncommon in pregnancy. It produces hormones that support the pregnancy until the placenta kicks in and keeps your endometrium lush. If you get pregnant, your cyst continues to function and remains intact. The problem was that mine was twisted on my fallopian tube.

Under general anesthesia, my doctor made an incision in my belly button. "I didn't believe there was such a thing as an ovarian torsion," she said. "But it was the coolest thing I've ever seen." She took pictures of it. After she made the incision, she lifted my ovary and it started unwinding. She wanted to make sure they didn't have to remove the cyst.

Six months along into my pregnancy, I felt fine. My back wasn't even bothering me. One day, Jay and I took a walk outside when it started raining. As I ran home, I tripped and fell right in the middle of the street.

I used a wheelchair for a little while because I couldn't walk. It was hard because I couldn't even lift Ethan. I couldn't do anything. I was totally ready for this pregnancy to be *over*. I think I had that mentality even before all these unexpected things happened—the novelty of being pregnant had worn off. I wasn't having the whole I-love-being-pregnant experience like I had the first time with Ethan.

Being an obstetrician definitely influenced my reasons for having natural birth the *first* time. I finished my residency at Parkland (a county hospital) because it offers one of the top-rated obstetrical and gynecological residencies in the country. Its clientele include many pregnant young girls ages twelve to twenty-two, and plenty of drug addicts. The hospital offered a midwifery program. The midwives took patients without birth complications to their wing.

Later as an obstetrician and gynecologist, I worked at a clinic in Stanford, then moved to Boulder, Colorado, to practice with a partner. When my partner moved away, I practiced solo for three years in a city filled with ardent soldiers of women's rights. I went from one extreme to the other and as a result, I found my own philosophy in the middle.

I was pregnant when I moved back to Dallas. I knew it would be a culture shock—in general and in my approach to medicine. In most hospitals, pregnancy or birth is not a disease. However, in a hospital, pregnant women are treated like they're sick. I didn't want to be treated that way. I looked through the Dallas newspaper for an alternative to a hospital, a birth center, to have our first baby.

My joints are fused in the hips and upper back. I had back surgery for a pinched nerve once, which was a mild injury, but with excruciating pain. That was why I didn't want to have an epidural.

I wasn't so worried about myself; I was concerned about the baby. In choosing childbirth classes, I didn't want Bradley because I felt it was too hard on doctors. I decided on *Birthing from Within* classes, taught by a midwife. My husband practiced with me performing pain-control techniques, such as keep your hands in ice water for as long as possible. I liked the art exercises and painted several watercolors.

BIRTH OF ETHAN, 10 pounds

I had taken Friday off. At 6:30 a.m., I had mild contractions. My father went back home and my mom stayed. I felt peaceful and excited.

The backup doctor, Margaret Christensen, M.D., planned to deliver our son at the Birth & Women's Center. We talked about the possibility of working together, professionally.

At my appointment Saturday, I was dilated to 3 centimeters. "Don't you want to burst my bag so I won't keep you up all night? I know how it is," I asked.

"Melissa, aren't we doing a *natural* birth? Go out and do stuff," she said. So we went to Dream Cafe for lunch and shopping. We returned at 5 p.m. before her office closed and then went home.

At 9:30 that night, I said to Jay, "I can't labor at the house any longer." I ate something, tried to meditate and threw up, so we went to the birth center.

At 10:30, I worried that the birth would keep Margaret up all night. "Don't worry about it," she reassured. We walked in the park. I went to another place, trying to get my feet moving in front of one another.

Jay lit candles, brought lavender spritzer, and put on music.

In the tub I could relax. Labor was slow. Everyone was calm, constantly reassuring me, "You can do this."

Then my water broke. The baby wasn't coming down. I could tell that there wasn't any pressure at all. Contractions came. But I stayed calm.

I tried sitting on the birthing ball as Jay pushed on my back. With the last contraction, I was getting angry at the pain. I thought, *you're not going to get me. I'm going to be fine. My baby's fine.*

The baby was posterior, though. The baby rotates as it comes down the birth canal but when the baby's spine is against a mother's spine, known as a posterior position, it can create lots of back pain. It felt like my pelvis was going to rip apart. Bad menstrual cramps doesn't explain it. It felt like searing hot pain and hurts more than I can describe. I felt a little bit deceived; no one told me. There came a point when I totally thought I couldn't handle labor anymore.

I pushed sitting on the toilet, facing the back. I felt free to push, bear down and grunt. I pushed only a half hour with small tears. Margaret got Ethan's head. "It's a big ol' baby," she said.

My brother videotaped us. He's kind of squeamish so I never thought he'd make it through the delivery. But he did fine. And so did I.

I felt I'm now a member of the club. If I can do that labor and delivery of a 10-pound baby who's healthy and vigorous, I can do anything.

My doula gave me a *soothing* full body massage afterwards.

Because Ethan was 10 pounds, I became nervous about delivering a bigger baby the next time. There's a tendency for each baby to get bigger than the previous one. Complications can also arise like shoulder dystocia. So, when I got pregnant again, I was careful about my weight. I walked a lot. I wanted him to come a little early, hoping he'd be smaller. Even if he was the same size as Ethan, he would be about nine pounds. That would be easy.

With the ovary torsion surgery at ten weeks and the fall at six months, I was also ready to be done at the end of nine months. I carefully scheduled my time off from work. My medical partners had already taken up the slack when Ethan was born. I truly was not anticipating being pregnant again so soon. They were doing it again seventeen months later. I felt time conscious of keeping everyone happy.

BIRTH OF JOSHUA, 8 1/2 pounds

My husband and I tried stimulating labor with sex and evening primrose. A day of natural induction might include sex, a lot of walking and a cervical exam. Then we'd try something more medicinal the next day. After a day of trying to induce labor, I was exhausted. I decided to use a cervical ripening tampon called Cervidil.

I didn't get much sleep though. Every half hour I checked the baby's heart rate to make sure all was okay. About 4:30 a.m., heavy contractions began. I didn't want to wake my husband because I knew what we had in store. So I was lying in bed listening to our baby's heartbeat and coping with contractions until 6:30 a.m. At that point, I couldn't take it anymore.

I got up and took a bath. I knew I was moving along because I didn't even feel like drying my hair or putting on make-up.

At 9 a.m., my husband and I went to an appointment with my midwife, Cherie. I was dilated to 5 centimeters by the time we arrived. I was excited because it took me all day to get to 5 centimeters in my first pregnancy.

The most painful part of my labor involved labial varicosities. (The labial lips become swollen from engorged blood vessels and can subside after delivery.) Every time I had a contraction, the blood would squeeze. I felt like it was just ripping my labia open outside. I thought I was gonna die. I wanted to push something up against it, like ice. When I got to the birth center, I had an ice pack crammed against my underwear. I was trying to stay active. I wanted to sit on a ball for counter pressure.

The midwife told me to walk a little. I walked for an hour. But, I was ready for the baby to be born. "Break my water in about an hour," I told Cherie. "I want this over."

At 9:30, we alerted everybody that the baby would soon be born. My brother videotaped the birth. One of our friends, Marty, took photos. Marty's hysterical. He and my brother had been in Europe with us—the same group that was going to be present for Josh's birth.

The midwife broke my bag and I was shocked by the amount of amniotic fluid. In my lap was a pool. "Can you get me some towels?" With that much fluid, I though, *maybe the baby would be smaller than anticipated*. I was relieved.

I went walking again for another hour. All of a sudden, I couldn't go farther. I hit a wall I never hit with Ethan's labor because his was long and slow. I hadn't eaten since dinner the night before. I hadn't been drinking fluids. Suddenly, I switched from vulvar pain to nausea. I was so nauseated, I couldn't think. I couldn't breathe.

I stopped dilating at 7 centimeters. Joshua wasn't coming down the birth canal, leaving me fatigued and nauseous. I couldn't get beyond it. I kept saying to them, "I can't. I know that I'm going to pass out. I think my blood pressure must be extremely low." My pressure was fine. My pulse was just kind of weak. The midwives gave me a liter of glucose through an IV. After I got it, the lights came back on. Okay, I was ready to work again. By that time it was 1:00 p.m.

The midwife decided to see if I could push past my cervix and get him to move down. My cervix was *extremely* sensitive and inflamed after the Cervadil. I needed to sit on the ball. I bounced softly back and forth on the edge of the sofa leaning on the ball. Afterwards, I tried to push my baby down my cervix. I walked a little around the room.

The birth assistant arrived. "Let me get in the tub to regroup because I feel like I'm just going to lose some focus here," I said. I was paying attention to the fact that I was 5 centimeters at 9:00 a.m. I was thinking I was zooming right along, then nothing. That was disappointing. And that, on top of the nausea, was not helping. In the tub I told myself, *I'm so close to being done with this.* It had been 24 hours. My body was tired, and the pain was sharper. I just wanted to go to another place.

After 15 minutes, I said, "I have to get out of the tub."

"I really think you need to walk," the midwife said.

"I really think not. I just want to get this baby out."

"Well, push," she said. I squatted on the bathroom floor, and they both held me up. I gave a *not*-so-subtle scream and pushed. "Well, he's right there," I said.

"Yeah, he is," she said.

I had to hold him inside me and get to the bed. He came with just one push.

Everybody was sitting in the living room talking. "Camera, video, get over here," Cherie said. They all flew in. With Ethan, I had enough time to get myself covered up. Now I was just butt naked. You know, with those big pregnant boobs, the huge pregnant nipples. And in walked Marty. I can't believe he had the nerve. I thought he would have been *so appalled* by what he was seeing, he'd say "Do you mind if I *don't* come in?" He was just doing the camera. My brother, it didn't bother me. But I could hear Marty's voice coordinating with Jay, "Okay you get over here..."

Here I was, sitting with Josh's head about to come out. Cherie kept saying, "Well, deliver him into your hand. Deliver him." All I could feel was my bottom stretching. I thought, *you know what? If I have to get stitches after all of this, I'm going to be really annoyed.*

"I don't want to," I said in a demonic voice. Jay was beside me.

I didn't want to deliver him myself. I do that every day. I wanted somebody else to. "Take him out of there! Get this baby *@## out of there." Cheri finally got her gloves on. He came flying out.

Jay actually did the whole delivery this time. Yeah, he had delivered Ethan after his shoulders were out. But this time Jay pulled the head down and did the whole delivery.

At 2:23 p.m., Joshua was born. I felt great, relieved and peaceful.

"I'm sorry, Marty, that I didn't have any clothes on. "

"That's okay," he said.

Josh weighed 8 1/2 pounds—a marked improvement. I thought he looked exactly like Ethan. But within ten minutes he looked different.

I told Cherie the placenta had delivered. She massaged my uterus and everything was fine. A few minutes later, blood was just gushing out. "Why don't I give you some Pitocin?" she asked. It nipped the bleeding in the bud. With Joshua, I already knew that my blood count could get extremely low. My hematocrit was 20 percent after Ethan's delivery. (Hematocrit means the ratio of red blood cells to the volume of whole blood measured by an instrument, also called a hematocrit.) Once the bleeding slowed down, I took a shower.

If I could have waited and *allowed natural labor*, I'd have had a better birth experience with Joshua. Emotionally and physically at the end of that pregnancy, I had been through enough.

Ethan arrived with my mom and dad, who picked him up from Mother's Day Out. He entered the room a little intimidated at first, a little scared. He came over to the bed as I was breastfeeding Josh, smiling. He wore a shirt that said "I'm a Big Brother." I picked up Ethan and held him by Josh. His face lit up, "Beebee. It's a beebee." He wanted to kiss him. It was really very sweet—the highlight of the experience, sharing Josh with Ethan for the first time.

We didn't stay long. I tried to eat little snacks afterward and enjoy the environment. We left at dusk.

I knew I needed to take the full six weeks off work. I couldn't just take time off while I was waiting to go into labor. I had to maximize the time that I had. I think that contributed to scheduling my birth and using Cervadil to get labor going.

I had my practice going and was not as settled in. I tried to find my place in the practice with people whose belief system was a little bit different than mine. I would have felt more accepted and supported if I had been with partners who encouraged natural birth. But I don't need that. It would have been nice, but *I know what my reasons are. I don't need it from the outside.*

I had this little psychological need to make up for the fact that I'd *evicted* Josh. For the first two weeks of his life, I don't think I put him down. I held him. I had this need, and he loved it. He would sleep right at my heart. I'd wear him and he was on me all the time. That was the least I could do because he's still supposed to be *in* me.

I weaned him when I went back to work. I didn't have the level of commitment to continue breastfeeding. It was hard to go back to work. I was only off for four weeks and felt exhausted. With everything considered, it was the right thing to do. I try to respect my partners' time.

Now I can compare our sons. Ethan was a hard baby yet an easy pregnancy. To this day, you still have to work to get him to laugh. Josh was a hard pregnancy, then an easy baby, just such a sweetheart. He's such a ball of sunshine…a fat smiley blue-eyed baby. You look at him and he laughs. It's interesting to see their differences.

What I Tell My Patients

I used to let them delude themselves. If they said, "Why don't we see how it goes? If I'm doing okay, I'm not going to get any drugs."

Now, I look them straight in the eye and say, "You're getting an epidural. If you want natural birth, you need to take some classes. You have to commit and feel deeply about it. I strongly suggest a doula because it's possible that you'll get little support from the nursing staff."

My husband was not sure about the birth center, an unmedicated birth, and classes. I encourage women to get birth support while they are in early labor—friends, family, doulas—to help keep them at home as long as they can. I remind them, they are healthy. "Take a lot of pictures of your pregnant belly," I say. I share guidelines to keep them feeling good about being pregnant.

Healthy women in uncomplicated pregnancies who want to natural childbirth should consider birth centers or private hospitals that support natural birth. With a private hospital, there are fewer exams, less invasion of your vaginal area. I would like to see more time for a normal birth. Not every birth is complicated. But you still have the dang monitors in the rooms; you hear the beeping. A hospital is a very sterile place.

For women facing family pressure *not* to go a natural birth route, they need to become a bit militant, get a little radical.

There's a push for "elective cesareans." It disconnects the role of a woman as a mother and undermines the family. [1]

Some believe they can control birth. Natural birth is accepting that you are *not* in control. Inside and outside of the birth you are going to be out of control. If you go with it, you go to another place.

Natural birth allows better psychological adjustment with newborns.

With a natural process, however, there's no need to call me every five minutes to tell me about a sharp pain in your left side, that your feet are swelling or that you want to be allowed to stop working on a certain date.

My philosophy of health care in general is that you need to *take responsibility* for your life and your body. Accepting natural birth is the ultimate in taking responsibility for your own pain and your birth experience. Women do this every day and it's not an illness.

One of the biggest benefits of natural birth is that it prepares you to become a mom. And motherhood is tremendous.

Note: Interesting to read how the physician "induced" herself for her second birth out of concern for the convenience of her fellow colleagues. Sometimes too much knowledge is detrimental and interferes with the birth process.

Hypnobirthing
Chantel's Story

My mom was knocked out before her first birth. She felt robbed. However, she was thrilled with the natural birth of my brother. "It's the greatest thing," she said.

My husband, Ed, and I took Hypnobirth classes, which I heard about from my sister-in-law. The name is misleading because many people think it's hypnosis. Instead, it's a combination of breathing, meditation and relaxation exercises. I also took prenatal yoga classes. We chose a hospital in Atlanta where midwives practice.

My friends thought I was crazy. "Gee, you don't have much faith," I said. My plan was to hold our son as soon as he came out of my body.

On a Saturday in May, my husband and I went to a movie. It was long. I had to go to the bathroom badly. After I finished using the restroom, I still had bladder cramps, which I thought was from holding my urine too long.

We headed home at 6:30 p.m. I started having gas pain. I didn't think I was in labor, although I was already one day past my due date. While Ed made dinner, I lay down hoping the gas pains would go away. Instead, they began to come and go. About 8 p.m., Ed timed the contractions which were one-and-a-half minutes long and two minutes apart, yet very tolerable.

We called our midwife, Laura. "Sometimes they start out real close and then space out before they get stronger and closer again. Call me back in one hour," she said. The contractions got stronger. I began using relaxation and breathing techniques I learned in hypnobirthing and yoga.

Ed called Laura back. "They're speeding up, not slowing down."

The move from the house to the car to the hospital broke my concentration. We arrived after 9:30 p.m. By the time we got a room, I was really having to focus on my breathing. When Laura checked me, I was five centimeters, 100 percent effaced and the baby's head was at station +1.

The contractions became so close, I couldn't tell one from the next. I found it difficult to focus, relax and regroup. That continued for two hours. "If they stay this way, I'm going to need something to help with the pain," I told Ed. I wasn't able to rest in between and that was making it impossible to use the techniques we had practiced. He reminded me to breathe and let Laura know how I was feeling. When she came over, I asked her to check me. I was at nine. I decided that I *could* go the rest of the way on my own.

"You can start bearing down with each contraction if you feel like it," she said.

I did and that felt much better. The next three hours, I breathed the baby down the birth canal.

At 4:30 a.m., I felt like pushing. My water broke and the *real* work began. I got so hot. My husband fanned me and put cold wash cloths on my head, which felt good. I spent the next hour trying to push our baby's head out. Every time I felt his head getting close to coming, the contraction ended and I felt him slip back in. I felt frustrated.

Finally, his head crowned and I began to feel a burning sensation. I may have been tearing a bit which was the most uncomfortable part of the whole experience. We massaged the perineum every few days, but I wish we'd done it daily. It took three more really good pushes and out popped his head. One more good one and out came the shoulders. The last easy push delivered the rest of his body.

Our newborn son, Hayden, was placed on my chest. Nothing could be better than to have Hayden next to my heart and Ed by my side.

The benefit of natural birth was to actually *feel* my son move down through my body. Not being numb was a huge blessing. I felt total bliss after Hayden's birth.

Don't Mess with Mother Nature
Becky's Story

A good friend birthed naturally with her midwife, Susan, and appreciated the experience. I wanted that too—the feelings she described.

If I hadn't heard her birth story, I don't know if I would have gone that route. I was never aware of that option—a midwife in the hospital.

Natural birth intrigued me. I read books and decided I wanted to try. The stories, especially of non-medicated births, told of the babies coming out and inching their way up to their mother's breasts to start nursing. They're so aware, eyes are open and clear.

It also helped to know that women have been giving birth naturally for thousands of years. I had such a great pregnancy. I knew I could do it.

Susan's the only midwife in Dallas with hospital privileges. That was comforting for my husband, Mike. He helped me make the decision. But he wasn't crazy about the birth center, because it was out-of-hospital.

The birthing class was honest about pain. We talked about it a lot, about relaxing through it as much as you could. I was nervous about the pain, but I never focused on it.

For my first birth, the unknown of it all was nerve-wracking. I talked to the few people who have gone through natural birth, and they were reassuring. Even with my friend's first long and nightmarish birth, she still talked positively about it. She said the end result is a wonderful thing.

I had other concerns. Am I going to have a healthy baby? I am only thirty-one, but all the news coming out these days says that the older you are, there may be more problems for your child. The bigger fear for me was *after* birth, bringing the baby home. What was I going to *do* with this child? I need lots of sleep and that was the hardest—the sleep deprivation. That's what I'm going through now. That scared me more than the actual birth.

BIRTH OF CHRISTOPHER, 9 pounds, 2 ounces

Labor lasted seventeen hours. We labored at home from noon until about 8 p.m. Our doula came to our house about 4 p.m. She was wonderful. We walked and eased labor.

We got to the hospital after 8 p.m. We checked in and walked that hospital for about five hours. I worked on their birthing ball. I threw up at one point. I ended up in the bathtub and shower for about an hour.

Quickly, I was ready to push. I pushed for about twenty minutes before our baby was born at 2:30 a.m.

Christopher was a big boy—over nine pounds with a big head. I tore quite a bit. That was the worse part, the stitching. The midwife gave me a local anesthetic for the stitches. I remember the pain. But the end result is a beautiful baby. The baby is healthy.

I had concerns that the nurses weren't going to do what I wanted with my baby. I didn't want eye drops, shots or a pacifier for him. They were accommodating. We never battled, but my husband and I had to make our desires known. That was frustrating. When they took Christopher, my husband went with him. I said, "No more than ten minutes." We shared a lot of early bonding. I'm sure the nurses go back and laugh, "These ladies."

BIRTH OF AVERY (21 Months Later) 8 pounds, 10 ounces

My first was less than a year old when I got pregnant with Avery. I was in *denial* for about four months. I was already in my second trimester. I had one period, but I didn't have a period the next month. I thought, *maybe it's just late.* Around Christmas, I was moody, nothing tasted right, all those signs. I had a meltdown.

I went to my mom's house to help her with holiday baking. I started crying, "Mom, I think I'm pregnant, and I really don't want to be pregnant right now." On my way home I bought a pregnancy test. It confirmed I was pregnant. I had so many friends who had been trying for months and months, *years* even, to get pregnant. I felt so guilty at the time for feeling upset. But today I can't imagine life without Avery. She's a blessing.

We used Susan, my first midwife, again. My level of comfort with her and the whole process was so high that I never anticipated any problems.

We did a sonogram at twenty-two weeks to pinpoint the due date.

When the technician measured, she said, "Now when did you say the first day of your last period was?" I knew exactly when. I had been charting.

"Well, honey, I'm measuring this child *four weeks bigger* than what you said," she said.

Apparently I had that period, but had gotten pregnant the month *before.* Susan says that sometimes happens. My due date of August 9 was moved to July 11. I was in a major panic. We were trying to get Christopher ready for the new baby, deciding on beds and rooms.

Other than the date moving up, the pregnancy went smooth. As we got down to the wire, we did another sonogram because the midwife couldn't tell if the baby had turned or not. She was concerned that the baby might be breech. It turned out that the baby was so high up in my diaphragm that Susan wasn't feeling it right. The baby was turned okay, though.

Susan had joined a bigger practice, and I met only one of the male doctors for one appointment. Had I been with Margaret, the physician I liked, I think I would have felt much more comfortable. She hired another midwife, Elizabeth, whom I also liked. But I wasn't comfortable with any of the male doctors in this new practice. One doctor had great bedside manner, but I just didn't get the feeling that he would give me the chance I needed. *Would they support me?* I was leery.

Susan was going out of town the next Monday for a week. I was due on the eleventh and had an appointment for her to check me. I was three centimeters already. *Okay, this could happen any day now,* I thought.

Friday came and she called, saying, "Becky, what do you think?" I told her I was nervous with the other doctors and wanted her there. She scheduled me for prostaglandin to induce labor that morning at 9 a.m. I got home around noon and started having regular contractions. Everything was going as it should.

We had the same doula. She was *against* me doing the prostaglandin. I should have listened to her, but I went ahead and did it. She came over about 5 p.m., when the contractions were long and close together. We walked the neighborhood. By 11 p.m. the contractions were lasting over a minute, a minute apart. We got to the hospital and I was only six centimeters dilated, so we walked and walked. The contractions started slowing down, lessening in intensity. Finally at 4 a.m., I was dead tired. Christopher had been sick the night before so we had been up with him. Now I faced a night of laboring.

"Susan, if I go into labor now, I don't have the energy to push this child out," I said.

"Ok, let's just rest," she said. So I lay down and the contractions stopped. I slept, but they wouldn't release me from the hospital because I was six centimeters dilated. "Well, we can break your water and that can get things along," she suggested.

Mike and I are analytical. He's an accountant and I'm in finance. We debated back and forth about what we were going to do. I didn't want any more drugs, didn't want my water broken, or any interventions.

At 7 a.m., the next morning, I started having these *puny* contractions. The doctor who was on call in Susan's practice came in and checked me. "There's no way we're releasing you," she said. "You can leave against doctor's orders if you want," our doula said. At that point, she was getting kind of militant about her natural childbirth beliefs. That was turning me off because I wanted my *options*. I think she realized that when I said, "I don't feel like going against Susan's wishes." I trusted Susan and felt she had my best interest at heart. Had it been a doctor, I might have said, "Ok, we're going home." We were all tired. Susan had been there since I arrived at the hospital.

Our options: Break the water, start Pitocin, get an epidural, or do another prostaglandin.

About 10 a.m., we *caved*. A doctor administered the epidural and the Pitocin. Avery was born at 5:30 that afternoon.

Susan came by the next day. We had a little counseling session because I was disappointed in myself. She thought the baby was *early*. The prostaglandin didn't take because my cervix wasn't ready. Even when the doctor came in, she said, "I can't believe that you're this dilated and your contractions were so close together and lasting like they were."

The end result was wonderful and beautiful. My advice to everyone is, *"Don't f- - - with Mother Nature,"* pardon my language. Had we waited for Mother Nature to do her thing, it would have been a much different story. The baby and my body could have triggered labor. I *know* I could have done it. It's hard. I didn't want to do it because it's convenient for everybody. But I wanted Susan there.

The epidural was a beautiful thing once it kicked in. I was able to rest and get some energy. Once I was ready to push, I was able to feel that sensation to push. The worst part for me was the IV. I hated that.

I didn't notice a big difference between Avery and Christopher when they were first born, but my husband did. "When Christopher came out, he was much more alert." When Mike started talking, the baby just turned and looked up at him. With Avery, he didn't think she was as alert as Christopher.

I birthed both ways but the second time was harder on me internally. Emotionally, I felt like a *failure*. That sounds very dramatic, and I don't mean for it to, because I got over it once our baby, Avery, was born. She was perfect and everyone was healthy. I was able to *let it go*.

See Chapter 2: Calculating Due Dates

Native American Births

Lois, an RN at the Public Health Indian Hospital in Santa Fe, New Mexico, shares her fifteen years of experience working with Native Americans. At her hospital, they deliver about 240 babies a year. No epidural service exists. The nurses and midwives know how to give more individual attention than other private hospitals that offer pain management.

Lois describes a sitting position the midwives have used successfully for laboring women. "The midwife sits on a stool with the laboring woman sitting on her lap facing out, wrapping her legs around the midwife's. The midwife has suggested another woman to sit on the lap of her partner. The midwife catches the baby from underneath."

"At another hospital, I witnessed a Navajo family that called in a Medicine Man for a difficult labor. The baby's heartbeat was weakening and the baby needed help during birth. The Medicine Man came in, played a flute, smoked a pipe, and announced, 'The cord is wrapped three times. The baby cannot be born vaginally.' The woman was wheeled down the hall to the operating room. 'I couldn't believe it,' the surgeon said. The cord was indeed wrapped three times around the baby's neck."

The more isolated that the Navajo live, the more traditional they are. The women use rituals for pregnancy and birth. For example, during pregnancy, they do no weaving to avoid coming across any knots in the string, which symbolize knots in the umbilical cord. And during labor, they hang sash belts used to help push. No knots are in them.

The hospital in Chinley, Arizona, honors the native culture with a hexagonal room. A Hogan house has six sides with the door facing east. Traditional healing is facing east in a building—to greet the rising sun. They also face east for delivery.

Navajo women have a high pain tolerance. They're stoic giving birth. Afterward, they take the placenta home. They bury their baby's cord portion of the stump at their home, which is in the Four Sacred Mountains: between Mt. Taylor, Mt. Blanco, Navajo Mountain and San Francisco Peak. They wish for the future generations to live in their homeland and not be dispersed. Harmony of life-with-nature is important to the them, and walking in beauty is one of their values.

"For whatever reason, Navajo women are at high risk in Obstetrics. Whether it's nutrition or genetics, I've seen weaker tissue, more hemorrhaging and lacerations," says Lois.

"One elderly woman I saw in Alaska used to be a midwife. She knew when someone carried twins. I asked her, 'Can you feel them?' 'I can hear the two heartbeats by listening with my ear to the woman's belly,' she said.

"Eskimo women in Alaska give birth quickly. Perhaps it is because they are more broad-hipped and shorter or it may be because they eat mostly fish and whale blubber," says Lois.

Using Mantras for Lotus Birth

Elizabeth's Second Birth Story

In the middle of the night I awoke and waddled my pregnant self outside into the darkness. I shouldn't have, but I wanted to be alone. I loved being outside on the quiet street in our neighborhood. I felt safe. *Something may be going on.* I'd been leaking. I noticed there had been some leaking right before I went to bed.

My first labor didn't happen naturally. I wanted to do prelabor for this second birth by myself. *Okay, does my body remember how to do this?* I was doubting. I was worried about getting Pitocin again to make my contractions start. I wondered, if I go more than one week over my due date, whether Dinah, our midwife, would still be able to assist my baby's birth. Or, would I have to go to the hospital again? I faced my fears alone in the stillness.

I kept saying to myself, *so what, who cares?* That was a meditation that a friend of mine came up with. I adopted it as my own. *So what who cares.* That mantra helped me overcome my worries.

I continued walking for several more blocks, *"So what if I have to go to the hospital and I can't have Dinah as my midwife? So what who cares? So what if my water is leaking, but I have no contractions? So what, who cares?* I was trying to get control of my mind. At some point in every woman's pregnancy, she can slip into a negative place. Or she can prepare and get ready for what she's about to experience. I had to get centered, to get ready. My mantra helped me do that.

I walked back home and slept soundly.

I went into my second birth with a new attitude that *anything* that happens is okay. My *preference* would be a natural birth that goes quickly and efficiently, resulting in a safe delivery and a healthy baby. But I told myself, *whatever* unfolds is okay. That's what I didn't have with the first birth, that open-mindedness. My attitude wasn't about "I've gotta have a natural birth." It was, "I'm going to do whatever."

It's like how you create:

You plant a garden. You pick the best spot. You cultivate the soil.

You make sure it's a good spot, well-drained and that it gets sun.

You plant what you want, and you nurture it.

You send love, you let the sun shine on it. You make sure it gets water.

You create an environment so that it can thrive.

Whatever comes after that is okay. You did what you could.

Enjoy the fruits of your labor.

How could that be wrong?

If you approach birth from that perspective, then whatever unfolds is *fine.*

Dan and I got pregnant on purpose this time, which was exciting. Nathaniel, our first son, was a surprise and has been my teacher in many ways ever since he was born. I always say that he's my little guru. I believe our children are our greatest teachers.

With this second pregnancy, I taught prenatal yoga all through it.

I purposely did not take any childbirth classes. I didn't even want to give Bradley any energy. I thought about doing a *Birthing from Within* refresher class, but the woman who taught the class had her baby early, and the class was cancelled.

What I did was undergo hypnosis a couple of times. I cried the first time because I had such a release. You visualize the type of birth you want. Being able to do that cleansed me. Maybe the act of visualizing what I wanted and letting myself see that and savor it helped. I thought, *there's no more room for any negative thoughts with birth.*

I went to Los Angeles for a week during my first trimester to study with Gurmukh, a woman who teaches prenatal and postnatal yoga. She produces yoga videos, too. She gave a Women's Teacher Training. She employs a number of outstanding women to work with her, including the women attending her workshop. We took many of the prenatal classes she teaches. There are so many people into prenatal classes in L.A. These women show their bellies comfortably. They think it's beautiful. Soon, I started to think my belly was beautiful, too.

I started thinking, *why don't we show our beauty while we're pregnant? Why do we hide it?* I was exploring. I started showing my belly. I wouldn't go to church doing that. But I celebrated my pregnancy.

I chose a different midwife, one who attended my yoga classes. We had a business relationship. I wasn't sure how it would work out but I decided to give it a try. Quickly, we clicked. It's important to have someone you relate with, someone who influences you in a positive way. But, I realized it wasn't just about the midwife. It was about how I approached my child's upcoming birth.

Dinah, who's British, helped me overcome some anxieties I had about Nathaniel's birth. "Oh, it will never happen the same way the second time," she said. "The really great thing is that you know a baby can go through there."

Okay, I believed her. But I thought, *Will it be 30 hours again?* It won't? Okay, alright. I felt different, so I knew I was going to create something different. I believe we create what we live, to an extent.

I did one ultrasound. Dinah kept telling me my baby's head was down but I needed to go get it confirmed.

A few days before Liam was born, I started leaking fluid. Unless there is a lot of water, Dinah is very flexible about leaking fluid. "Okay, it's alright, a little bit of water. Some activity, that's good. That's a change, we'll just watch," she said.

"Are you going to check me?" I asked with curiosity. She checked vital signs. She listened to the baby's heartbeat.

Lotus Birth

"Lotus Birth" is new to a lot of people. I heard about it from Jeanine Parvati Baker, an author in New Mexico. A friend told me about some of her books I found at a home schooling conference. On her website she offers a Lotus Birth packet. What it means is you don't cut the cord. You let it fall off on its own. That idea felt true for me; I thought it made so much sense. I ordered her Lotus Birth packet long before we conceived.

I thought, *I don't know if I can do Lotus Birth, but I want to know about it.* The newborn, cord and placenta stay intact. You carry the baby and placenta together until the cord dries up and falls off, usually within a week. The placenta air-dries covered with salt and some mothers cover it in a cloth bag or diaper. I worried what other people would think.

This was the first Lotus Birth that Dinah had done. I asked if she had ever heard about it? She said, "No, but if you want to do that, it's fine with me." She wasn't against it. She had just never heard of it.

Dinah prepared me about the due date. "Usually if you're late the first time, it'll happen that way the next time. That's what I've noticed," she said. It felt so different because the baby was not breech. I was grateful that she didn't start micro-managing me. I told her I didn't want anybody massaging my cervix or doing any interventions.

Toward the end, though, I asked, "Are you going to check me?"

"I don't check until you're at your due date. I can check you today and you might be one centimeter dilated. Several weeks later, you could still be one centimeter dilated, or you could have your baby tonight. It does not tell me anything. The truth is, you're going to have your baby when it's ready. That's just the way it works."

I *loved* that. She focused on the moment.

I woke up that morning after my walk in the dark and noticed more water leaking out. I waited until 6 a.m. to call Dinah to let her know.

"How much?" she asked. I told her.

"I'm not alarmed," Dinah said. "But if you don't have some contractions going by so-and-so time, you should come in and let me check the baby's heart rate and see how things are going."

"If nothing is happening, we can start being more aggressive in terms of nipple stimulation and some walking," I said.

Today was going to be the day.

I relaxed. Dinah wasn't rigid. I went to the bathroom not long after I talked to Dinah and had some bloody show. After that I had a mild contraction and they kept coming.

I called my friend who asked me to when I went into labor. "Just calling to let you know...it'll happen by tonight."

"That's close together, Elizabeth. A couple of minutes apart. You just had a contraction."

"Yeah. You know what? I'm going to throw up. I've got to go." That's what happens when you really get going. *Why am I throwing up already?* That was another thing I was worried about, being out of control the second time around. *Oh, God, here we go again.*

Dan took Nathaniel to school for picture day. We wanted Nathaniel at the birth so he could come later.

I couldn't find a comfortable position. Before they left, I said, "I want to get in the bathtub." Dan drew me a bath. I got in. I poured water on my belly during contractions. Dan left. I was by myself.

I didn't realize how close I was to delivery. I had no idea. Unlike my first labor, I was making a lot of noise, "Uuuuuuughhhhhha." I was getting louder and louder. "Aaaah, ah, aaaaaaahh." Dan called Dinah again. He frantically packed the car while explaining the contractions were getting closer. "Put her on the phone," she said.

"I can't get her on the phone."

"Get her out of the tub, in the car and don't go anywhere else but here. Right now!"

"Really?" We were thinking hours. I was pouring water on my belly, making sounds and thinking, *how am I going to do this for 30 hours?*

Something else I did besides making noises, was saying little mantras. I didn't plan it or even think about them in advance. They came to me while I was birthing. My mind said, *I cannot do this.* But the mantra that came out was, "I *can* do it. I can do it." During the contractions my mind said, *no.* So the mantra that came out was, "Yes." So I kept saying, "I can do it. I can do it. Yes, yes, yes-yes-yes." I kept saying those things over and over again. My mind didn't believe that at all, but for some reason that birthing side of my brain *knew* that I needed to say, "Yes. I can do it." The mantras eased contractions. "I can do it. I can do it. Yes, yes."

Dan said in the car on the way to the birth center that's all I said, "Yes, yes, yes. I can do it I can do it."

We arrived at the birth center and Dinah wanted to check me.

"No," I said. I couldn't lay down. There was no way.

"This is the one time I *really* need to check you, to see where you are," she insisted. I didn't want to, but I let her check me.

"You're at a five to six." I felt excited because that was much further along than I was last time.

"I want to get in the water right now," I said. As I sat down, I had the most intense contraction I've ever had. I screamed bloody murder. I had never screamed like that before. A deep release. Part of my cervix opening was letting that sound happen. There was no resistance. I just allowed my body to do what it needed to do. I got out of the way. The water helped my body relax. My cervix opened, doing the work it needed to do. I went from five to complete in that one contraction.

We were glad Nathaniel wasn't with us yet because it would have scared him. He had seen several quiet births on tape. I was very quiet the first time. I didn't realize I was going to be so noisy this time, though.

After my contraction, I said, "I need to poop."

"The potty's right here. You can just come over," Dinah said. It was literally three steps away from the bathtub, but it looked like Mt. Everest to me. I thought, *No way in hell am I ever getting over there.*

"You know what? I have a scoop if it happens in the water. But it's probably the baby," she said. All of a sudden I remembered all of my yoga students telling me they needed to poop right before the baby was born. It's the baby.

"Don't worry about it," Dinah said. I thought, *I'm not getting in the way of this energy. I'm going to let this happen. If I have to poop to get it to happen, that's what I'll do.* Another contraction came and I screamed again. Then it opened up. A little poop floated to the surface. Dinah tried to scoop it, but it broke apart.

"Elizabeth, I'm really sorry. I know you want to have a waterbirth. But I don't think this is a good idea for the baby to be born in the water now."

"Let the water out and put some more water in," I said.

"I don't think you have time."

"Just do it. Just do it."

"Elizabeth, I want you to get out."

"Why? We're going to change the water."

She knew there wasn't time. She'd seen this kind of birth before and the baby was coming fast. I was still thinking we were a couple more hours away. I didn't realize I was complete at that point. The water drained out.

"I still want you to get out of the tub," she said. I balked. I started to put my leg over the side, and contracted right then. I was standing. No way. I put my leg back in and I started to sit back down.

Dinah didn't want me to sit in that last little bit of water. She told me later she did that for two reasons: because that usually slows things down, and I shouldn't be in the poopy water. I got on my hands and knees and had a really big contraction.

"I see some eyes." Dinah started slipping in the water on the floor. She was leaning over the edge of the tub to catch the baby.

"Oh my God, I'm having this baby right now." I pushed him out and sat down. She handed me Liam, our sweet newborn.

I felt lightweight with a rush of emotion. I said, "Oh my God. We really did it!" I wanted it to happen in the water, but it was right up there under the heading *"Whatever unfolds is okay."* It wasn't the perfect in-the-water, let-him-float-slowly-up-to-the-top birth. But, Liam was born and it was great.

He breastfed. He lifted up his head and looked around, looked at us. Nursed. Very attentive and so sweet.

A friend brought our son, Nathaniel, just when we were walking to the bed with our newborn.

Liam's birth was not nearly as hard as it was with Nathaniel. It's easier when it goes faster. Liam was born at 10:51, twenty-one minutes after we got there.

Dan commented about his two sons. "How was the second birth compared to the first: three-and-a-half hours versus thirty-six hours of labor? Labor started at 7:30, birth at 10:30, and back home at 3:30."

It's not about being a martyr and enduring it. It's about tuning in to it and respecting the awesome power that moves through your body.

I *believe* those mantras now, *Yes, I can do it.* That's exciting. When a woman is empowered, she becomes a better mother. If we start off knowing our strength, we have a better place to nurture our motherhood.

It's better for the baby, too. The baby has a gentler welcome into the world.

Others want to rush children out of the womb, rush the placenta, rush to wean off the breast, hurry out of diapers, get kids to sleep, and more. After birth, babies need a decompression chamber, one place to be calm and quiet for a week. It requires patience to let the cord fall off. Yet Liam remains calm to this day. Have you seen the "Tree of Life" art? It's a placenta print, like a tree with veins on one side.

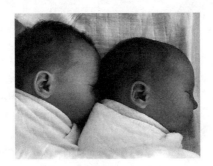

SECRET 10:

Transform Life's Challenges

Twins, Breech, VBAC, Episiotomy, Wanting Normal, When Natural Doesn't Work Out, and Down Syndrome

Twins Born Naturally
Kimberly's Story

On a Tuesday night I went to a friend's house to play Bunco. "Oh, I can have wine tonight because on Saturday I'm getting pregnant," I said. And just like that I was. I used the rhythm method.

My husband, Bob, and I have a four-year-old son, Max. With this second pregnancy beginning, I said to the ladies that I walk with one morning, "You know I better not be having twins 'cause that's not okay with me." I was worried.

I called the birth center where Max was born. "I'm pregnant," I said. Since it's not my first they said, "We'll see you at thirteen weeks." They assume you know how to take care of yourself through the first trimester during your second pregnancy.

At my appointment, I said, "Tell me I'm not having twins."

The midwife laughed. "Why would you think you're having twins? Do they run in your family?" she asked.

"No." We weren't on fertility treatments either. She heard one heartbeat, but you have to search to find two heartbeats because they're tiny.

"You're fine."

"Okay, I'm not having twins, good."

I never asked about it again. During my fifth month, I gardened and started bleeding. I called, worried. "I'm bleeding. What should I do?"

"Lie flat. I have a lady who is coming in," the midwife said, "Meet me at the birth center afterwards."

Bob was working at a Rangers game as a radio announcer.

I called a friend, "Could you take me along with Max down to the birth center?"

She did. The midwife listened to my baby's heartbeat. "Okay. Your baby is fine," she said. That calmed me down. "Now we need to find out what's causing this bleeding. Get an ultrasound tomorrow," she said.

The next day, the technician performing the ultrasound said, "Oh, look! See the two heads? You're having twins."

"I had a feeling that I was," I said.

I tried to hide my tears from her. I didn't want her to think I was an ungrateful mother.

I'm reluctant to say I've been psychic my whole life. I *knew* I was having twins. It's not like what you see on TV. I'm just more in tune with people. I think my brother, sister, and I grew up trying to read my mom's mind. Or maybe it was natural, I don't know. I suffered with depression growing up. If I would walk by an angry person, I'd get angry. Walk by a sad person, I'd absorb that energy.

At twenty-six, I saw a psychic who told me, "You're as psychic as I am. What are you doing here? You should be doing my job." That comment confirmed that I'm not nuts.

"When you leave the house everyday, turn the volume down," she said. I quit having everyone else's feelings and my depression went away.

Now that I was having twins, I thought, *why did I ever plan this pregnancy?* It would have been better if this had been an accident. Instead, I did this to myself. I felt devastated. I thought, *poor Max* because I had started thinking about how to integrate a second baby. Let's not dethrone the King. We were happy and we loved our son. Should we even have another? To find out we're having two more was a major upheaval.

With my first pregnancy of Max, I felt nervous and sad because my family lived back in California. I looked up which obstetrician was on our insurance plan and close to home in Texas. I called and said, "I'd like to make an appointment, because I'm pregnant."

"You can come in on this day and have our test done," the doctor's receptionist said.

"I already did a test." I could tell, they doubted I was pregnant unless I did *their* test. I made the appointment, but I knew I would cancel it.

I looked through the phone book, saw the birth center and called. "Of course you know you're pregnant. Come on in, we'll do an exam and see how far along you are," the receptionist said. They sounded friendly—a good sign that made me feel excited about my pregnancy.

Bob got a new radio job in Dallas and we moved mid-pregnancy. I contacted the only birth center in town at that time. It hosts a MaternaTea, where all the mothers who gave birth in that month come back and talk. It struck me how that's your rite of *initiation* as a new mom, the telling of your birth story. The women get emotional. All of us have heard it before. But we're all on the edge of our seats listening to the story again and crying. Even if you never see these people again, you share something intimate, something that honors our passage into motherhood.

Instead of birth classes, I read the Bradley book and I meditated.

If people tried to talk me out of natural birth, I nodded and smiled. I never felt I had to defend myself. I felt this is my decision and it's *personal*. I wondered, though, why they feel they need to put their ideas on me? They're not pregnant. Why in the world would they care?

I come from an athletic family, and started competitive swimming when I was four. I already knew that I had a high pain tolerance. Still, I wondered, *how much was it going to hurt?*

The only person I wanted to talk to about my decision was my aunt, who went to Berkeley in the 1960s. They moved out to the country and her best friend, who lived across the creek, was a midwife. She had both my cousins Ryan and Lucas naturally. When I went home for a baby shower, she offered one piece of advice: "When it starts to hurt so bad that you think you're going to *die*, have the presence of mind that you are in *transition*. You *will* be able to do this. It's only a few more contractions that will help you through," she said.

At the birth center, I started to have a few contractions right around ten centimeters where I thought I couldn't do it.

Sitting in the bath, I said to my husband, "Go get the midwife."

"Okay, come on. Let's get out of the tub," she said. I did not want a waterbirth. They took me to the bed. Within ten minutes, she said, "Here comes the head." "Why don't you get up and hold on to the post of the bed and squat as you have contractions," she suggested. I was in good shape from walking every day and the squatting helped.

"Did you hear that?" I asked. Suddenly a gunshot sound went straight through my body. I stood straight up. No one else heard it because it was inside of me. "Something popped. I don't know what it is."

"You've had back trouble, maybe it's that. Get back in the bed," the midwife said. Within ten to fifteen minutes in bed, I pushed Max out. My first baby was born. He weighed 8 pounds, 12 ounces.

We did not know that his arm was up. He came so fast with one arm by his head. "He looks like the Heisman Trophy," my husband said. But his elbow broke my tailbone. The tailbone repairs itself.

If I had given birth to Max at the hospital, though, they would have said, "You're going in for an emergency C-section. Let's go." There would have been no way they'd let me push him for two hours.

When I was born at Laguna Beach, California, my mother had a progressive doctor for that time. "You need certain foods and avoid eating other kinds. Don't smoke and don't drink," he advised because many did back then through their pregnancies. He helped her at a time when she didn't have a network of women, including her mother and grandmother, to help her with personal issues.

Even though I'm in a Moms Club of sixty women, only two gave natural childbirth. One is from Germany who uses homeopathic remedies. The other mom had all four of her kids naturally. If I tell most women I had natural birth, they'll say, "That's kooky Kimberly. I would never do that. I walked in and said, 'give me the epidural now.'" I keep a lid on it because it's my private decision and I don't want people to think I'm bragging.

Some women tell me their doctor encouraged them to schedule a day for a C-section or induction. Others express dismay at their medicated experience they had in the hospital.

Pregnant women in their late thirties, like me, are treated like our eggs have already grayed. I ovulated two eggs because I'm getting to that point in my cycle where you either skip a month, have more trouble with infertility, or, are more likely to have twins.

Doctors prefer to deliver twins by cesarean. It's perceived as safer, even though it's major surgery. It's easier for physicians to schedule and say, "Come in and we'll take them." From reading, I got the impression that they expect one twin to get bigger than the other. They monitor so closely, that as soon as there's a red flag, "Yep, we gotta take them now." They assume you're going to have premature twins and trouble with pregnancy and delivery. *They don't ever assume that you'll have healthy full-term babies.*

I felt *over* monitoring with the twins—eight ultrasounds. I had none with Max. Even though they swear it's safe, are they going to find later, "You know, ultrasound isn't good for the fetus." You can refuse a test.

After the sonogram confirmed twins, I asked the midwife, "Okay, what do we do now?"

"You can't have them here because it's high risk at your age and we don't deliver twins," she said gently. She has five children with her second pregnancy resulting in an undiagnosed twin. In the middle of birth, out came the second baby. I was in my second pregnancy, but at least I knew I carried twins.

The midwife took a personal interest in me. "I'll be at your birth, no matter what," she said. She would attend the way a doula would, and walk the hospital halls with me when I went into labor.

I needed to switch to the Birth Center's back-up physician. Bob and Max went with me to my first appointment. I was still not happy with having twins. The doctor was brusque.

In reading, I found out that it's important to know if the twins are fraternal or identical because later in life, they might need to donate blood or bone marrow. It's expensive and troublesome to find out when they're grown. But when they are born, a doctor can look at the sac and know.

As I started asking a question from my list, the doctor asked, "Why would you want to know that?" Her response rattled me. I started to cry. I thought, *I don't know her at all. Why did the midwife send me to her?* I hit a panic button: Now I *have* to go to the hospital. It has wrecked everything. As I cried, the doctor became gentler. She was pregnant herself.

As I set up my next appointment at the reception counter, I couldn't stop crying. Someone would need to mop up the floor.

The next month I got myself together. I took care to avoid confrontation because I needed to forge a relationship with the doctor. Secretly, however, I carried a chip on my shoulder. I was upset I had to deal with a new doctor and being pregnant with *twins.*

They wanted me to have an amniocentisis, but I didn't do it. I negotiated for a 3-D ultrasound, instead. I had to fight with the clinic at the hospital. The perinatologist who does the in-depth ultrasound made me sign all these waivers. The deal I cut was to do the detailed 3-D ultrasound. If there's a reason to suspect trouble, then do the amnio.

"Our counselor will have to talk to you first before you get this done," he said. If I had the ultrasound and the amnio, I would have been finished in half an hour. Instead, it was drawn out because they had a "kook" who didn't want the amnio.

I hated the hospital. It was hard on me. I learned that the chance of losing your baby with an amnio increases. "If we have to stick a needle in, does it double the chance of losing one or the other of these babies?" I asked.

"Absolutely," said the ultrasound technician.

"There's already a risk with one baby. Why would I want to lose twins? If I lose one, does it die inside me and the other one remains viable?"

"Yeah, we could take the dead one out," he explained.

Thankfully, the scan turned out fine and I didn't need the amnio.

Before thirty-six weeks I felt fine. But after that, I couldn't walk. I was out of breath because of the pressure on my lungs. And I was nauseous as well. Blood volume increases double with one baby, but with twins it's more than double. It's more tiring and more weighty. My blood pressure suddenly went up. If I sat up it rose to 160 or 170, but if I lay down it would returned to a tolerable 120.

"You need to go home and be on bed rest," the doctor said. Even though I felt bad, I didn't want to go on bed rest.

"We can induce," she said.

"No," I said.

She made me angry sometimes. She could be intimidating. But my midwife trusted her. She never took over. "There's birth center ways," she said. I wanted as much time as possible for the twins' lungs to develop. Her idea was to use gel to stimulate contractions. But other ways work like power walking, nipple stimulation.

The physician worked with the midwife and called her saying, "This is the situation, her blood pressure is way up. What I want to do is this... Kimberly calmly said 'no', she wants to wait. What do you think?" And the midwife had told me two days earlier at my appointment that she wanted me to get to thirty-eight weeks. I was mad we couldn't go to forty.

The doctor told me, "We want a healthy mom and healthy babies. And I know you want to do this naturally. I'm afraid if we wait another week or two that your health is compromised and you won't be able to have the babies naturally. You'll have a C-section."

"Can we at least go to thirty-seven weeks?" I asked.

"If you go home and lie down. You can't sit in bed. You have to be lying down, because as soon as you sit up your blood pressure goes up."

And I could feel it, like someone squeezing me, my head tingly. Your heart races and you can't breathe well.

"I'll see you Monday morning at the Birth Center. You and Bob go down and power walk around the park for an hour, starting at 9:00 a.m."

I called my mom for help. That night she took a midnight flight out from California because my husband had to broadcast the baseball game on the radio. I knew I could sit in bed and color with Max, but I could not feed and entertain him day after day for a week. She had planned to come when the twins were born anyway. She just came early.

Monday morning felt like the first day of fall, cool with a crisp sunny sky. We went to the birth center and I started power walking. They gave us a room to do nipple stimulation, which hurts. It's supposed to mimic a baby nursing and stimulate your hormones to trigger labor. But your teeth are on edge as you keep trying to concentrate on the larger goal of getting your labor going. I was visualizing contractions. With Max, I took black cohosh, an herb, to get labor going.

Contractions finally started. The midwife came in at 10:30 a.m. She examined me to see if I was progressing or if the doctor needed to meet me at the hospital to stimulate labor with gel. I was in labor. "Do this another hour or two and maybe 12 noon or 1 p.m. I'll call you again and we'll see how it's going." My contractions began intensifying to the point where I had to stop when I was walking and concentrate on them. They were starting to hurt. My blood pressure was high, but as long as I didn't pass out, I was fine.

At 1:00 p.m., the midwife said, "Okay, I'll meet you at the hospital."

I thought, *what a difference from my first labor with the drive in the middle of the night already at seven centimeters.* This time I can deal with it, even walk and talk. We drove, parked and I waddled in with my huge stomach into the maternity ward.

"What are you here for?" the nursing staff asked.

"To give birth."

"Oh, who's your doctor?" The nurse still had a nonchalant tone. I guess I looked fine and they thought, *your doctor is going to send you home.*

"I talked to my doctor twenty minutes ago and she's meeting us here. I'm dilated to 6 centimeters and oh, by the way, we're having twins."

I had a contraction and couldn't talk. They realized I was serious.

They all hustled around like, *we need to find her doctor before the twins are born in the lobby.*

It was awful at the hospital. They put me in the bed and strapped me with a monitor for each baby and for me. I felt trapped. I couldn't breathe. "Don't move," the nurse ordered. I thought, *there's no way I can have my babies without drugs because I'm getting scared and bossed around.*

Can I do this? I felt nervous. *What else are they going to do?*

A guy came in and drew out five vials of blood. All the protocol, none of it unusual, was the hospital's procedures. I felt uptight. It was hard to be calm and relaxed. When the doctor arrived at 1:30 p.m., my contractions had diminished to cramps.

"You're still dilated. That's okay, we'll break your water." That helped me immensely. She was calm, "Big deal, you're fine." I had an ally now against all the idiots. "Get her off all this stuff," she told the nurse.

"Carry your IV with you and walk the halls," she said to me. My contractions started to roar. I walked with the midwife and my husband. While we walked the halls, the doctor delivered four babies in an hour-and-a-half. I was up for a while, but because it was going fast, I became uncomfortable within a short time. As soon as the midwife left and we went by our room, I went to lay down because it was too painful. The floor of my pelvis, being upright with all that weight, hurt too much.

The twins were positioned differently. Nicholas' head was down and engaged, and Jackson was transverse (horizontal). We knew that from my latest ultrasound. My doctor has delivered many twins. "You know, it's okay if he's breech. I'll reach up and help," she confidently said. I wanted that rather than a C-section.

The circus act that I had read and heard about with twins delivered in a hospital started to happen. I didn't want the 15 other people in the room. I wanted only my midwife, my doctor and my husband. To tell you the truth, in the middle of having the twins, I could have had 400 people and I couldn't have cared less.

I scooted into the room and lay down. They could deal with it. I was going to start having these babies. I felt like I couldn't breathe or talk or stand upright anymore.

"You need to get with the program because I'm ready," I said. My nurse appeared. Suddenly my whole body started shaking.

With Max I didn't shake. I was more calm during those transition contractions.

This was painful but I was determined to ride it out. The midwife came in saying, "It's okay." I thought, *here I am, flat on my back.* That's *not* how you push a baby out! All this equipment hooked up to me. I had birthed before, but now I worried.

"I can only do this a little while longer. How much longer do I have?"

She stroked my leg. "Oh you've got only another twenty minutes."

"I've got two contractions left, not twenty minutes."

"It won't be that long," she said calmly. I knew she told me little white lies, but it was what I needed to hear. Somebody to reassure me and tell me *you can do this.* You did this before. You're fine. I felt like, *you're right.*

"Let me go see how the doctor is coming with this other lady," she said. She went and told her, "Come on now." In a couple of minutes, she came back with the doctor. The room filled up with staff and I heard a lot of commotion. A team of five persons for each twin waited. All I knew was Bob, the midwife, and the doctor. I focused on them.

I gave a half-hearted first push. I didn't feel the contraction yet and I didn't remember how to push. I thought I would, but I wasn't into it. I pushed to see what this is going to feel like because last time I broke my tailbone. Nobody could say whether it was going to happen again or not.

"You're not going to push a baby out like *that*," the doctor said. I love her. I laughed and gave a big push. Two more and Nicholas came out. He had the cord around his neck and looked a bit blue. Nicholas weighed 6 pounds, 9 ounces. A team rushed in and took him. He got whisked away. Nobody asked me. I was glad I was at the hospital. I was impressed by how everyone had a job to do. When their time came, they did it.

They used an ultrasound to see the second twin, Jack, and observed that he started to be distressed because the cord was around his neck. We didn't have twenty minutes to wait for my water to break and for him to be born. They needed to get him out. As they discussed whether or not to break the water, all of a sudden a bursting sound, *shhhhhhhhhhh*, happened. A shower of amniotic fluid sprayed out of me.

The doctor reached up and pulled Jack's head down. "Okay push him out," she said. He was out in one or two pushes. Jack weighed 6 pounds, 2 ounces. They whisked him away, too. Both twins had their lungs checked, to make sure they were okay. The twins were born before 5 p.m.

The staff burst into applause. My nurse bragged, "Did you see that?"

Strangers were talking about it and coming up to me, patting me. "That was incredible." What I did—deliver twins naturally—was *not* something that happens routinely in a hospital. They don't even think it's possible. The doctors, interns and nurses were all *stunned.*

I thought, *how silly*. Their applause didn't matter; I had my healthy babies. My midwife patted me and leaned down whispering, "*You did the best thing for your babies.*" That was the moment...for me. She was proud, there's one for the birth center. I did it without the screaming and agony. A woman lay there and birthed her babies. I was proud of myself.

Two days later the doctor visited me in my room. "I'm sorry about all the people at your birth," she apologized.

"I didn't even realize they were all there," I said.

"With twins natural, I couldn't keep 'em out. I needed to concentrate on you," she said.

It was a bit of a freak show. They needed to come see. That's okay and fine with me if it helps other people know it's possible. They didn't invade my space. I focused on having the babies and the obstetrician did what she promised to do.

My main complaint with the hospital is their literature states, "We support breastfeeding." Then they gave each baby bottles. Nobody ever asked me if I wanted to pump milk. Jackson couldn't latch on properly for five weeks. Try to imagine breastfeeding *two* babies and one of them will fool around and can't quite get on the nipple for five minutes every time you need to breastfeed.

We paid a lot for the twins. Our insurance was a nightmare. My husband is still working it out. Here I didn't have all these expensive procedures and I'm the type of person who thinks the insurance company should care about that. I thought, *Hey, I could have checked into the hospital and had my double cost C-section. How come you won't cover the fact that Jackson had an extra test?* They spent three hours having their lungs monitored in ICU. They could have been in for eight weeks if I had listened to all the doctors.

Twins did change life for all of us for the first six months. I simply did not have enough hours in the day. So it goes: babies and Max, and we try to rotate who's on top. I'm last. It was hard to keep it from rocking Max's world. We've come through it okay, though. I might write a book on raising twins since I haven't found much to read.

A young girl at the hospital, possibly an intern, looked at me after the twins were born. I got the feeling that she was inspired to have her babies naturally. To see someone do it helps you realize you can, too.

Teacher Learns from First Birth and Delivers Twins Vaginally

Cara's Story

Meet Cara, a teacher who birthed her first son naturally and then found out she was pregnant with twin girls. She delivered them vaginally—a rarity today. (Nearly all doctors perform a C-section for twins.) The blonde tousled-hair toddler twins bounce in and out of the living room with abandon. One girl wears a wide dog collar around her neck. Cara says, "She has a leash and she wants me to walk her." Her elementary-aged son, Samuel, sits and remains oblivious to us as he plays his Game Boy.

Our kids were all a surprise, and I wouldn't change a thing. We started thinking about starting our family, but it happened quickly in the middle of my teaching contract. I assumed that you go to the hospital, whatever your doctor says, you do, as if only one option exists.

As my pregnancy with Samuel went along, I talked to people and read a lot. I had more of an opportunity to learn about natural birth. A couple at our church delivered three children naturally, the last two at home. That made me think, *I don't want to do this in my home, but maybe we'll consider the natural option.* Now looking back, home birth would have been a *wonderful* thing.

My husband, Keith, and I took a hospital class taught by a nurse, who encouraged natural birth. They learned about all that could happen in labor with drugs and surgery. The R.N. talked about a focal point during labor: to bring a picture of your first child or a beautiful place. That focal point takes your mind off everything else that is going on. Having a *professional* recommend natural birth solidified my decision to try.

When I told my doctor, I felt comfortable that he would honor my wishes. He was a D.O. (Doctor of Osteopathy), and their pediatrician. I even asked him why he chose Osteopathy over the M.D. route.

"Because of my holistic practice, I look at the big picture rather than the symptoms," he said.

I can't say that I was 100 percent committed to doing natural childbirth and nothing else. I felt like I could handle it, even though it may be painful and even scary. Between my husband and me, we can make it happen. I thought about fear and pain with an open mind since I had never given birth. Let's take this in steps. Instead of fear, I felt a sense of *calm.*

Our faith played into our experience, knowing that God is in control and He created us to do this. Women throughout history have given birth without all of the perks we get these days...the extra attention, the extra comforts. Births happened throughout history with higher mortality rates. What took the fear away from me was knowing that my body was created for giving birth by God's design.

We expect a lot these days, like our comfort. Why shouldn't we have to suffer a little bit to do something this great? Not that I look to suffer; I don't want to bring pain upon myself. For something this incredible, though, why should we expect it to be a piece of cake? I also knew that it's not without complication to have all of the interventions. You take risks in getting an epidural.

We ate a big dinner with my husband's parents and went back to the hotel with them. The whole time, I was shifting my feet. Samuel was about ten days early. I was not quite expecting him yet.

Back home at 11:00 p.m., it dawned on me that this was something I should start watching. I couldn't do anything about being awake, but my husband could sleep. If we were having this baby tomorrow, he needed his rest. I got out of bed. Labor started as discomfort at first, not pain. I went to the couch to sleep, but I was more curious about keeping track of time. By morning, the contractions were closer together but still not painful. I called the doctor.

"Keep me informed," he said. "Try to relax and take a walk." We walked and walked. When I came back, juice sounded good. Keith went to buy it.

I got in the tub. And that's when it *really* started happening. By the time he got back, I got out of the tub and thought, *we need to go. We need something.* I quickly called the doctor back and I couldn't talk to him.

"If you want to go to the hospital that would be fine, but if you can hold out, stay home for a while," he said. It hurt, so we decided to go.

The doctor's office called the hospital to pre-admit us. I got there at 10:30 a.m. and was dilated to seven centimeters.

"You are going to have this baby right now," the nurse said. She asked me about an epidural.

"I don't know...how much longer?" I asked.

"You are so far along, why don't you hold off? We would have to do it this instant, if you wanted it. But, you're doing great. You're going to do fine. It's not much longer." That was my opportunity to make a decision. And because I had the encouragement, I was *pleased.*

The nurse immediately took over in a kind way. "What would you like?" she asked. "I'd like for you to sit in the tub. Do you feel like sitting in the tub? Okay. What else can we get you?" She became attentive and wanted me to be comfortable, no fetal monitor either. "Now, how do you feel? I'm going to leave you two for a moment." She allowed a special couple moment.

I got in the tub for twenty minutes. Suddenly, I needed to push.

Keith became uncomfortable with my pain. "Hold on, now I don't know what to do."

"Honey, I think I need to push. What do I *do?*"

"I don't know." He called the nurse. A few minutes passed before she came. She got me out of the tub and into the bed.

The whole time, I thought, *I need to push now.* My inclination was to squat, like I wanted to kneel. She asked me not to push yet; they needed my doctor to get here.

We had only spent an hour and a half at the hospital when Samuel was born at 12:08 p.m.

After it's all done, you have this sense of *I-am-woman.* Doing it without drugs, knowing you've actually experienced the *true* process as it was meant to be, is inspiring.

A lot of women think, *my doctor knows best, he's done it hundreds of times, who am I to question him? I'm much better off and safer going with what the doctor is comfortable with than my own needs. I want to put it in his hands.*

We make the switch through *education.*

I don't know if a doctor would ever admit this, but I wonder if it is easier for them to make birth more *uniform.* It's easier to put in that IV. It's easier for the doctor dealing with this mom and her husband watching his wife in pain to lessen that pain and give her some help.

I tell others to get informed. Look at all the information on both sides. I encourage them to read books to help them make informed choices. Chances are they will have a healthy pregnancy and healthy baby.

For the next pregnancy, my husband and I started talking about home birth or the birth center. But my mom was not comfortable. Thirty years ago, my mom was out cold during her births and she admits this is all new to her. I don't know if I would listen to anybody else. But I thought, *if she is uncomfortable and something happens, I don't think I could live with myself.*

We moved, and I called a doctor's office closer to our new home. I found her practice through La Leche League. She gave me a book, *While Waiting* by George E. Verrilli.

"Are you interested in one of our midwives?" she asked me. Yes, I was. I came in and did the blood work. At my next appointment, they did a sonogram and saw *two* babies. So I was back with a doctor.

When we found out that we were having twins, Margaret and Jane, we were excited. For me, I felt 70 percent excitement and 30 percent of *oh-my-goodness, what are we going to do?* It wasn't so much the pregnancy that I was concerned about, but the twins' health in the womb. With this pregnancy, the decision of where to birth was made for us. I was more comfortable knowing I'd give birth in a hospital.

"Let's take this from one appointment to the next and not make any major decisions. Let's look at how you are progressing," the doctor said. She knew I gave birth naturally with Sam.

With twins there are other things to consider which she prepared me for. We were fortunate to have her. I didn't take classes. Now, I wish I had. I think you can read, but with your second you are busy. You read the basics about the technical parts, and skip the spiritual and all the preparation you have to go through.

My doctor asked me to think about the epidural in my last few visits. She brought this up because the babies might come early on their own. She wanted me to know that Margaret was already in position first (head down) and Jane was breech. She explained that Margaret would be born and Jane would turn and follow her out. Or, they could try to turn her manually, using external manipulation.

For me a cesarean would be a last-case scenario. I wanted to try vaginal first. I asked many questions and felt if the doctor recommended something strongly that's what we would do. If she was leaving the decision up to me, I would have asked even more questions. I felt she thought this would be the safest.

I liked her style and agreed with her values. She made decisions that could work for her children in a professional setting. For example, she had her own child or two in her office suite with an au pair (nanny) taking care of them. A friend of mine who went to her remembers the physician coming in and examining her while nursing her own baby. That's the way it's supposed to be. I thought that was great. Showing us that as a professional woman, she's taking care of her family.

I had been to see my doctor that morning.

"How are you doing?" she asked.

"I'm uncomfortable," I said. "I'm ready for these babies to be born."

She did a "vigorous" exam. Someone told me later, she stripped my membranes. After my appointment, we went shopping. I bought curtains, hung them, and got ready for my in-laws coming over for a big dinner.

By that time my contractions started. They felt like menstrual cramps at first. After we ate, we decided to go to the hospital.

Upon arriving, we were placed in the operating room. I wondered if the doctor was concerned. I had an epidural at 5 centimeters. *Now is the time you do it?* My thought at the time was I can be relaxed for them to get a needle in my back. I didn't want to see it. I had the epidural long before I started pushing.

I psyched myself up. We had talked about what it meant to "be a real woman." Part of me felt like, I was going to miss out. But the other part of me knew I was doing what I felt was right for my babies. In the long run, you're doing the right thing. You can have an epidural and still be a real woman. This is what we have to do in this case. They still are my babies. I felt what other women go through when they try to give birth naturally and it doesn't work out.

Physically it felt other-worldly. It was uncomfortable. My husband, Keith, held my hand. We listened to the radio and laughed. I remember being fearful since I couldn't move. The epidural felt painful going in my back. They taped it down. After it was in, it didn't feel bad at all. Losing sensation in my legs was worrisome, though. I had to have a catheter to empty my bladder. I had a fetal monitor, too. I felt frustrated, like I wasn't pushing correctly. I didn't feel the urgency to push.

"Try to push, stomach crunches instead of having a bowel movement," the doctor directed.

This time around, it didn't hurt to push. The first twin was born.

I was holding her while pushing the other twin out. I wondered, *who is going to get the second baby?* They checked her on the screen. They tried to move her, but she didn't turn. Six minutes later, they had done all their stuff to try to turn her with some urgency to get her out. The doctor reached up and grabbed a foot and carefully pulled her out. I had to push that head out. It all happened fast.

I didn't realize this was uncommon.

Later, one of the nurses said, "Thank you." She had never seen a vaginal twin birth before.

Unexpected Twins
Katherine's Story

I had no idea that my husband, Martin, was going to be a priest when we met. He worked at a bank and played in a rock band. After college I went back to the beautiful Episcopal Church in Beacon Hill in Boston where my parents married and where I was baptized.

There he was.

We both come from small families. We have only one brother each. Before we married, we talked about how fun it would be to have a big family. We didn't want to use any contraceptives. Not because of our religion, but because we didn't want drugs or anything artificial in my body.

My mother had cesareans with both my brother and me. She had diabetes, but she gave me books to read that helped. My husband was induced so that his mom's doctor could go on vacation.

When I became pregnant, I started reading about medical childbirths. The most shocking thing was the episiotomy. You know you don't want that cut to happen to you. You discover how it isn't necessary. That was when I started questioning modern methods of delivery.

I read the Bradley book, *Husband Assisted Childbirth*. We went to the Bradley childbirth classes. We found a midwife just as they were starting to become fashionable again—around 1995.

Mass General Hospital, for instance, had redone their whole maternity ward. They had midwives and were trying to integrate them. I started out there, but after a while, I realized that the midwives *didn't have any power*. It was superficial. The fetal monitor, for example, is put on you the minute you arrive. You were not to allowed to drink water, either.

I decided I didn't want to go, even though it was convenient—less than a mile from my house, at Beacon Hill. Instead, I ended up going 45 minutes away to Wellesley Women's Care. We didn't even have a car, so I took the subway and walked for over half an hour. They had midwives who were into natural birth and low technology. I agree that if something goes wrong, I am grateful to have modern medicine. They practiced out of the Wellesley Hospital, a small hospital, but a good one.

Michael's birth, my first, was extremely long. It started a couple of days before with contractions. I was leaking fluid. I was determined not to go in because if you're leaking, sometimes they induce you because of their rules. I was going to go in at the last minute. I lasted twenty-four hours, walking around Beacon Hill with my husband. He is a calm and strong man.

I moved into hard labor during the night. The contractions were strong and painful. I tried to relax. I do not deal with pain well though.

We drove to the hospital. It was only a short time and I began pushing. It was a profound experience. I was in pain, but I was still excited. My husband helped. When you push the baby out it's a moment of intensity and a thrill. When the baby's head comes out and you can feel his hair as he's making his way into the world, it's like Christmas morning.

Maria was born in the same hospital. I pushed it to the last moment—only twenty minutes with her.

Peter was born in Wisconsin because, by then, Martin was in seminary. I found midwives a half hour away. They worked out of a hospital. I had a wonderful midwife and I discovered how great hot water is for birthing. Halfway through my labor the hot water in the hospital gave out. I was under the shower in agony and the water started to go lukewarm. I discovered the water with my second child, doing most of the labor at home, which I've always done. Laboring at home is safer than going to the hospital too early because of their rules regarding interventions.

Seminary can be hard, financially. Our insurance ran out and for my fourth pregnancy I didn't go to the doctor. But, my neighbor was a nurse and she took my blood pressure.

We moved to Dallas when I was seven months pregnant, and found the Women's Birth Center. They don't do sonograms. I had a diabetes test. I knew I was fine physically. But I have the lowest pain tolerance of any one that I know. However if you know that you are going to get through it, you know that the outcome is beautiful, it's worth it. It's your journey.

The midwives were wonderful. It worked out in the most miraculous way. I was three days overdue when I went in for an appointment. The midwife said, "Do you want to have this baby right away?"

"Yes."

"Call your husband and go home and do these things," she said. We tried sex to help start labor. I got contractions, but they weren't going. They'd stop.

I went back in and asked her to break my water. I was exhausted and huge. I stayed because labor finally started. It took only a few hours, but it was hard. I tried going in water and the birth ball, but I couldn't get comfortable. I coped using hot water, moving around, and walking. Sometimes unexpected things work. The only contractions that worked were a few when I was leaning back on my husband's arm and he was holding me. I arched my back. It was a rubber band pull. It stretched my front.

Baby Anna was head down. I did a lot of squatting. But toward the end, I was reclining. She was born. I was smiling but still had a lot of contractions. I didn't think anything about it.

"I guess I'm pushing the placenta out, right?" I asked the midwife.

"These should not be as severe."

She felt and pushed around, "I think another baby is inside you."

Excitement broke out.

The back-up doctor happened to stop by when I was giving birth. I think she was worried about my having these twins.

"Put your gloves on. We need to get in and get that baby out," she said.

The midwife calmed her down. "No. We've got this. It is fine."

Sarah, the second twin, came out completely naturally, head first.

No one knew I was having twins. If they had, I would not have been able to birth there. Who knows what would have happened. I can't imagine how freaked out they'd get about twins at the hospital.

I felt humbled and grateful about receiving an extra gift. I secretly imagined having twins. When I got big, people said, "I bet you're having twins."

Since having my babies, I've been emotional, likely to cry and become sentimental. That's a good thing. There's nothing wrong with getting down on your knees and weeping while you look at your baby. Crying on your husband's shoulder, wanting to be held. Those are appropriate for having had a baby. You're more likely to become depressed if you don't go *with* those hormonal changes. If you need to cry, you need to get it *out*.

I'm learning how to juggle five children. We aren't perfect. I look at parenting from a Christian view, like I'm being tested beyond my capability. Having one kid tests you beyond your limits. That's how you become more like the person God wants, that's what I'm trusting.

Breech Birth
Ann's Story

Ann, a friendly, tall and athletically built mom, has three children. On a full moon, Ann labored with her first daughter in Bloomington, Indiana, where her husband, Ken, was in school.

My water broke at home. For a couple of hours, I anticipated a slow process. Contractions were four minutes apart. I walked. I was excited and nervous, yet had no fear. Sports prepared me the most with mental visualizations, goals, and cheering. I've played basketball, field hockey, and walked two-and-a-half miles a day. I heard, "At one point, labor is like an out-of-body experience. Hang on to it." I never felt that I couldn't do it, never felt out of control, and never felt scared of birth.

Ken and I drove to the hospital. The nurse checked me and discovered that our baby was breech: the baby's bottom presents first instead of the head. Between three to five percent of births are breech.

[The baby's heart rate dipped during labor. Normal fetal heart rate is between 120 to 160 beats per minute bpm. During the second stage of labor the baby's heart rate can decelerate to 80 and 90 bpm during contractions and while squeezing through the birth canal. That's normal. An unusual dip, though, may mean fetal distress. Sometimes changing position and drinking fluids helps alleviate the baby lying on its own cord, which can restrict oxygen. As long as the fetal heart rate rebounds and the deceleration, known as bradycardia, does not last an unusual amount of time, vaginal birth can happen.]

I thought, *is my baby going to die?* The doctor gave us our odds and risk factors. I was scared of a C-section, but dilated quickly. My husband didn't freak out about the heart rate.

No empty bed existed in the labor ward. Was it because of the full moon? The only room available was the operating room for C-sections with a whole team of spectators. I was hurting and fully dilated. I kept telling myself, *you can do this. I'm going to push this baby out.* I became more determined and I focused. *This is going to come.*

The baby's heart rate dipped again in the middle of birth. I didn't like the monitor; it felt horribly uncomfortable. They whipped out the oxygen and I had to turn over. I'd relax, then okay—here comes another contraction. I was happy that the pushing lasted for only twenty-five minutes. Our baby daughter, Claire, was born.

I was thankful that I could birth vaginally and didn't require surgery. In comparing my first two births, the breech birth hurt *less* than the second with the baby's head coming out first.

I didn't want the effect of drugs on me and didn't want to pass on the drugs to the baby. I had read up on it and wanted to go natural. I knew that my mom birthed me naturally and I came quickly. She tried drugs with her other births and she didn't like it.

Most women walk into pregnancy blind. They tell their obstetrician, "I think I'm pregnant." If the doctor says, "We can always induce you." NO. Make your own choice. My friends let doctors tell them what to do and don't research for themselves. My sister-in-law didn't even know having an IV was *optional*. When women hear my story, they say, "Oh my God, *why?*"

I say, "That's part of my experience; having my baby, the way it's meant to be. It's healthiest for me as a person. I made all the decisions. But if it turned out otherwise, that would have been okay."

A friend, with her first baby, said, "I was thinking of going naturally."

"That's great. You can do it. It's not a failure if you try and don't go natural," I said.

She later told me, "When I talked with my doctor, he said, 'You can always change your mind.'"

I loved my doctor, but had to rotate to the other physicians in the group which I hated. They all had different opinions. I took a class taught by a midwife which was informative, though.

Epidurals and scheduled inductions baffle me. I would like to see women consider natural birth as an option. If they have even an inkling, go ahead and explore it. They can say, "That's not for me." It's their own decision.

For my next pregnancy, I toured two hospitals in Dallas. One was more on the medical side of birth. At the other one, I asked, "Who encourages natural?" They mentioned Dr. Margaret Christensen and another practice on the floor below them.

At eight weeks, I was at my mother's house in Colorado and started bleeding. I miscarried. It was painful, emotionally. I called both practices. Elizabeth Fairchild, a midwife at the first one, was nice and understanding.

The nurse practitioner in the other one, though, was not empathetic. "You'll be fine," she said. I didn't want her for my next pregnancy.

I chose Dr. Christensen's practice and saw another midwife, Susan, was available. We really connected.

The due date fell on the holidays. We had a house full of family and I had false labor for a day. It stopped, the midwife swiped my membranes to stimulate the cervix and I went into labor that night. It was a charged atmosphere at home. I had not done any childbirth classes and did not address fetal heart rate issues. I took for granted that I could do it. I didn't remember the pain from the first birth because I focused on the fact that it was breech. I was not prepared at all.

At 8 p.m., Ken and I entered the hospital. I was four centimeters dilated. As I used the birth ball, my water broke. Susan the midwife was with me. The baby's heart rate dipped. I became overwhelmed with fear again and I couldn't let go of it. I got on my back because it was more familiar, but that position increased the pain.

I said to myself, *you have got to let it go*. I went out of my body. I let it happen. Everything went fine, although I tore. At 1:20 a.m. our newborn son, Duncan, was born. He had the cord wrapped around his neck twice and looked blue, but he recovered. I needed some stitches.

"If we have another baby, we'll be more prepared," I told Ken.

I took a one-day refresher class for my next birth. In preparing for labor, ask yourself, "If the heart rate dips, what would you do?" It can scare you, so get informed.

At nine months, I started with false labor from midnight to 7 a.m. When I saw Susan that morning, I said, 'I'm having this baby by noon tomorrow.' Back at home at 10 a.m., my water broke. I felt gushes and leaking when I moved. Your body keeps making more fluid, though, so keep sipping on fluids. I felt relaxed and my husband participated more.

"You can hang out for a while 'til contractions come about four minutes apart," Susan said. I had tested positive for Strep B, but I felt fine. Antibiotics were required before birth: two rounds, four hours apart.

"As fast as you go, know how long you should stay home?" Ken said.

We left. At the hospital, the nurse was great. "I'll hook you up for the antibiotics. It takes a second, no big deal. Then walk around," she said. We were left alone together as a couple. I sat on the birth ball and walked around the halls. I dilated in two-and-a-half hours. Contractions were five minutes apart. Susan suggested a shower. I sat on the birth ball in the shower. I switched to different positions which helped me to continue laboring.

When the nurse did a doppler check, I said, "I need to sit down. It's starting to hurt." Moaning, "Oh, those sound good." Feeling of contractions wrap around your body, from the rib cage down, squeezing.

"Remember, every contraction helps. It's a good thing," Susan said.

Midwives allow you to feel in control of what you are doing. In my mind I thought, *release, don't hold. Let my muscles work. It's working, it's working, it's working.* Oh no, it's two right in a row. I think the baby is coming. Could feel it coming down the birth canal. I was fully dilated in 20 minutes.

Susan punched the button for the nurse, but it didn't work. "Could you punch the button on the wall, Ken?" she asked. A funny moment.

I wanted to lie on my side. He's coming. *He's coming.* Everyone scrambled as I put my foot on Susan's shoulder.

"Yes, looks like you are going to have this baby. Easy, slow-and-easy," Susan said to lessen the risk of tearing.

Four pushes. *Aah, I did it.* This beautiful little baby, Lou. I would have 20 children for that feeling. The first birth was exciting, but the third was the easiest of all—stress-free.

I breastfed all of my children. But, I was not aware that they check out the newborn for 45 minutes.

I'm grateful to Susan, my midwife. She allowed something special to happen. Susan hand-picks her nurses for each labor. I felt very thankful.

Moxibustion Used for Breech Presentations
Eric Jacoby, M.D.

Practicing obstetrics for six-and-a-half years, Dr. Jacoby respects a woman's right to choose her birth. If she wants natural birth, he suggests a doula and he hand picks the nurses for labor. "I'm here to make it safe. I choose nurses who are compassionate. Yet, I need to have control, no waterbirths. I don't know how women do it. I'd get an epidural."

This Californian worked for Pritikin, was interested in exercise, kinesiology, holistic and chiropractic healing. Yet, his own children were born by cesarean. I notice a statue of an old doctor holding a baby upside down (a practice no longer used) behind his desk.

"I look forward to my work every Monday. I attend 95 percent of our 250 births a year. Women don't wait more than fifteen minutes in the reception area. I used to have a 10 percent C-section rate. Now many women ask for inductions for logistical reasons at thirty-nine to forty weeks and they're dilated."

Dr. Jacoby brings out a bag of herbs, instructing how women can use them to turn their breech baby. He shows a medical article[1] that endorses this natural, but not often known method. An ancient Chinese practice, though still widely used, is moxibustion for the turning of breech babies. At thirty-four weeks of pregnancy, a bag of dried Artemesia (*Artemesia vulgaris*) is given to moms with breech presentations. The mom takes home the herbs with these instructions:
- Roll into two cigar-shaped burning sticks,
- On stone or tile, burn rolls close to (not touching) outside corner of pinky toes, an acupuncture point,
- The heat at a point on the little toe stimulates turning of breech babies
- Expose for thirty minutes, twice a day, for seven days.

Results of a randomized controlled study confirm that at thirty-five weeks, 75 percent of fetuses in the moxibustion group were in cephalic position (head down), compared to 48 percent of the control group. There were no adverse effects.

Breech Babies
Margaret Christensen, M.D.

Because of the medical-legal climate, the standard now for breech presentation, especially if it's your first baby, is a cesarean section. Whether or not a breech baby is born vaginally or by C-section, a higher rate of having neurological deficits is possible. Physicians are not willing to be blamed for adverse neurological outcomes if they were born vaginally, even though the neurological problems may not have anything to do with the mode of birth.

Which begs the question: are they breech in the first place because the neurological *signal is not there* to tell the baby to turn around?

There is a slightly higher risk of birth trauma or birth injury from delivering vaginally with a breech. In rare cases, babies can get stuck. The bottom can come through and the head can't. A doctor uses forceps and hopes to get the baby out. It's scary, although I've never had that happen.

Criteria for having a *vaginal* breech birth are:

1. The baby hopefully doesn't weigh more than 8 pounds.

2. The baby is in frank presentation (bottom down).

3. No footling presentation, because you have a higher incidence of cord prolapse.

4. A "proven pelvis," in other words you delivered vaginally before. You can have CT scans done that can measure the dimensions in the pelvis and to see whether or not there is enough room to accommodate the baby's head. An ultrasound doesn't show. One needs to get the bone dimensions.

5. You have to have a physician who is willing.

6. You go into labor on your own.

7. You have no augmentation (or Pitocin) of your labor, you have to labor on your own.

Facilitating a vaginal breech birth is becoming a lost art. Very few physicians in training now ever get to do them. This is the one time having an older obstetrician helps.

When I had women who wanted vaginal breech delivery, I sat them down and said, "I'm willing to do this. However, you need to be willing to have full cooperation and take responsibility for these things."

I would run an ultrasound ahead of time to have an estimated fetal weight. Whether it's accurate or not, for medical-legal purposes, I wanted to show the baby is 8 pounds or less. I didn't use the CT scans a lot, but I would now. They had to meet all the other criteria.

"This is what to expect: We're going to have extra people around and I may need to use forceps," I'd explain to women.

I did most of the breech deliveries in the operating room, in case we needed anything. I'd turn down the lights, put on the music and avoid a circus atmosphere. I had fifteen to twenty vaginal breech births in ten years, including some of the birth center patients.

The other thing to expect is breech babies come out "floppier" and bluer because the umbilical cord is compressed for a little bit longer time because of how they are coming through. You stimulate them and give them a little oxygen. I'd place the baby on the mom's tummy, put a mask on the baby and leave them connected to the umbilical cord. You can do all the stimulation right there.

The first couple of years I was in practice, we had a high-risk maternal-fetal medicine guy who used to do home births with midwives in Louisiana, where he was from. He was cool with doing breech births. He would come hang out in the room with me and I would feel supported.

A friend of mine, an operating room tech, was the first of ten children of a hispanic mom, born in Mexico. She was her mother's first baby and breech at ten pounds. Her small mother was in labor for days and days, forty years ago. They thought the baby was not going to make it, but Maria was born fine. Nobody would do that these days.

With a breech baby, you can ask to have an ***external version***, meaning manipulating the baby externally by hand. If you're going to do that, it's helpful to use visualization and relaxation techniques.

When I tried to turn a breech baby, I did a guided meditation with the moms, trying to get them to relax as much as possible. I'd ask them to think about their baby as a little dolphin swimming around in the ocean and they were going to do little flips. It's fairly uncomfortable to have it done because it involves a lot of pressure. Sometimes it's not how hard you do it, but it's almost a *coaxing*, like you are asking the baby to turn. The mom needs to be relaxed enough on her part.

When considering an external version, one thing that can help is to get some terbutaline, an intravenous medication given for preterm labor, because that helps to relax the uterus and prevent a contraction.

You can have external versions without extensive monitoring, but very few doctors would do that these days. The current procedure generally requires coming in to the hospital without eating anything, so your stomach is empty, having an IV placed, and being monitored first for twenty minutes, making sure the baby is okay. Then I attempted the version. Afterwards whether or not it was successful, the baby is monitored for thirty minutes to an hour.

An emergency during the external version is rare. But theoretically, you could cause abruption of the placenta or the baby may get tangled in the cord and the heart rate goes down. I'd send the woman home to monitor the baby's movements for the rest of the day with fetal kick counts, at least ten movements per hour.

Success varies depending on the person doing it. Having experience helps. It's fifty/fifty. They are easier to do in "multips" (women who have had multiple births). If you've had a baby before, and your uterus and abdominal muscles are more relaxed and stretchy, it's easier to move around.

Pelvic tilts can be helpful: elevating your pelvis, three times a day for fifteen minutes. Talk to your baby and use visualization techniques. Some chiropractors do manipulation. Acupuncture meridians can help as well.

Often with *twins,* the first baby will be head down and the second will be breech. Because twins generally are smaller, many times you can deliver the breech one easily. You can do a "breech extraction," where the first baby comes out and you reach up and grab the feet of the second baby and pull her out. New obstetricians don't have experience with that.

One of the great things about training at Baylor Hospital was learning from guys who had been practicing for years. We had good forceps experience and breech experiences. It was better than being in a large county hospital program where it's the senior residents teaching the junior residents. You don't have a lot of staff supervision in places like that.

Forceps can be safe when used appropriately. But they can be a problem with serious consequences. Many obstetricians have not been trained well with forceps. They would do a C-section.

The key to breech birth is when a woman is pushing, I tried to keep my hands *off.* She had to deliver as much of the baby herself as possible. Once I saw the shoulder blades there's a series of manipulations I could do to help deliver. All the babies that I've assisted with just popped out.

I've heard disaster stories, where the head gets stuck. You can understand why physicians are reluctant to do breech births because of that. Unless you have parents who are motivated and understand the risks, most obstetricians won't do vaginal breech deliveries.

Two Vaginal Births After Cesarean (VBAC)

Shelly's Story

"Oh, Shelly," the technician said at my first sonogram, "Your baby's going to be big."

In April, the doctor gave me the news. "This baby is breech."

"Is there anything I can do?" I asked nervously.

"No, no. We're going to schedule a cesarean."

"Shouldn't I go into labor? Wouldn't that be better? Is there a way for this baby to be born breech? Why can't we do that?"

"Oh, cesareans for these babies are safer," he said.

I was young, only in my twenties, when I read about midwives in *Mothering* magazine. I was afraid to try it, though. Plus, I didn't know any midwives.

My husband, Danny, and I took Lamaze classes at the hospital. I was scared of the pain, or of something going wrong. I remember hearing, "Oh gosh, you've got to have the epidural" stories. But I've always been against drugs. I thought, *I'm not going to use drugs.*

One evening at home, Danny and I had a little disagreement after dinner. I walked outside and went down this little country lane with a canopy of trees overhead. I saw a beautiful dusk sky. The most incredible, spiritual moment happened. I've never had this kind of experience before or since, but I felt completely surrounded by spirits. It was amazing. I felt a presence. I got a little bit scared; *what's happening?* At first, I was afraid maybe I had eaten something bad at supper.

It was like a whole bunch of voices, but I wasn't hearing them with my ears. I knew some sort of discussion was going on. Then a decision was made. Something changed. Only one Being—a spirit, a soul—was present. That Being entered my body and from that moment on I knew my baby. I didn't know if it was a boy or girl. She came to me because she chose me as her mother. Before, I was pregnant and getting a little fat. Now, I was amazed. I had a sense of her presence with me.

I didn't tell anyone about that moment until years later. Another woman told me she had experienced it as well. I almost fell on the ground. "It happened to me, too."

On the scheduled cesarean day, I wanted my husband with me.

"No. He can't be in surgery," they said at the hospital. That was their rule back then.

Danny had been with me through my pregnancy and I wanted him with me when our child came into this world. I cried.

I was awake, though, and completely aware for the entire birth. I felt, in that sense, that part of the birth was a gift. I heard Hanna's first breath, saw her when she was blue, and watched her turn pink.

They took her away, put her in this incubator, and placed her face down. She cried. I couldn't reach out to her. I wanted to hold her, bring her to my breast to nurse. For years, I mourned that loss of bonding.

Before stitching me up, the doctor said, "Oh, you've got a cyst on one of your ovaries. I'm going to remove it."

"Okay, whatever." I was looking at my baby across the room.

Later at an appointment, the doctor admitted, "Not much of your ovary was left, so I took it out."

I stared at him in disbelief, "You what?" I felt violated.

"It's a good thing we scheduled the cesarean because you're a small person. You couldn't have had this baby vaginally. She weighed 8 1/2 pounds. We did the right thing," he said.

As soon as I got pregnant with my second child, Naomi, I started reading everything I could get my hands on, including information about vaginal birth after cesarean (VBAC). I was inspired; I could do that. I thought, *I'm going to do it completely differently this time.*

I found a VBAC group with a lot of women who were grieving deeper than I because they were completely sedated during birth. At least I got to see our daughter, Hanna. That was something for me to cling to. These other women woke up, and everybody knew their baby except them. "How do you know that's my baby? I didn't see that baby come from my body." It was a foreign feeling for them. I thought, *oh, I'm thankful that I don't have that to deal with.* Talking to other women helped me.

I wanted to feel healed after my first birth of Hanna. We brought our children to go through a process where we symbolically "gave birth" to them again, like the way we had wanted to make it. I get chills thinking about it. I get choked up, even now. I held Hanna, who was three and a-half years old at the time, and told her everything that happened when she was born plus what I had missed. She looked at me and said, "Okay, Mommy." I cried and then I was ready to move on.

Hanna is grown now. I'll talk to her more when she prepares to have her own children.

I read about all the statistics about VBACs. To me, if you have a scar on your uterus, it is going to be stronger, not weaker. In my mind I said, *my body is stronger there; I'm going to be fine.*

But, there was still that fear factor. People asked me, "Oh my gosh, aren't you afraid of something bad happening?" I went to every VBAC meeting to hear every single detail of those births. That encouraged me. A lot of women had great natural births. I thought, *I'm going to pursue a home birth. That is what I want.* I envisioned it.

Danny supported me, too. "Whatever you need to do," he said.

The parenting philosophy of "let the baby scream in the crib until they give up," didn't work for us. I was adamant about breastfeeding, too. I started making decisions to take control of my second birth.

I talked to people, trying to find a midwife who did home birth. I even went to several births and said, "Oh, this is what I want."

"We don't do VBACs," the midwife said. I became disheartened.

Someone in the group found Dr. Bullock, who supported VBACs. He said, "This is the way it needs to be. Women need to take charge of their births. I don't do fetal monitors. We do heparin locks (or hep lock, small tubes attached to a catheter, inserted into the arm and held with tape in for quick access in case drugs or fluids are needed) so you don't have to be tied to the bed with your IV. There are all kinds of things we can do."

I got a great intuitive feeling about him. He even supported midwives. He was in this small community hospital in Wiley, Texas. I asked him about delivering our baby vaginally. "Great. Fine with me," he said.

At two weeks past my due date, I woke up at 6 a.m. and my labor had begun. *This is it. This is going to be hard.* But, all along I knew I could do it. It wasn't anything I couldn't handle, but it got a little bit harder. I moved around a lot and walked at the mall. Later, I did lots of squatting until my legs couldn't squat anymore.

Looking back, it would have been better to have somebody with me who had given birth naturally, or a doula. But it didn't matter in the end because it was great. I could breathe...slowly.

I remember thinking that this was exactly like mountain climbing in Colorado. You don't ever look up at the peak. You look down and you take one more step.

I could take one more contraction. If you look up at the mountain, it looks too overwhelming. I'd never make it. But, I could always take another step. That visualization enabled me to deal with the next contraction.

I never looked at a watch. They didn't even have clocks in the room and I lost my sense of time. I took the next contraction. They slowly increased and became stronger.

Eventually, I got the urge. "I've got to push." Pushing for me was the greatest thing in the world. I loved it because I was *doing* something. I pushed and tried different positions. Hours went by. I felt exhausted.

Dr. Bullock was not like a regular doctor. I knew he was there, but he didn't interfere. He didn't have that worried look on his face. "Shelly, if you push a couple of more times like that, she's going to be born." I pushed with my all of my might. "Now, there's one other thing, because you're having a large baby. I know you don't want an episiotomy, but you might want to consider it. What do you think about the episiotomy?" he said.

At that point of exhaustion, I resigned, "Yes, I want you to do it."

He didn't say I had to do it. He said "It's up to you." *He let me decide.* As soon as he did the episiotomy, our baby was born.

They turned the lights off, and she opened her eyes real big. We had this huge baby. Fat, fat fat. Rolls of fat. Dr. Bullock handed the baby to Danny. He didn't tell us the sex. He smiled and said, "Dad, tell us what we've got."

"Let me look; oh, it's a girl." Danny said. She was 19 inches long and 10 pounds, 10 ounces, a butterball. That whole birth was awesome. Dr. Bullock stitched me up quickly, cleanly, and perfectly.

I felt completely empowered. My body did it. What a great moment. With an episiotomy and everything, it was such a success to me. I felt euphoric and that feeling stayed with me for days.

I'll never forget the doctor, standing back with a smile like, *this is what it's all about.* He was silent in the background, observing the beautiful moment. He was an answer to our prayer.

I nursed Naomi immediately. She completely latched on in the first five minutes. The doctor let me birth the placenta and he showed it to me, which was important because I didn't see it last time. He let the cord stop pulsing, like a midwife does, which was a request I laid out ahead of time.

Hanna was four, and I talked to her about the birth. She looked at the baby and said, "Oh, she's so fat." She was concerned about the vernix on her.

"This is what we rub in," I said. Hanna had this funny little habit of cleaning her own toes before she put her shoes on. She was checking the baby's toes and getting vernix out. We have a video of it, a cute moment.

Labor began at 6 a.m., and she was born at 6 p.m. I attribute the good birth to lots of information on my part and talking about it beforehand. If, for whatever reason, a cesarean happened again, this is how I want it. I prepared for that, too. I kept an open mind because it could go either way. The doctor said he even delivered breech babies.

I was involved in LaLeche League. The best time to read their book about breastfeeding is *before* birth. Go to their meetings for a full series of four times. It gives you all of the important points. Everyone in LaLeche who had had a cesarean was referred to me about VBACs and I gave them Dr. Bullock's name. Many had births with him after that.

Our third child was actually a surprise. At the time my husband and I...well, we grew further and further apart. It was a hard time in our marriage. Lo and behold, I got pregnant. I couldn't believe this was happening. This wasn't something I was ready for. Then we accepted it.

I knew I was going to birth at home, but who was I going to choose to help me? I started talking to women in my VBAC group. I went to see several midwives and loved Susan Whisman, who delivered VBAC babies. She felt comfortable. "Of course your uterus is strong," she said.

Two things I worried about: hemorrhaging and having a large baby, resulting in shoulder dystocia [where a large baby's shoulders get stuck on the mom's pelvic bone]. I had been anemic the first time after hemorrhaging, so that was a concern of mine.

"What would you do if I was pushing this long?" I asked.

"You figure out positions that feel best to push like mammals do," she said. She was calm and relaxed. A quiet sense of absolute certainty. She was empowering. When I brought up my concerns, she said, "Okay, let's talk about it." She listens to the woman's intuition.

Throughout that pregnancy, I exercised more, ate completely macrobiotic (vegetarian, brown rice, no night shade veggies—like eggplant, no dairy, no eggs). Since then, I've needed meat. My mother taught us to do that: to eat when we were hungry, not necessarily eat at meal time. We learned young to listen to our bodies. That was a real gift from her. I felt better during that pregnancy than I did in the other two. Maybe it was the diet. Maybe it was because I was exercising a little more, but I had no swelling in my legs.

I prepared myself for the eventuality of anything that could happen. I tried not to have any expectations. As much as I wanted this home birth, the perfect way I envisioned it, I had let go. The way this birth happened was up to the baby. I'd think, you know, baby, I want you to come exactly the way you're *supposed* to. That's how I felt. I was going to do everything I could to create it, but whatever happened was meant to be. It's the way I accept my life, and I was focusing on that for the baby.

I was five days overdue with great Braxton Hicks contractions. I knew I was getting ready.

At 1 a.m., I was sound asleep in a dream, and vawooom. The baby kicked and my water wishhhhhed right off the bed. I rolled over and said, "Um, Danny, okay."

"Okay," he murmured sleepily.

I called Susan (the midwife), "Hey Susan..." I had a contraction that was so strong, I couldn't talk.

"Okay Shelly, I'm going to head that way." she said.

No slow and steady mountain climbing this time. This was like in the middle of hard labor. Ha-ha breathing. I kept having strong contractions, and I freaked out a bit. It was too much at the beginning.

I needed to go to the bathroom and as I sat on the toilet, I had another strong contraction. I was alarmed because I thought I needed to push or I had to have a bowel movement.

I looked at Danny, "I...I think I have to push."

"What?" He went to the front door, unbeknownst to me, and let my sister, Shannon, in the house telling her, "Okay, she's panicking. We have to remain calm."

Back in bed, I hummed this little tune, a happy song. Shannon and Danny were gabbing, talking. *I want quiet.* I didn't want them talking because I was trying hard to focus and get through these contractions which got very strong. I got the urge to push again. It started to come on. When I got it full force, the midwife walked in. I've never been so relieved to see anyone in my life.

All the lights were dimmed. The bed was ready. Danny gave me little pieces of crushed up ice to eat, which helped. I started pushing. Susan held my legs and told me, "Push right here, push right here." She touched my perineum, "Push at your bottom." She instructed. She supported the perineum with a soaked cloth.

I pushed and pushed.

"Maybe with this next one we can get you up a little bit forward and maybe get the baby to pass under your pelvic bone," Susan said. I didn't want to move, so they helped me get in a squat on my feet. They had me leaning slightly forward, like I was going to fall. "We've got you." I pushed and man,—the baby went under the pelvic bone like that. I felt it immediately. I knew right then the baby was crowning.

I wanted to get back in a reclining position. I told her that she could do an episiotomy, because we knew it was going to be a big baby.

"Okay, with the next contraction, Shelley, I don't want you to push, I want you to breathe. *Breathe* the baby's head out." She was supporting my perineum [slight pressure with a cloth on the area between the vagina and anus] the whole time. One little tiny layer of skin tore. It stung a bit. Caleb, our son, was born weighing 11 pounds, 5 ounces. No stitches. No shoulder dystocia. No hemorrhaging. I bled less than a half cup of blood.

My sister was in the other room watching a movie with the kids, prepared for twelve hours of labor. All of a sudden, they heard a baby crying.

Everyone walked in. Naomi, our four-year-old, didn't want to look at him. Danny had to carry her in. She peeked and went back on his shoulder. "That's the baby." Hanna, at eight, was sweet and so excited.

It couldn't have been anything more perfect. It was a fast birth and a little bit hard at first. It was over like *that* and I had a baby. It was easy with the comforts of home. My body knew what to do.

The midwife waited for the placenta and for the cord to stop pulsing. Danny cut the cord. Caleb was the biggest baby she delivered at home for years after that.

After Caleb was born, we got up. I didn't want to get up much because, after my second birth, I had this woosey sensation. I asked the midwife if I could crawl to the bathroom. I felt much better on my hands and knees than standing up. "Oh a lot of people crawl," she said.

We got a warm bath. Susan put herbs in the water. It was just me, our newborn son and Danny with candles lit. A sacred space. The herbs from that bath were rejuvenating.

For me, comfort during labor involved the ability to move around in the early stages, and not move in the later stage. Once I got situated, I could deal with the contractions better if I wasn't moving. I thought maybe I'd want to get in the water because I love hot baths. I found that I didn't want to do that, though. Pressure on my back and a warm cloth felt good. I loved chewing on crushed fruit juice ice cubes; so refreshing. Midwives encouraged moms to eat during labor, but I never could. You have to take in something to maintain your energy, though.

Some people think you are putting the baby in harm's way by giving birth at home, but I was prepared. I believe that good midwives know things ahead of time. The signs show up. If you have placenta previa [a 1 in 200 chance that the placenta is too low in utero covering the cervix and preventing the baby an exit through the birth canal], you need transport to a hospital. You're prepared to transport in an emergency situation. We had a doctor who was prepared to accept us at a hospital, who supported Susan in her work. You prepare for *any* kind of birth.

Women have been giving birth for years. Things that happened in the past, when babies died, can now be found out ahead of time. A midwife would know those things.

For breastfeeding, be around women who are nursing before your baby is born. It's the greatest gift you can give yourself and your own baby. Giving the baby access to the breast in the first few moments after birth helps tremendously. Allow no artificial nipples. Let the baby experience the breast.

Later, I wrote a letter to the first doctor, who did the cesarean, after my son was born. "Boy, were you wrong. I birthed vaginally, naturally and had a eleven pound, four ounce baby boy at home."

I've experienced birth both ways. I surrendered control to a doctor and had little to do with Hanna's birth. Then to do the ultimate of what I wanted, to give birth at home, there's no describing it. The most important thing I say about birth: believe in yourself. Believe in your body and surround yourself with women who do the same.

Her Gut and the Doctor's Cut

"Labor and delivery are a natural part of women's physiology, not a medical condition. Pregnant women are not sick. Pregnant women are doing what they are supposed to do. Let's not deal with a doctor who's trying to diagnose something that doesn't exist."
— Kristen, a High School Biology Teacher

When I watched *Baby Story* and *Birthday* TV shows, I noted how many births ended up with C-sections. That scared me. I read that some of the ways to avoid C-sections are to avoid epidurals and inductions. I decided I wanted to labor without anything so I could avoid having a C-section.

My best friend and I were pregnant at the same time. I had already planted a seed in her head about natural birth. We went to the bookstore together. *The Thinking Woman's Guide to a Better Birth*, by Henci Goer, popped out at me because I consider myself as a thinking woman. "I've got to get this book." It scared the daylights out of me after reading it.

I started to question my choice of having an obstetrician, too. It seems to me that most obstetricians have that mindset that pregnancy is a medical condition. The whole time I was pregnant, I kept saying to my husband, "I don't feel comfortable with this doctor."

"Oh, she's cool and receptive to what you're saying," he said. Still I never felt comfortable up to the end. I was a slave to the insurance.

Last year I miscarried at ten weeks along. The baby died in utero. Another doctor ended up giving me a uterine procedure called a D&C (dilation and curettage, or scraping) and didn't get everything. Seventeen weeks later, I passed this huge chunk of tissue. I was in labor, my cervix was dilating and I didn't know what was wrong. When I called the doctor, she didn't believe me when I told her what it was.

"This is tissue. It's got a blood vessel on it," I said. As a biology teacher, I know what a blood vessel looks like.

"Are you sure it's not a blood clot?"

"It's not a blood clot."

She asked me bring it in to show her. "Okay, it's not."

"Why is this happening to me?" I asked.

"You've been chosen for special suffering by God," she said.

My friend recommended another obstetrician to me saying, "She's good." At one of my prenatal visits, fifteen weeks along, I asked, "What are some of the procedures done during labor?"

"If your water breaks, twelve hours later we give you Pitocin."

"Is that routine?" I didn't like the "this is what we do here" attitude. A lot of it was what I read you *don't* want. I asked about natural birth.

I could tell she thought it was strange. "The *few* that go natural...blah blah blah." Every time I left an appointment, I said, "Mike I don't feel good about this. I don't get good vibes."

"Honey, she's cool. She's going to let you do what you want to do."

"Okay." I was listening to *him* instead of to my *intuition*.

I prepared the best I knew how. I read anything I could get my hands on, the internet, pregnancy books. That's the only thing I did. Everything for me is *mental*. I'm brainy...bookish. I didn't exercise enough, though. Spiritually speaking, one thing that I did to train myself was to think: *This is the power of the woman. A woman's power is to have children. A woman's purpose is to have children. Women throughout time have been doing this and I will too.*

Nothing could have prepared me for what happened. Nothing. I knew that if my water broke before I went into labor I was in trouble, but I never read any stories about that. I needed a story of a girl who wanted to have natural labor in a hospital with people trying to fight her about it. That would have helped a lot.

My glucose tolerance testing time came. I rushed to make it to the doctor's office on time. Rushing makes you stressed; that can cause your glucose to increase. When they gave me the one hour glucose test, of course my glucose was a little high.

They made me do the three-hour test next. I *knew* I didn't have gestational diabetes. In my gut I knew I was not. And I'm a hard stick. I had to get stuck four times, before it and every hour after drinking a sticky, super-sweet orange soda.

Afterwards the paperwork never got faxed to the lab. The doctor's office called, "Guess what, they threw away your blood."

"Okay, why don't you put me on the diabetic diet because it can't hurt me. I don't want to go through all of that testing again," I said. My eating habits are good; I eat like a rabbit.

"No, we want you to redo the test." I had to do *another* three-hour glucose test for something I didn't have. They were trying to diagnose something that didn't exist. It was a nightmare. I felt naive to stay with them because I wanted to quit that doctor many times.

The childbirth classes at the hospital were Lamaze. I looked for a more "natural" one, but I couldn't find any. So I didn't take birth classes.

I had a lot of Braxton Hicks [mild contractions prior to labor]. I worked hard at school and was tired. I took off the 2nd of November.

As I lay in bed at home, I wondered, *oh my God, am I peeing on myself?* My water broke. I was going to the hospital to catch the baby. No episiotomy. I'd go home as soon as possible. That was my plan.

My husband and I took our time and ate lunch first before going in. My doula, Jane, came with us.

We got to the hospital at 1:30. I had *no* contractions. I was only three centimeters dilated, with the baby at station -1 in the birth canal. A new nurse seemed shocked that I didn't want an epidural. She asked me interview questions which seemed stupid. I started to eat a spinach veggie sandwich that I brought. "Just crackers," she said.

They told me I was Group Strep B positive. I had taken the test five weeks earlier. "Why didn't I already know?" I had antibiotics by IV.

Nothing happened. That nurse left at her shift change. I didn't want Pitocin. I walked for an hour and got checked.

My doctor went off of her shift, and Dr. Capman came on.

"Okay we're doing natural," I told him. *Leave us alone, please.*

I could tell the new obstetrician didn't like natural birth. He came in, talked to the nurses and left. I didn't see him for a long time.

Finally, we had a good experienced nurse. Roseanne, in her fifties, came in. She brought the birthing ball, the squatting bar, all the tools that the hospital had in the closet collecting dust. She was awesome. My attitude changed from "fight, fight, fight" to "someone's here to let me do it."

The next nurse, Christy, came on, who Roseanne had hand-picked for me before she left work.

The doctor entered. "It's been thirty-six hours. You aren't progressing, Five centimeters is progressing. Let's do a slow drip of Pitocin," he said.

I felt like a caged animal. If I had been in a birthing center, I would not have had anything. Mentally, I got through it. I'm stubborn.

I thought, *Oh good, I'll have this baby by 8 p.m., Friday night. Let's do it.* Three hours later...nothing. The doctor came later and checked me. *He's going to say my labor's stalled out and do a C-section,* I feared.

However, he said, "I think you are in transition."

I felt happy. The doula and I squatted with each contraction. We had been rocking. I had continuous fetal monitoring, so space was limited.

I started out sitting up in bed. But the nurse inched my bed down while I pushed. They broke down the bed and suddenly my feet were in stirrups. The doctor laid out all his instruments. *I'm going to get cut.*

"I'll give you one more push before I give you an episiotomy," he said. I was *crazily* trying to push to avoid that. I trained my husband, "If you see scissors coming anywhere near my perineum, say 'NO'."

Baby Zoie was born.

The doctor stitched me up. "Why are you stitching me? Did I tear?"

"No."

"What are you stitching then?" I asked, puzzled.

"Your episiotomy."

My husband was powerless. We all were. He never told me that he did that to me. He cut me even though I said *not* to.

"I need to give you some Pitocin," he said. "Because your placenta is not detaching."

"Why don't we let my baby breastfeed and do it that way?"

"That's not good enough. We don't have time for that."

He reached back in me to get the placenta. He stuck his hand up and pushed down with force. It felt awful. That became the most abusive part of the birth. I got brutalized for a half-hour. I felt angry. I asked if I could see the placenta, but they left it in a container and I never got to see it. Everyone was too busy fussing over our baby.

I couldn't lift up my arms because they were sore. I had to have the IV replaced so I had two IV sticks in one part of my arm and the IV on the other side. I was out of it. I couldn't even lift my seven pound, fourteen ounce baby girl, Zoie. (*She cries.*) People had to pick her up for me.

My mother came...to comfort me, which I appreciated.

In retrospect, I would have changed my birth. I felt like I had been *raped* with that episiotomy. The thing that sucks is it's a screwed up medical system that needs to change. If I ask for natural labor, I shouldn't be fighting the staff. I will never *ever* give birth in a hospital again.

Nursing Zoie helped heal what we went through. I can't even imagine not breastfeeding. It's the perfect food for a newborn.

I would like to share with women to take charge of their prenatal care, their labor and delivery care. Go with your instinct. If your gut is telling you not to stay with an obstetrician, don't.

Note: Ignoring intuition makes birth harder. Birth classes might have empowered Kristen to change doctors, and helped to know other natural couples, and inform her husband.

Sam and Her Sisters

Linda's Story

On Easter Sunday three days before my due date, my water broke at 8:30 a.m. I wasn't having contractions. But I noticed meconium in the water which means the baby is in distress. [Meconium is from the baby's bowel movement in utero. It varies from watery to thick and is not usually an emergency unless it is thick, like pea soup. Then, the baby is in distress.] We went to the hospital within the hour. A fetal monitor was strapped on me and I was checked for dilation. When I reached five centimeters, I received Pitocin. I got an epidural next. I pushed for one hour and at 6 p.m., Samantha was born, weighing six pounds, two ounces. However, our joy soon turned to concern.

She looked *ashen*. Apparently, she had a lack of blood for two hours before another hospital's neonatal team was called to transfer her. We were told she had fetal-maternal bleeding—blood loss through the umbilical cord into my system. Her hemoglobin was seven, with normal as thirty to forty. "She has brain damage," the doctor told us. We were devastated. Our newborn spent twenty days in the hospital. I cried and coped the best I could.

At an appointment later, my obstetrician said to me, "When you do this again, we'll schedule a C-section." Her comment turned me off. Keila, my chiropractor, had all three of her children at home and I took Samantha to her for therapy. Reading *Brushed by an Angel's Wing*, stories of how God intervenes in our lives, helped me.

It was tough because Sam wasn't reaching developmental milestones. At age three and a-half, she still didn't sit up or roll over. It was hard, not to compare her with other children. Our whole life was Sam—her doctors and medicine, her therapy, her feeding, her sleeping or not, and her seizures. Dan and I needed a relationship again. We needed a relationship with other children. I wanted a normal baby experience.

Moms with children like Sam say, "Wow, you sure were brave to do it again. " I know every mother worries about her children. But when you have a child with disabilities, many areas of concern come up, including medical things. If you have a healthy child, you fear that he might fall off the playground equipment or injure himself. But when you start with a child that's *already* injured, things we worry about are feeding tubes and the surgery involved with that. How will she react to the anesthesia? I can see where people would not want to go through birth again.

With Samantha, I had all the interventions. But we found out in the Bradley class how *unprepared* we were when we had her. Like first-time mothers, a lot of us go into pregnancy and walk into the hospital thinking, *Oh we're going to have a baby*. We had no idea what that meant.

Now, I wanted a natural vaginal childbirth with a midwife and *no* intervention. The only way of having a *prayer* of doing that is to be prepared. It *is* an emotional, physical, and spiritual process. You have to draw all of that from inside yourself in order to do it.

I was determined, however. Toward the end of my pregnancy, I started getting scared. I told Dan, "I don't know if I can do this." Because he had gone through the classes with me, he knew what to say. He knew that I would have doubts and there would be fears. He said, "Sure you can. Why wouldn't you be able to do it? You're strong. We took the classes. You're prepared. You know what to expect. I will be with you."

I'm a researcher at heart. That's what I did in my job. It amazed me when I look back that I didn't do more research with having Samantha. When I got pregnant again, I needed to understand the process of labor and what happens. We found out about the different stages of labor and what you can expect: things you might say, how you'll feel physically, or how you'll feel emotionally. Knowing removed the *mystery* and prepared us for the experience ahead of us.

My mother told me that when she was pregnant for the first time with my sister, Debbie, she had no one to talk to and knew nothing about having a baby. She visualized birth in a dream, though. She saw every step and what happened. When the time came to have Debbie, she felt prepared. She had no fear; she *knew* what was going to happen.

I was at peace, but I know that the Bradley Childbirth class helped. Knowing the stages and what was to come helped me. It helped Dan, too. In class, I said to Dan, "Since this is my second child, I may not have that putzy waiting stage. We might not have that kind of time. And I might not feel like working on a photo album during labor."

I was right. When labor started, it came on strong. I'm glad I warned him. We skipped a lot of steps.

I gained twenty pounds during pregnancy. I wanted to get out and walk all the time. In reality, I decided housework and taking care of

Samantha was enough exercise. Toward the end, I did walk more because I felt like it would help progress labor and bring it on more quickly.

I felt comfortable with my midwife, Susan. My sister even said, "Linda, you don't need another soul. You can do this by yourself. You don't need the midwife. You don't need the nurses. You don't even need Dan. You can do it. Women have been doing this for centuries." That kick-in-the-pants gave me confidence that I could do it. But if I had the midwife, that's a plus. If Dan was there, that's another plus. I didn't need anybody else. Mom decided to help by staying at home with Sam.

On Monday morning while still in bed, I realized I felt the same kind of pain every ten minutes. I was irritable and I hadn't slept well. What could be worse than waking up and feeling lousy, but having a baby on top of that? I knew the baby was coming.

I remember in the Bradley class, they said that the first signpost was excitement. But I wasn't excited at all.

By 9:00 a.m., I got in the shower, had to stop when a contraction came, stand there, hold the wall for a minute, breathe and try to relax. Remember that sensation. You don't want to call it pain; it's what moves the baby out. Your baby out is your ultimate goal. I called Dan at work.

In the Bradley class, you learn not to go to the hospital too soon, but that wasn't my intention. Because of the problems with Samantha, I wanted to be at the hospital sooner, where I could be monitored. I knew that if anything went wrong, we would have professionals to help.

After showering, I sat at the kitchen table and I threw up, which was new for me, although we had learned it could happen.

My dad sat down with a watch, a pen and a piece of paper. He started timing my contractions. He said, "I've never been this close to a birth before." He was excited to participate even though I was fussing at him when the contractions started.

My contractions kept getting stronger. I said to dad, "Okay, shut up. I can't listen to you talk. You have to be quiet." It was during that period of time I realized I was in that *serious* stage.

At 10 a.m., I called Dan. He answered the phone, which was not good because that meant he hadn't left the office yet. He said, "I'll be home in ten minutes." We went to Baylor at 11:00 a.m. I was dilated six centimeters and fully effaced, I had done most of my laboring at home.

The contractions were painful. They felt like bad menstrual cramps. I remember when I was younger having really bad menstrual cramps. You learn to breathe through them and relax. They hurt *worse* if you tense your body, which is what I did with Samantha. I knew I had to clear my head, breathe deeply and *will* my body. That's the one thing that got me through the birth process. The breathing and the relaxation made a big difference.

I needed to go to the bathroom. Susan encouraged me to get up. That was horrible. I thought that I would be walking the halls, standing up and doing all the positions. Yet, all I wanted to do was sit on the edge of the bed and try to relax. That's all I could do. As the labor progressed, Susan encouraged me to get in different positions and I tried to, but I kept coming back to sitting.

After sitting for many hours and not moving around, Susan gave me a suggestion, "Roll over on your left side." I wanted to do it but my legs were going to sleep. She and Dan physically rolled me over. As soon as they did, I yelled out, "I have to *push*."

"Let me check you," Susan said. As soon as she did, my water broke.

I pushed for about thirty minutes. Pushing was hard, scary, and painful. During the contractions, I knew that I couldn't fight against it. I knew I needed to relax. I knew I needed to let my body work on getting the baby out. That's how the process works. Susan had my number. She said, "Linda, I know that you are scared, but the baby is going to come out today. The baby is going to come now, and you need to push through it."

And I did. I never once thought I needed pain medication. I knew it was better for me if I felt everything, experienced everything. Those sensations I was having were normal. They didn't scare me. I knew it was best for the baby not to expose her to any chemicals.

I remember I said to my husband earlier after one of our classes, "Okay, Dan, this is my birth plan: I start my labor. The labor progresses rapidly. My water stays intact until the baby's born."

In that period during the pregnancy, I dreamed about water almost every night. I dreamed not only about water, but *fast*-moving water. I would be in a boat, or in a raft. There would be a waterfall. Water was moving quickly around me.

Dan said, "When Megan came out, it was almost like she was riding on a wave." My water broke and more water followed her. The labor progressed quickly. My water did stay intact.

My envisioned goal became my actual birth.

Megan was born at 3:59 p.m. and weighed eight pounds, nine ounces. I was proud of myself. I was thrilled. I looked at Dan and said, "I did it."

When Megan was born, our first thought was, *We're not going to vaccinate*. We gave ourselves time to do more research. I insisted only on those manufacturers that did not use mercury or Thymerosol. I found that on a *Mothering* magazine's website. Megan has her polio and Hib (Haemophilus influenzae type b). Most babies get vaccinated at two months. That's too young for their immune systems.

Bringing Megan into our family gave us a new perspective. We see what life could have been like. Instead of feeling sad about what Samantha didn't have an opportunity to do, we're joyful that we're able to see Megan develop, learn new things, and discover her world. Megan is healthy, inquisitive, and quite active with tummy time. She's doing great with milestones, at nine-and-a-half months old.

Our third daughter, Emma Grace, was born naturally two years later. She weighed eight pounds, eleven ounces and came after only twenty minutes of pushing.

Two categories of moms-to-be that I've met are: Women either don't have a clue, or they've already decided to have an epidural. Either they don't realize they have a choice, or a choice has been made by a doctor. Be in the smart, third group. You need to know what your rights are, not only in childbirth, but with *everything*. Trust your instincts.

Author comment: When I met Linda and Sam, I found out that Linda had gone to the same obstetrician that I had switched from to another physician/midwifery practice (see A Birth Quest). I recommended my midwife to Linda. Her other two healthy daughters were delivered naturally without any complications. Besides mentoring pregnant women who wanted to birth naturally, meeting Sam was another impetus for this book.

When Natural Birth Doesn't Work Out
Elizabeth's First Birth Story

I went into therapy for several years and did a lot of healing about leaving an acting career behind me. I had majored in theater. People try to get me to act again and I'm good at it, but because you're good at something doesn't mean that's what you're meant to do.

When I took a new yoga class one day, I suddenly realized that I could heal myself. I could continue my *own* integration, learning how to find my center, process things, and balance my life. I didn't need therapy anymore. I fell in love with yoga because it was part of my personal transformation.

After beginning a yoga teacher training seminar that summer, the instructor said to me, "You know, you'd be a great yoga teacher."

"Wow, that sounds interesting," I said.

In the middle of that training, she urgently called me one day, "I need you to teach class for me tonight."

"Noooo, I need to finish the teacher training first," I said.

"I'm sick. No one else can teach the class. I need your help. You're the only one who's ready."

"I can't do it. I...really can't."

"I'll talk you through it," she insisted. I wrote it down. I felt scared and excited at the same time as I taught the class timidly. When I walked out the door that night, the sky looked expansive and the ground felt solid. I knew that I had begun something important. I felt a defining moment.

I've been teaching yoga for ten years and prenatal yoga for five. I teach postnatal baby yoga where the moms and their babies do it together. I even taught through my own pregnancy.

My quest is to become natural. On some level we express ourselves in this society from a unnatural place that we're not even aware of. We doubt ourselves. We don't listen to our inner guidance.

I don't want to take the power away from an experience that could be potentially life-giving for me. How can I empower myself as a woman? Stepping into the birth experience is a way to do that. I thought if anyone can do it, I can—with my yoga, my breathing and my commitment.

I remember a party we went to before having our first baby. A friend, who is a labor and delivery nurse, told us a few stories from work like how they get the forceps out every now and then at the hospital so doctors can *practice,* whether it's needed or not. I felt repulsed. *Gross.*

Our son, Nathaniel, was a surprise. Dan and I lived together, and planned on getting married, but Nathaniel inspired us to go ahead. There was a whirlwind of activity for us to get married before the baby came.

After I became pregnant, I thought of a strategy: *If I had a midwife, the birth wouldn't be at a hospital.* I called and asked our nurse friend, "How do I find a midwife?" She told us about a birth center, so we made an appointment and took a tour. As I looked around and listened to the midwife, I decided *this is where I want to have my baby.* My insurance would cover it. I didn't need to look anywhere else.

We enrolled in a Bradley childbirth class, but they talked about all the things that could go *wrong* in labor. They give you a heads up, but I did not like that part of it. That threw me off and lots of things ended up going wrong. I focused on bad outcomes during my pregnancy. On an energetic level, I *attracted* them.

At eight months into pregnancy, my baby was breech. We went to have him turned after trying everything else. That was emotional because no one would help give me the chance to consider regular birth. If you have a breech baby, it was a C-section right away. I felt incredibly frustrated. When we had him turned, it was successful, thank God.

At two weeks past due, I went to see the midwife because my water was leaking. She massaged my cervix with gel, without asking me. She made the mucous plug come out and I started having contractions. Technically, she got me going. That's not a *natural* birth. I didn't like somebody messing with me. I didn't know then what I know now: The apple falls from the tree when it's ready.

I labored all that day and threw up. Nathaniel was posterior. He got kind of stuck which made the birthing hard. My body was trying, but because of his position, the head wasn't pressing just right to help the cervix open.

When we called the midwife, she said, "Okay, I think you should come in." We had been doing all kinds of stuff all day long, walking, nipple stimulation, the whole nine yards. At 8 p.m., we arrived at the birth center with me throwing up. We thought we'd have the baby by midnight.

She checked me. "I think that you're having trouble progressing. You should be further along than two centimeters. I've been in this business for a long time and I've seen 'failure to progress.' I think you should go to the hospital and get some Pitocin to help your contractions," she said. We had just gotten there and she was telling us to go to the hospital.

"I don't need any help with my contractions. I have plenty of them."

"When people get Pitocin they almost always get an epidural. You might as well get one," she said.

Stunned, I looked at her like she spoke a foreign language. I could not believe it. I thought I would hear something else than, "Go to the hospital and give up." I was taken aback that there was no other solution than succumb to all the medical treatment that I didn't want.

There are explanations for labor not progressing like posterior position of the baby and my first birth. On an emotional level, I was afraid. Perhaps my ego was *way* too invested in the outcome being a certain way. I didn't want to tell people that I had medical interventions after being almost holier-than-thou about having a natural birth. I talked about it, read a lot, and had been a good Bradley student. To think that I would have to say, "Oh, we had a regular medicated birth like what everybody else does," to admit that I wasn't strong enough, was *failing* in some way. Failure was quite scary for me.

I've heard my students say, "Oh, I cratered." Some other women say, "I'm going to try to have a natural birth." You don't say I'm going to *try*.

"Isn't there some other solution? Isn't there something else that can be done besides going to the hospital?" we asked.

"I've seen this. We can try some things, but..." She said that the other options weren't going to work.

"Let us try the rest of the night, please," we pleaded. At that point I was dehydrated, still throwing up. They put an IV in me immediately when I arrived. She saw that I was tired and having a hard time.

"I don't see how you're going to be able to do it." She let us stay.

In the morning, she did everything from stretching my cervix to things I would never wish on anyone. That hurt so bad.

"Okay, we tried, but I think that you have to go," she said. At that point my contractions petered out. In retrospect, I needed to rest.

We drove over to the hospital. I got Pitocin for two hours without an epidural. They turned it on full blast right away. I started throwing up all over again because the contractions became intense. They didn't ease me into it. I've heard of students that have gotten a small Pitocin drip and they were rested. They hadn't even been in labor, so they were able to handle the Pitocin without an epidural. It can be done, but not in this instance. I already had been laboring for 24 hours intensely and throwing up on top of it.

It felt as if I was treading water in turbulent waters and I could not keep my head up. I couldn't even get a breath. Forget about being a yoga teacher who knows how to breathe deeply. I thought that was my ticket. I know how to relax, how to breathe deeply, how to feel connected to the earth. I thought those things were going to carry me through my birth and the Bradley classes were to simply be informed. Before, I felt like I could do it. Not now. Not at this point, I did not.

After two hours, the doctor who did the breech turning came in. They wanted to put a fetal monitor on the baby, but I didn't.

"If something doesn't happen by so-and-so time, we need to start scheduling the C-section room," the doctor said.

Alarmed, I thought, *Oh my God.*

The midwife was not there, but she sent over one of her birth assistants. She had come by at one point, but didn't stay.

I'm going through contractions that are hard to handle because of the Pitocin. I finally agreed to an epidural. However, we asked for the *lowest* dose they could possibly give. I could still feel the contractions. It was enough to help me relax. I progressed to being complete right after that. My cervix finally opened. The baby could turn into the right position. They told me to start pushing which was exciting. In a short time, I pushed him out.

They tried to take the baby away. We wouldn't let them. As soon as they would let us go, we went back to the birth center for recovery.

Afterward, I felt a great sense of failure. Women at my work wouldn't have chosen natural, were probably laughing behind my back. Like, "Uh-huh, she had to do it with drugs." There was a lack of support. One friend had a baby naturally at the same time. A woman at her church asked her about it and she said, "It was challenging for me."

"And you didn't get a medal, did ya?" the lady said sarcastically. Like, you don't get anything for it, why in the world would you choose that? For several years I processed a lot of disappointed feelings.

I had been a vegetarian for years and was militant about it. If you did not eat vegetarian, you were either uninformed or wrong. But, something happened where it didn't feel *right* to be pushy. I realized that everybody makes their own choice and no choice is wrong. That was insightful.

With birth, I thought the best choice that you could make is to have a natural birth. And I didn't even doubt. I was not saying, "I'll try." It's what I wanted more than anything. I thought of the irony of somebody who has a natural birth because she doesn't get to the hospital in time, versus me, wanting one so badly and not being able to actually manifest it.

Now, I'm thankful. If I had had a blissful natural first birth, I don't think I would be flexible and *understanding* with all of my yoga students. I can help others who want a natural birth, help them work through some of those feelings when it doesn't work out. I think that if you are *so* attached to it, there's a chance that you can "funk it up." When you're not flexible, if you have to be one way or it's *wrong*, that's when we get into trouble. Having the kind of birth you want is no exception.

It's better to keep natural birth to yourself. Telling others is like an invitation for criticism. That's what I teach my students now: *Create a sacred space* for yourselves during your pregnancy. *Only* share with people who are going to *support you* and uplift you into what you're wanting for yourself in your pregnancy and in your birth. It may be someone you meet in birth class, or somebody who has made that choice before and has been successful.

People that don't know are going to misinform. They're going to tell you about the horror stories. When somebody starts one, I teach my students to look at their watch and say, "Oh, I gotta go." Whatever you do, get the hell out of there.

I love this quote: *A mother's best friend is another mother having a better day.* If that's true, a pregnant mother's best friend is another pregnant mother who has done what she wants to do, a mentor. If you don't know somebody like that go to LaLeche League meetings, or a birth center. Ask about someone who's had a good birth recently and see if it's okay to call them. Find a mentor and absorb their inspiration.

Unexpected Down Syndrome
Celia's Story

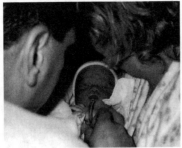

Photo: Helen Simonsen

"I'm worried that I'll ask for an epidural."

"That's not the end of the world," my cousin said. I had grown concerned as my due date approached. A few days later, my cousin gave me an article called, "Epidural Epidemics," from *Mothering Magazine*. The article strengthened and confirmed my choice of having natural childbirth.

I wanted a drug-free baby and the best birth experience possible. I took Bradley classes, read books, walked and talked with other moms. Others who gave birth naturally motivated me. I worked through my anxiety and nervousness, and fear of pain. *How was I going to handle it? Would I forget or freak out?* I imagined the worst.

Rick, my husband, reminded me to relax. I knew that fighting the process and getting tense would not do any good. Let go of your body and let it do what it needs to do.

During birth, my doula encouraged me. "You're doing great. You are doing good for this baby. Sing those songs of labor." The pain was intense. Then it left.

My mom was amazed at how well I did. I was positioned on my side when our son, Michael, came into the world.

I didn't like birthing Michael in the hospital. I remember at Michael's birth I was singing what I call my "birthing song." Making rhythmic sounds comforted me. A young nurse, who I'm guessing had never given birth or even been around birth that much, told me, "You know you'd better be quiet."

"I'm going to do what I'm doing." I said. "I have to do it."

My mom recalls that when she birthed my brother, the staff said, "You're disturbing the other patients."

"That's too bad," she said.

As soon as I had Michael, the nurses came in. They took him and measured him. I didn't like them taking him, period. I didn't like those bright lights, either. What a total invasion for a brand new baby. I thought, *He's been protected inside, where it is dark and safe.* This is why I chose a birth center for my second birth.

The birth center feels more personal because we know everybody. At the hospital, we were met by strangers. They didn't know what our plan was. They had procedures and policies that they had to follow.

For my next birth, we took a two-hour "Refresher" course. Rick teased me, "You only did one hour because you had to go somewhere. You missed 50 percent."

"What did I miss? I got to relax on the floor and breathe."

"You knew how to do that before you went," he said.

Women at my church gave me a wonderful baby shower. It felt sacred. They even said a prayer for the future wife of my second son.

I invited my cousin to the birth and asked her to remind me to relax and breathe. Rick, my mom and I arrived at 2:20 a.m. I got a shot for Strep B. The midwife checked and confirmed dilation at four centimeters, 80 percent effaced, 0 station. They listened to the baby's heartbeat with a Doppler [a hand held device that amplifies the baby's heartbeat, which is waterproof for using when a mom is in the tub, also].

We walked for two hours, with stops back at the birth center for a drink of water or to use the bathroom. Toward the end, I bent over on the walks and stretched my lower back. That felt good.

At 4:30 a.m. I returned and found a rocking chair. Rick timed the contractions. I rocked with my eyes closed. I was in active labor. The midwife came in and checked me at 7:15. I was at six centimeters. The hospital expects around one centimeter per hour, which meant I should have been about eight centimeters.

At 8:00 a.m., my cousin went to get breakfast for those who were hungry. As I draped over the birth ball on the bed, my water broke. It felt like all of a sudden, boom, and I was close to giving birth. I was groaning. A combination of hot and cool cloths on my head and neck was soothing.

At 8:40 a.m., my midwife asked me to turn over. I didn't want to. I was comfortable pushing, but the baby's heart rate dropped. I hollered out as I got off the birth ball and over on the bed. I pushed the baby out in one push. His head in the sac was blue and the cord was bleeding. My baby son, Garrett, had arrived. But a flurry of activity erupted.

Oxygen was given to the baby to stimulate him. The midwives suggested to Rick to bathe the baby and then used a heating pad afterwards to bring up his temperature. Shortly, I was able to hold him and breastfeed. I studied his face.

This birth felt comfortable, relaxed and safe. They had the equipment they needed and the hospital was right around the corner if necessary.

My midwife retreated to her office alone and returned with startling news: she suspected possible Down Syndrome. One recognizable sign she shared is that Garrett was sticking his tongue out a lot. The other signs had to do with a crease on his hand, and his big toe went out at a forty-five degree angle on one foot. Nobody knew any of this ahead of time.

We were ready to go home, but instead the baby was transported to Baylor Hospital's Neonatal ICU, or NICU. I felt utterly exhausted and heartsick. Rick called my cousin, who already left, to explain the turn of events. Rick drove me home to recover and rest. Besides, there was nowhere for me to stay in the hospital near the NICU.

It was my first time to see a NICU at the hospital. Nobody is allowed visitation except parents and grandparents. But my cousin got to take the place of Rick's family since they lived out of town. I experienced breastfeeding separation from that Sunday until Monday afternoon—over twenty-four hours. Garrett was fed with a tube. I promptly obtained a breastfeeding pump Monday morning. I visited my baby for three hours that afternoon. My cousin found information from the Down Syndrome site that encouraged breastfeeding, which I did.

Breastfeeding is even more important for babies with Down syndrome. They have a greater susceptibility to infection than typical babies. That's why the immune factors present in colostrum and breast milk are especially valuable. Breastmilk encourages growth of intestinal flora, reduces respiratory infections and helps with optimal brain development through fatty acids in breast milk [not available in formula].

Mothers need patience, regular scheduled feedings every two hours, lots of skin contact and lots of time to feed.

When my cousin came to visit Garrett on Tuesday morning, she rocked and held him for an hour and a half. He received a bottle of Enfamil from the nurses, which he threw up. It bloated his tummy. He was rooting for the breast.

When I got there my mothering instincts pulled strongly. I wanted to hold my baby. I immediately breastfed him discreetly in a chair. Garrett held his head up when over my shoulder and sucked his thumb strongly. He was trying to focus his eyes and made noise. He seemed okay. I felt relieved. My heart yearned to heal him somehow.

One nurse told us that he seemed stable enough and could be moved to "intermediate," a step closer to release. That gave us hope. In NICU, the babies were only touched for routine work, not cuddled. "Kangaroo" care is vital by the mother—holding, rocking and breastfeeding her infant. I wanted to take him home and take care of him myself.

Garrett's development was delayed. Instead of feeling sorry for him, I dealt with trying to get him the help he would need. As he became a toddler, I learned to communicate with him and teach him sign language. Like I would ask, "Thirsty?" Or, "Drink?" while mimicking bringing an invisible glass in my hand to my mouth. He understood that.

NICU Recommendations:

Don't be afraid to ask questions. Use kangaroo care (holding your newborn to your chest in your arms) which is extremely important to the survival of your baby. Bring pictures of your family and place around the bed of your child. Request a stay overnight to sleep with your baby. Stay with your baby as much as possible. Breastfeed. Pump if you need to supplement milk bottles. Request a sign stating you want your baby to have your breastmilk. Check to see if there is a milk bank in your area that supplies to ICU babies if needed. Enlist the support of family, friends, church and neighbors.

Down Syndrome happens in one out of 800 live births. It is caused by an error in cell division resulting in a third chromosome 21, or "trisomy 21." Named after John L. Down, M.D., some of the physical features are: Flat facial profile, upward slant to the eye, short neck, abnormally shaped ears, white spots on the iris of the eye (Brushfield spots), a single deep transverse crease on the palm of the hand, protruding tongue, and a wide gap between first and second toe.[2]

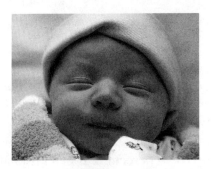

SECRET 11:

Go Confidently with Expert Encouragement

Ina May Gaskin, C.P.M.

Founder and Director of The Farm Midwifery Center, Author and Founding Member of Midwives Alliance of North America

Spiritual Midwifery, by midwife Ina May Gaskin, inspired the collecting of natural birth stories from women of *today* for this book.

The Farm's Midwifery Center delivered 1723 births over a nineteen-year period with an outstanding safety record: zero maternal mortality and only ten neonatal mortalities, three of which being lethal abnormalities. The majority were home births with 4.2 percent in a hospital. Only 1.4 percent of the births were C-sections.

So far, Ina May Gaskin is the only midwife that a birth maneuver has been named after. The Gaskin Maneuver is a position of the mom on all fours—hands and knees—for assisting shoulder dystocia. If a baby's shoulder becomes stuck during delivery, moving the mom into this positioning allows gravity to open the way for the gentle birth.

Another term coined by Ina May is the "Sphincter Law." The circular muscles of our body stay closed until they need to release the contents of the organ. "You can't order a sphincter to open. Why don't we call the *cervix* a sphincter?" Ina May asks. In dilation for labor, the Sphincter Law explains when a woman may be dilated but suddenly closes to a smaller opening because of being afraid or sensing the anxiety of someone in the room. Understanding how much the setting and her vulnerability affects the birthing mom means offering privacy, access to food and drink, and allowing her to labor with love instead of fear for the best outcomes.

Penny Simkin

Childbirth Educator, Counselor, Author and
Founder of Doulas of North America (DONA)

Right now, I'm writing an article about three epidemics in childbirth:
1. Epidurals are up to 90 percent in urban hospitals.
2. Induction of labor is increasing rapidly.
3. Cesarean rates are higher than they've ever been in the U.S.

In order to have natural birth, women usually have to take a lot of responsibility on themselves. They need a lot of courage to do it. The midwifery model fosters natural birth.

Epidurals

As a childbirth educator, I don't think that facts, risks or benefits are the most effective way to have people think about epidurals. Yet most people who want an epidural try to resist people who use scare tactics. They bring up, which is true, more instrumental deliveries, more fever, more septic (a toxic condition from the spread of bacteria or infection) work-up on the baby.

What people fail to realize is that in order to keep the epidural *safe*, you have to have a lot of interventions. Epidurals cause a slow down in labor, which means 80 percent of the time you have to have Pitocin. In order to keep the epidural safe, you have to have IV fluids running. You have continuous monitoring because the epidural can plunge the woman's blood pressure and cause problems for the baby. These are things that come with the epidural that every anesthesiologist knows, every obstetrician knows, every nurse knows—but most women *don't*.

They say, "Oh, darn. The epidural slowed my labor and I had Pitocin."

The epidural *always* slows labor. Almost everyone has to have Pitocin. It's a *package*. It involves a lot of wires, tubes and devices. This is what people don't realize. I think many women hear, "You must have an IV running, you must have continuous monitoring." It is a package that many women are willing to accept.

"As long as it doesn't hurt, I don't care," they say.

But others say, "Oh my gosh, I had *no* idea it's that complex."

My goal isn't to persuade people not to have an epidural. That may be one reason I'm effective. I believe the most effective way of teaching is this: *I want you to be fully informed, so you don't have surprises.*

Another myth is this: If a woman is free of pain, she has no stress. Many people believe this, including most caregivers like nurses and doulas, as well as most pregnant women. There have been studies that show it is not true. *The stress shifts for the mom.* They are delighted to have the freedom from pain, but then they think, *why is it taking so long?* All the technology. When the fever starts—which is common, especially the longer the epidural is in—there's a lot of buzzing activity. The woman thinks, *what's wrong here?* The staff talks about getting labor going, because they're on a time clock now. They don't have time to fool around. The woman feels a sense of urgency, but often people aren't telling her exactly why. A lot of her creature comforts are gone, like not being able to drink.

The decision to have an epidural is the <u>last</u> decision that you get to make. What I mean is you can't even roll over without the permission of the nurse. You can't have anything in your mouth. The position that you're in is dictated by the nurse. The smallest things are not your decision from that point. A lot of people are startled by that. A lot of couples with birth plans don't realize that now it's up to the nurse and staff what's going to happen. If you didn't want forceps or a vacuum, you have *no choice* if the baby won't come out and you can't push well enough. Before the epidural, you may have had more *ability* to push your baby out. Suddenly, you're not in charge.

Many women will say, "Whatever you want to do." But they are turning over their entire labor, their bodies, and their baby's well being to complete strangers.

When women search on the internet, they get a polarized, scary picture of an epidural. The risks may be tiny, but what is more compelling is that you're *totally* dependent on the staff and on all these machines. You feel helpless.

Inductions

There was disapproval of inductions in the late '70s for three main reasons:

- Iatrogenic (doctor induced) prematurity of newborns
- Overcrowded Neonatal Intensive Care Units (NICU)
- Huge unnecessary costs

For a first-time mother, an *elective induction* will double or quadruple the need for cesarean. I give a talk called, "The Seduction of Induction" for La Leche League. Induction interferes with the intricate and marvelous hormonal cocktail that starts labor. I wonder, if there is no medical reason, could we be giving up something that we don't even understand by cutting short a pregnancy by three days or a week? Does a baby benefit by a few more days in utero?

We certainly know that "term" is defined as thirty-seven to forty-two weeks. Yet thirty-seven-week-old babies are not able to calm themselves. Their ability to suckle, their ability to habituate to others, their cuddliness, and their consolability are all affected.

"Oh, why don't we go ahead and induce?" I'm the first to say, that if there is a medical problem, yes, let's induce. But if there isn't, I believe our babies miss out. Plus parenting is harder.

Michele Odent, a researcher and obstetrician who introduced birthing pools in the 1960s in a hospital in France wrote, "According to traditional wisdom in rural France, a baby in the womb should be compared to fruit on the tree. In other words, we must accept that some babies need a longer time than others before they are ready to be born."

An induced labor is more difficult than a labor that has started spontaneously. It usually leads to the need for epidural anesthesia and an oxytocin drip, which more often than not precedes a cascade of interventions, culminating in a vacuum, forceps delivery or an emergency cesarean. The "labor induction epidemic" helps to explain the rising cesarean rates all over the world.

Natural birth rates are about 10 percent or less, including in rural areas where they don't have epidurals. Many certified nurse midwifery practices are not natural childbirth oriented. They are in big urban hospitals and have a medical approach because that's what is expected of them.

In my childbirth classes, I draw people who want to have minimal medication and intervention, virtually all first-time moms. I have 40–50 percent natural childbirth. I teach a home birth class where 70 percent birth at home, but 25–30 percent are transferred to hospitals. It's a high transfer rate, although we have a good climate in Washington State to still support a vaginal birth in the hospital compared to other parts of the U.S.

For second births, the transfer rate is only 10 percent.

My main accomplishment in promoting normal birth is establishing DONA (Doulas of North America). In my opinion, DONA has been the best thing that has happened in maternity care in the last twenty years.

My work with abused women is in a book called, *When Survivors Give Birth*, co-authored by Phyllis Klaus. I think I have helped enhance the understanding of the special needs of the abuse survivor, especially with sexual abuse and helped caregivers understand how to be more respectful, more kind and more sensitive.

Cesareans

I've been in the field for thirty-five years working hard to promote normalcy. I see the cesarean rates higher than ever and ask myself *what have I accomplished?* Things are getting worse. It's depressing to me.

Regarding hospitals, I was just over at Evergreen Hospital for a vaginal twin birth. The nurses were lovely and the doctors could not have been more supportive.

I regret that they refuse home birth transfers, though. Right across their parking lot is a birth center that has to take people all the way into Seattle for transfers, about sixteen miles away.

The fear of malpractice is often an excuse. Doctors get paid more for doing a cesarean. They work for an hour or less and they get paid more than they would for a 14-hour vaginal birth. They may say, "I'll get sued if I don't do one." But what if they got paid *half* of what they get paid for a vaginal birth? I wonder if the cesarean rate would still be so high.

Mother Nature never thought that we needed 100 percent perfection. There is room for medical assistance. But, when a woman has a deep down confidence in her body, loves the pregnancy, loves the wiggling, when she starts contractions, even though they hurt, she allows the process to *unfold*. She needs encouragement and reassurance that it is unfolding well. She knows that if something *does* go wrong she's in good hands, but those things are rare. In my classes, I want to show them how well birth works.

Women who experience natural birth need to *talk* about it. Their personal testimonies make birth less scary. They can tell their friends, neighbors and co-workers what their birth was like and share what the many benefits of natural birth are.

Susan Akins, CPM

Pain Management for LDR Nurses
"Each one of us owes our life and breath to a woman.
To create life on this earth, some woman has opened
and has cried." —Birth, by Linda Christmas

Why do some women choose to give birth *without* medication?

Today, most women don't believe that they can give birth without technological or pharmacological help. This belief and overwhelming trust that Western women have put in clinical medicine for the last hundred years underlies acceptance of a model that seeks to obliterate or *control* pain rather than to approach it as a *catalyst* that can help women develop power to overcome a challenge and be strengthened by it.

In a biomedical framework, the obvious answer to pain is to *cure* it. That's a good and noble thing that we, as nurses, do.

But, pain is an essential element of life. We can learn to *face* pain. We can *use it* as an opportunity to grow. "Looking outward to avoid pain by turning to medication and technology is a cultural reflex," says Pam England, a childbirth educator, midwife and author. Our first reaction is, "I need to fix it."

Suzanne Arms, author of *Immaculate Deception*, talks about pain that leads to "growth and enlightenment versus affliction." Affliction is pain without end: pain without purpose, like thumb smashing. Pain is something that you can learn to deal with and something that you can manage.

Normal labor pain doesn't need fixing, and it can be a healthy sensation. Labor pain can serve as a warning that something is about to happen and we need to get someplace where it is safe for birth to occur. Pain is way of *warning* that birth is imminent and gives us time to *prepare* physically and psychologically.

I'm asked all the time, "Why are babies born in the middle of the night?" I think it's because in our days as hunters, gatherers, and wanderers, we were safer at night. We all stopped walking. We got to a place in a cave or under a tree or somewhere where it was okay and built a fire. The animals would not get our baby before we had a chance to hold it. That's probably why.

Fear is a cause of suffering. I'm sure you have all worked with women who were afraid. We experience pain in our mind, but it is shaped a lot by external factors: attitudes to pain, life philosophy, your age, nature of society and culture. It depends a lot on what people have come to expect, what they have heard, and how they have dealt with pain in their life.

Major injury, anxiety, and boredom increase the sensation of pain.

I talk to women who say, "Oh, I'm telling you, I could never make it without medication in childbirth, because my mother told me I have no pain tolerance." If you look at it in a different way, you might be more successful than you think.

Studies show that Scandinavian women describe labor as "good" pain, but Americans describe it as excruciating. They are terrified or they are in a situation where they don't feel in control. Women here don't have normal coping resources to deal with the experience that they're having. Look at the comparison:

	American Women	Dutch Women
Expected great pain in labor	54%	24%
Pain medication, thought needed	65%	20%
Successful with natural birth	16%	62%

Are Dutch women that much stronger than we are? Probably not. They have different expectations. American women see birth as a medical event, while Dutch women see birth as a social event. Their healthcare system provides for a "mother friendly" birth at home. They enjoy great afterbirth care, too.

Severe pain may not be seen as suffering if a person believes that it is *productive*, if it is getting you somewhere good.

In the 1930s, Grantly Dick Read wrote the book, *Fear Tension Pain*. He explained that if you are afraid, you tense up and you feel pain more.

We do women a disservice if we try to make them believe that labor doesn't hurt. But, if you expect something painful, it will be. The fear of something can make your anticipation of it a lot more difficult to deal with.

Robbie Davis Floyd, an anthropologist and author says, "Obstetric rituals transmit the values of society." Unfortunately, a lot of women in our society feel powerless. Many providers, whatever their training, think of women as powerless, too. We're dependent on science and technology, and stereotypes affect the care that we give and the care women receive.

A woman who's seeking a natural birth can feel tense when all her friends have had an epidural. She can feel under assault when others ask, "What are you thinking? Why in the world would you do that?"

Most people tell *bad* labor stories rather than good ones. Women who had a good labor are embarrassed. "I don't want to tell my friends that it only took me six hours and it didn't hurt that bad."

The great challenge of birth is the loss of voluntary control over basic functions. Women can be humiliated by actions they can't control. Does this sound like suffering? Yes. Or they can cope with the pain and feel more confident to meet other life challenges.

Autonomy is an important concept for us. It is the ability to make informed decisions and take responsibility for them. Women have to *understand* what they are deciding. It's hard if your mother is there saying, "Oh, please get an epidural. Please get it for me. This is hurting too much. I can't stand to watch you in pain." It happened to one of my patients during labor and I nearly threw her mother out of the room.

For lots of women, success in labor is not just the birth of a healthy baby; it is the sense of achievement that they get and a personal satisfaction that comes from choice, control, and support.

Going to a childbirth class does not decrease pain, but it helps the use of pain medication decrease because women feel in control. They feel they know what's going on with them. Focusing on pain doesn't help.

Women need preparation for the intensity of contractions without inducing fear. They need ways to cope. Remember: pain is *perception*.

"They are going to make me be quiet," a concerned mom said to me. That is an expectation and you know we've all been guilty of saying it ourselves. "Ah, that woman needs an epidural." Some women are quiet in labor and some are not.

Women need permission to do what helps them the most. Some women chant. If somebody is trying to keep their pain level lower, their labor will be slower. Strong labor requires power and aggression. Focus on this aggression and help them with chanting. If you don't like the cursing option, move to the moaning option. It's that "uuuuuuugh" kind of sound.

We all know how to moan. We've all done it, right? That's part of our work life—moaning and groaning. It releases endorphins. It helps women have a sense of control. I don't mean the high pitched sound. That doesn't help anyone. The low moan helps, growl like a momma bear. Humming or singing songs works, too.

"Nurses are the guardian angels of women and of birth." If we think a good patient is somebody who's quiet, controlled, and peaceful and women who are not like that are bad ones, remember: doctors view labor through *your eyes.*

If you are the labor and delivery nurse, or the postpartum nurse who's taking care of a mom, what the other providers know about that person is *what* you tell them and *how* you tell them. It makes a huge difference in what happens for that woman in her labor. Remember that your personality, your attitudes, your view of birth and pain, your support of women impact how a woman is treated in labor. That's why I say that nurses are the guardian angels of women and of birth.

Your brain's endorphins are ten times better than morphine. That's another reason women go without pain medication during labor: they get the best endorphin rush of their life after the birth is over. That's something we should SELL a little harder. Birth makes people go out of their minds. You all know that. You have to start using that bottom part of your brain. Where people get into trouble is intellectualizing too much. Patients that read 27 books before they come to labor sometimes do not do near as well as the young girls who are 16 who come in and do it. Sometimes our older moms that have worked hard to get to that point have studied a little *too* hard. They are cramming for the final.

The best ways to provide comfort? We use relaxation and distraction.

• Distraction therapy: Suggest to the mom to get in the shower for a little while. Walk in the hallway. Or, go lie down. Would they like to get in the tub?

• Environment: One important thing that we overlook is providing a safe *environment*. Turn the lights down. Bright lights increase performance anxiety. Get some soft music out. Encourage people to bring a few folks to their labor that support them. If you are having a birth without medication, though, it's not a big crowded party.

• Time interventions: Don't do painful interventions during a time that makes it more painful.

• Tune in to the woman.

Here's a scenario: "I'm afraid," she says.

"What are you thinking about?" (You don't want to ask what they are afraid of and do psychoanalysis). "What made you say that? What if that happens?"

Some want to have quiet all the time. I have some patients who don't ever want me to talk. And I have patients who don't want me to stop talking. That's where *tuning in* to the woman comes in.

• Aromatherapy: Lavender makes you feel calm.

• Touch is important. In our society we are afraid of touch. Some do not want touch at all. Or they don't want their husbands to touch them, but it's okay if *you* do. Nice, firm and long strokes in the direction of bringing the baby out. Water is wonderful, too.

• Understand your patient's satisfaction: Quick pain relief is not necessarily associated with greater *satisfaction* in childbirth. It's all about how women feel about their experience. How much participation or decision-making they had. What happened to them. What they were successful in doing themselves.

A 1993 study shows an important difference in outcomes between labor nurses who took the time to get to know their patients with an information sheet a bit better, versus the ones who did not.

• Only 5 percent C-section compared to 19 percent
• 50 percent less use of forceps
• Shorter labor

You can make a positive difference for a new mom, a newborn's life and obtain more satisfaction with your job as a nurse, too.

"My baby was born and suddenly there was no pain."

Bette Epstein
Director, Master Hypnotherapist and Hypnosis Instructor

My own births are much a part of the reason I do hypnosis work today. My first two babies, a year apart, came before I was twenty. At that time, the hospitals gave "twilight sleep" [a hallucinogenic] to laboring women. Do you know how horrible that is? I felt so out of it that I climbed out of the bed, even with the rails up, and ran down the hospital halls naked.

I hardly remember the births at all. I knew I had no control over myself. I thought, *I'm insane, it's okay, I'm having a baby.* All the medical students came in to look at me as I drifted out which was disconcerting. I didn't know if I was supposed to be gracious or not when the contractions came. It felt horribly cold; the room was freezing. When it was over, I didn't remember anything bad. I didn't remember pain or even what the doctor told me to do *or* not to do, either.

Ten years later, my husband and I decided to have our third child. We were so young when we had our first two babies that we wanted to do it again and enjoy the process. I found a new doctor, who taught at Southwestern Medical School in Dallas.

I liked him but, when my water broke, the obstetrician induced labor. He gave me Demerol. Did anybody tell you how awful Demerol is? You wake up for the contraction pain, doze off, and wake up for the next one, like they got it backwards. My birth canal never got ready to deliver and they used forceps. I was miserable with a terrible fever, too.

I knew the power of hypnosis for birth because it had a positive impact on my fourth birth. But, I didn't even know it was hypnosis.

When I decided to have our fourth and last child, I wanted it perfect. But, when the test confirmed my pregnancy, I panicked. *How am I going to get her out?* I cried every day. I even waited six months before going to the doctor. I chose not to have an amnio, which was required in 1982. Instead I went to a women's clinic to check the baby's growth. By then, I had read everything I could find.

Hesitantly, I ended up going back to the Demerol doctor.

"You're barely here in time to get an amnio test," he said.

"No, I'm not having an amnio," I told him. "I made a deal with God. I'm having a baby, and whatever kind I get, it's *my* baby."

"You don't have a right to bring a defective child into this perfect family."

How in the world could he assume I'm having an abnormal child? "You haven't even asked me if I have a cat in the house. Do I empty the litter box? If I exercise, take medications, or what I eat." Right then, I knew.

"So you can't possibly deliver my baby," I said.

"How could you make such a terrible decision?"

He wouldn't deliver my baby anyway if his partner was on call, whom I could not stand.

I started interviewing other obstetricians. I finally found one that supported my desire for a natural, drug-free birth.

"Fine, I'll encourage your natural birth," he said. "I'll do everything you need, whatever you want." He lied. He didn't do *anything* he promised.

One of the reasons I was able to go through with natural birth was because when I went for the childbirth classes, I looked around at women ten years younger than me. I thought, *if these little kiddos can do this, I know I can do it.*

I was in labor for the usual twenty hours. It was fine, except the physician made me lie flat on my back, forbidding other positions. I had severe back problems for *years* after that. He wanted to put a heart monitor on me.

"I'm healthy, I haven't taken a pill. I don't even take aspirin, nothing in years," I objected.

"Sorry, you have to..."

"Then I'm leaving. I'm going to walk out of this hospital *right now.*" I got away with denying the uncomfortable monitor in a traditional setting.

In stressful situations I practiced leaving my body. *I'm out of here.* I went up and watched from above what was going on. I rose above it until it was safe to return. With every contraction, I left. I heard my husband coaching me to relax, saw the green walls, felt the muscle ease up, and back into my body I'd go. I gave birth using self-hypnosis without knowing that's what I did. Later I learned this is a common hypnosis practice.

Our baby girl was born perfect. No drugs were used. My husband didn't pass out. He cried when he saw her because this was the first birth he had ever been able to be a part of. Together, we admired our child.

I saw a stage hypnotist's show once where my teenage daughter, Lorre, volunteered from the audience to take part in the show. She wasn't outgoing, but she was influenced to do things that were freeing. She danced on stage. She went into a total body catalepsy, which means stiff as a board, light as a feather. Her head was on one chair, her feet on another and the hypnotist sat on her. That's unwise, though, unless they ask you if you have back problems or if you're pregnant. But I was fascinated, and decided to research it.

I had a jogging accident where I fell and cut my face up in gravel. Despite the trauma, I put myself into hypnosis and didn't go into shock. I stopped the bleeding. I even walked home and called a plastic surgeon. In the hospital, I lay there for three-and-a-half hours while he worked on me. I had one hundred twenty-five stitches in my lips. I could have never done that without hypnosis.

Immediately after healing, I took a class in San Anselmo, California, to begin hypnotherapy training. After my first class, I was hooked. I'm ADD and it rescued me from Adult Attention Deficit Disorder.

Before that, my experience covered the arts and spiritual psychology such as grief, addiction and dying. My mother and aunts were midwives, taught by the elders in the family. They washed the bodies of the deceased in their rural community. My life journey was to take me back to my roots, all the things that were natural.

I opened my hypnotherapy practice in 1986. In 1990, I opened a school to train lay people how to become hypnotherapists. I trained psychologists and other healers about using this powerful tool in their practices.

I'm proud of the 500-hour course I teach. Only ten students attend class for twenty-seven days, from 9:00 a.m. to 6:00 p.m. I give a tremendous amount of homework, much more than the 200 hours I give credit for. I believe it is the best hypnotherapy training anywhere. We cover all aspects of hypnotherapy, from the things most commonly associated with hypnosis, like smoking and weight loss, to more complex issues.

Two-thirds of my students come from out-of-state. I include all of the esoteric practices, and how to develop your intuitive skills, subjects which can make you more in tune with your clients on every level. I bring in guest lecturers such as Timothy Trujillo, who gives a workshop on hypnosis for autoimmune diseases and HIV. He spoke at the United Nations on this subject.

I teach by example. Each day, a client comes in where I do the total session in front of the students, from the intake interview to the trance work and the after talk. When you have a new client, you can quickly look at their eyes, their eyebrows, their nose, the fullness of the lips, their chin and you know how to deal with them on a different level than going by what they tell you. What they tell you is not always what they need to tell you. Life is a like an onion, you peel away one layer at a time and sometimes you cry. Because of my own losses, I trained in Palliative Care and Grief counseling and even wrote a book about grief, *A Time to Mourn*.

Most pregnant women I see for hypnosis are preparing for their first birth and are anxious to do the right thing for their babies. The first thing I remind them is, "Your body knows how to give birth."

Next, I find out, "Where would you like to go? Where would you like to go in your mind?" You create your *own* visualization. I call it your "safe place." Nobody can come in unless they're invited in. It can be as awesome as a mountain top or simply their favorite room. For me, it was the ceiling so I could watch.

In trance, we practice an exercise over and over. In present tense, we project the *perfect birth experience*, which includes leaving the body during the contraction. You visualize it. The minute the first intense contraction starts, you're *out of there*. Immediately, go to your safe place. You'll know when it's time to come back. Okay, come back and go about your business. Next contraction, you're out of there because your body *knows* how to give birth. It doesn't need you to guide it. *Let* your body give birth. *Bless* that muscle that contracts and pushes your baby to life. Don't fight it. Don't try to control it because it's going to make it unpleasant.

I'd ask you, the client, to come in twice, once with the partner during the last six weeks of the pregnancy. You make a tape in your own voice because yours is much more powerful than mine. I give good instructions on how to make a self-hypnosis tape for a perfect, stress-free birth.

Hypnosis works because when you have an experience with your eyes closed, the brain receives that vision as an actual experience and the brain synapses begin to program in the new truth. You see birth as beautiful and you see yourself relaxed. You have no desire for tension.

A few years ago I took a workshop in Hypnobirthing. After completing it, I felt my own work was better. I didn't need to change my technique that had been successful for many years. With "hypnobirth," you must use its vernacular, but I'm not good at script. All of the work I do is spontaneous and unscripted.

Here's an example: Shortly before her due date, Amanda, a patient of a midwife volunteered for hypnosis in front of the class. She was a beautiful woman with an ethereal quality. Everyone liked her immediately.

During the interview, Amanda revealed that she had a bad experience with her first birth and she wanted to get over her fear. A thoughtless student talked about her *own* birth horrors. I kept telling her, "We don't need to hear this." But Amanda was determined that she must have ignored her.

Amanda suffered from a back condition and resigned herself to the fact that one day she would be an invalid. I suggested that when the baby delivered, she would have no more back pain. We talked about support from her family, her friends, her worthiness to have everyone around her contributing to the quality of her life. She mentioned that her husband had never been comfortable being a part of the birthing process.

After birth, she left me a message. "You changed my life, you're an angel. The delivery was perfect, the baby was perfect and my back does not hurt anymore." She couldn't say enough good things, how it brought her life together. Her husband was even more open and involved with her in the birthing.

This life-changing experience is not unusual with hypnosis. Once you're ready to make changes and own a plan, it is reprogramming. Your brain only knows what the sub-conscious tells it… the sub-conscious only knows what *you* tell it. All hypnosis is *self-hypnosis*. I can't change your way of thinking. *You* have to. I'm just a guide.

Aviva Romm, CPM, RH*

*Clinical Herbalist and Midwife, President of the American
Herbalist Guild and JAHG Executive Editor, Author*

Since 1986, I've practiced home births. I do what I do carefully and I do it well. If I ever practice where direct entry midwives are not recognized, I can say that I did it right. With home birth, there's a special level of relationship that midwives have with their clients. We get insight into when the women are well and when they're not. We train our *senses*. Our experience tells us *earlier* if things are going wrong. Not only do we have to make the call, get them ready, get them off to the hospital and drive, but we have more lead time.

For example, I had a mother with a large baby ten days overdue. There was a bit of meconium, slightly elevated blood pressure, and the parents were both a bit hyper. Nothing out of the ordinary alone, but combining all these factors, I suggested going to the hospital. The heart tones were going up and I noticed a certain smell around the mom. The mother had a chorionic infection, but it was something I noticed *way* earlier than the staff because I wasn't waiting for the *monitor* to tell me that the heart tones were up. I wasn't waiting for the temperature to tell me there was an infection. My experience of knowing what's normal told me something wasn't right. Hospital personnel said everything was fine, only to discover that it wasn't. That's not uncommon. It's not metaphysical understanding. It's a higher awareness because we, as midwives, don't rely solely on machines.

Home birth is a political issue. Whether doctors believe in home birth or not, mothers still have the right to safe care. Doctors should support that choice, even if they don't support the midwives themselves. I have a disclosure and consent form that parents sign. It spells out that there are no guarantees in birth and that parents understand the risks, the possible complications, and take full responsibility for the outcome.

My experience with midwifery is that if somebody is doing a home birth for the wrong reason—because their friends did it or it's the hip thing to do or because you saw it on the show, *Baby Story*—that's not the right intention. Their body will find some way to put them in the hospital because their own anxiety will prevent them from birthing. I try to make sure people are making the right choice for the right reasons.

My own births were vision quests. I wanted to *meet* each birth and find out what my body could do. I wanted to meet the challenge the way a mountain climber might approach a mountain. I did what I could to prepare physically, emotionally and spiritually.

I had never grown up with bad birth stories. All the women in my life had easy births. My own cultural orientation to birth was open and relaxed. I started studying midwifery when I was young. I was exposed to natural birth in the beginning instead of inculturated as an adult woman into the negativity of birth. I wasn't afraid of birth. I never thought about it any other way. I went into it open-minded.

I don't have a particularly high pain tolerance and I *don't* have great stamina. Physically I'm fit, trim and petite, but I'm not an athlete. But, I experienced a beautiful birth, seventeen years ago, when my son was born. Straight forward. Purely natural. There was no intervention. I wasn't afraid; I felt complete *trust*. I just birthed.

I never looked for something that was going to reduce my sensation of birth. I wanted to *feel* it. I wanted to experience it. I'm curious by nature, but I'm not a daredevil or risk-taking sort of person.

With my third baby, my labor was three times longer than my two others. I was afraid to let go. It felt like I was holding on to my muscles. A couple of comments made by other people, planted a little seed of terror that I never had with my first two, and I didn't have with my fourth. But, it gnawed at me. I had some self doubt.

Once I was able to let go of the fear in labor, I had her an hour and half later. It was *getting* there. That was one of my most powerful midwifery experiences because my other labors had been easy. They weren't challenging to me in that I never had a fear that I would have to go to the hospital. But that third birth was painful. It showed me how self-doubt gets in the way. Yet, it was more beneficial to me as a midwife than an easy birth because I learned *more* from it.

The benefits of natural birth at home are:
• You're able to call your own shots. It's not a matter of control over birth, because you *can't* control birth. You *can* control your environment, though. You don't have interruptions. You don't have people coming in literally 7–8 times in a row offering an epidural at the height of every contraction.
• It's more natural physiologically.
• You have more options: to eat, rest, or walk when you want.
• There is less exposure to pathogens at home than in a hospital.
It is important to prepare for birth and do some kind of spiritual

preparation that the woman can relate to. I'll have them do artwork, meditation, dance, or sing.

I give my clients postpartum support:
- Checking in on you regularly
- Making sure you are doing okay
- Reminding you to "take it easy" as a new mom
- Suggesting what to eat
- Listening to you.

Aviva Romm is author of *Botanical Medicine for Women's Health; Natural Health After Birth: The Complete Guide to Postpartum Wellness; Naturally Healthy Babies and Children: A Commonsense Guide to Herbal Remedies* (with William Sears, M.D.); *Vaccinations: A Thoughtful Parent's Guide: How to Make Safe, Sensible Decisions about the Risks, Benefits and Alternatives; Pocket Guide to Midwifery Care; The Natural Pregnancy Book: Herbs, Nutrition, and Other Holistic Choices;* and *ADHD Alternatives: A Natural Approach to Treating Attention Deficit Hyperactivity Disorder.*

* Certified Professional Midwife, Registered Herbalist

SIGNS REQUIRING IMMEDIATE TRANSPORT

The World Health Organization advises to go to the hospital/health center immediately[1], day or night, without waiting if any of the following are signs during pregnancy:
- vaginal bleeding.
- convulsions.
- severe headaches with blurred vision.
- fever and too weak to get out of bed.
- severe abdominal pain.
- fast or difficult breathing.

Doula Becomes a Midwife
Shana's Story

A Pastor along with his wife, a lay midwife, serve their community in a continuous circle—assisting those who are getting married, giving birth and facing death.

One of their members, Shana, invited her pastor's wife to be her doula at her birth. Since then, she has trained to be a doula herself, and continues her studies to become a certified nurse-midwife. This young lady was so inspired by her own birth that she has dedicated her life to helping as many women birth naturally as she can. Here is her story:

I always wanted natural birth. My stepmom had a birth center birth and a home birth. At a church in Oklahoma, the pastor's wife is a midwife. She delivered my brothers. I had great female role models to look up to growing up. I didn't want to have medications to *blur* the experience.

When I worked in the hospital, I'd seen other women who mostly had medicated births. They would take the epidural, but I knew it could be done without it. God created us to do it.

Now I'm trained as a doula and I help my clients with natural birth. I tell them that the hospital will try to intervene, even if you say "no" to drugs. Here's our strategy: We can ask the staff for *time* to talk about it. I tell the woman in labor, "Stay in there. You're doing fine."

Typically the nurse comes in asking why the epidural is being declined, "I have to tell the doctor why."

"Because I want to do the birth naturally," the mom says.

"I don't think your doctor will let you," the nurse says.

I'll intervene. "We've discussed it and want to stick to it naturally."

My own birth experience of having our daughter, Hanna, has inspired other women. "Wow, you're our inspiration," my friends say. I feel that it's not wrong to birth another way. However, Hanna's birth has influenced me to continue school to become a certified nurse-midwife.

When I was pregnant, I walked with my husband, Walter. I did prenatal yoga and enjoyed it. My diet is fairly healthy and I have major aversions to sweets and red meat. I prayed and meditated a lot, focusing on relaxation. I listened to spiritual music; I saved the tape.

I questioned, *am I going to be able to do this? Will I break at some point? What if my commitment wavers?*

Elizabeth, a lay midwife and our minister's wife, was my doula. At 5 a.m., I got in the tub and called out to Walter, "This is fast. Okay, this is hurting." I opened only to four centimeters and stayed at that dilation. I was mentally stopping the labor until my doula and my sister got there.

I labored in the tub for twelve hours. I tried different positions, but there were no breaks in between. I had to get from the tub to the toilet to the sink then to the bed on my hands and knees.

The pain was much more bearable than I thought it was going to be. Without talking, I went inward with my eyes closed and breathed deeply.

I'm not an out-of-body type, but I was not *in* my body. I was *above* my body watching. My body took over. We played music. My husband held my hand. He got right in my face, encouraging me. The doula and my sister rubbed my legs.

I pushed for one-and-a-half hours. They checked and opened me up...it hurt so bad I yelled. "Oh my God. I don't think I can do this." The baby's head had turned to one side. I was ready to push. I remembered what Linda, my doula trainer talked about "pushing against the pushing." That's what I was most afraid of, but I pushed baby Hanna out.

Birth gave me a feeling of empowerment and confidence. I'm proud of myself. It was what I wanted. After the birth, I felt good. People said, "You don't look like you've just had a baby." I felt high energy, but I had to watch for not overdoing it. I felt more connected to Hanna and Walter.

My husband said after Bradley classes, "Okay, I can handle this." He was so supportive after birth. He stepped up to the plate and handled it.

I breastfed, but pumping at work was a hassle. I continued for seventeen months and dropped the last few pounds of my weight.

Three friends who gave birth said to me, "We're inspired by you."

You'll do fine. Your body will let you know what you need. Learn ways to cope with the pain. How do you cope when you're sick? Some people like touch; that helped me through it. I say to other women, "You can do it. It's not as bad as you think."

Now, I know I can do it. *You* can do it, too.

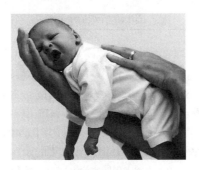

SECRET 12:

Prepare for Baby's Arrival

Beyond the Name and Nursery

Breastfeeding

*Breastmilk is alive and life-giving like a white
blood transfusion to your baby.*

The best time to begin breastfeeding is right after birth while your newborn is alert. Help your baby latch on properly by getting the whole areola (brown circle with the nipple) in your baby's mouth. The suction action of your baby helps to contract your uterus (along with external massage below your belly button) which is important to reduce bleeding. Colostrum, the clear fluid before your milk comes in, is the *perfect* food for a newborn.

Your milk comes in within a few days. The more often you feed, the less discomfort you'll have from engorgement, and the more milk you provide your baby. Engorgement, a normal fullness or swelling of the breasts, occurs when you first begin producing milk. Breastfeeding as often as possible relieves the pressure. Ice packs also offer relief. Don't give formula supplements or water to your baby for the first three to four weeks.

Watch for cues. Rooting, an instinctual turning of your baby's head toward you with mouth open, is a sign of hunger. Crying is a late sign and your baby's stomach may be empty and hurting. Feed your baby often rather than by a clock schedule.

Make a special place in your home to breastfeed—a comfortable place where you can sip water or an herbal tea or smoothie to stay hydrated. This will facilitate the milk your newborn needs. While breastfeeding, hold your newborn in varied positions—cradle, cross-cradle and football hold. The side-lying position in bed helps for feeding at night.

How do you know your baby is getting enough? Nurse for fifteen to twenty minutes on each breast to get the full fat content that comes toward the end, and nurse eight to twelve times in a twenty-four-hour period. Supply and demand happens with taking the time to feed, then you make more milk. If one supplements with formula, their supply goes down. Watch for between six to eight wet diapers a day while you are nursing. A baby loses an average half pound of fluid after forty-eight hours from birth which is normal before gaining weight within two weeks.

Top Ten Reasons to breastfeed your newborn:

1. Breasts are for feeding our young.
2. The bond between mother and child is strengthened by a hormonal release from breastfeeding.
3. Immunities in breastmilk fight infections, including ear infections.
4. Breastmilk is the perfect food, from the early colostrum or "liquid gold" to the high-fat milk.
5. A brain boost: Studies prove it increases children's IQ.
6. Breastfeeding reduces the chances of breast cancer in the mother.
7. Less waste in the environment by eliminating formula consumption.
8. It lowers the risk of SIDS.
9. Breastmilk tastes sweet and is freely available at the right temperature.
10. The milk soothes your baby's digestive system and their poop does not stink.

Breastfeeding is a *learned* art. First-time moms benefit from attending a LaLeche League meetings during pregnancy to learn how to breastfeed *before* the birth of their child. Watch educational videos showing the correct way to breastfeed. Be around women who support it.

Leave the hospital's "give-away" formula and bottles to avoid temptation. Keep at it through discomfort for the first six weeks. If you have problems, call a lactation consultant to answer your questions. Use lanolin on your nipples if needed. Together, you and your baby will learn.

If you breastfeed for six months, your baby will be better off than with formula. But the American Academy of Pediatrics recommends nursing for at least the first year of your baby's life. Babies who are breastfed for a year or more are less likely to need speech therapy or braces later in life. Enjoy this special time of nourishing your baby.

Note: Studies published in the *British Journal of Obstetrics and Gynecology* (BJOG) show that the use of oxytocin, known as Pitocin, to stimulate contractions or induce labor and other medications to reduce bleeding may *delay* a mother's milk from coming in during the crucial 48 hours causing mothers to give up in frustration. www.lalecheleague.org, Breastfeeding.com, youtube.com videos

The Case Against Circumcision

By Margaret Christensen, M.D.

As a second-year resident, I was moonlighting by getting paid to do circumcisions. But, I was getting sicker doing it; I would physically shake. Strapping the baby down, I questioned, *why are we cutting off the most sensitive part of his body?*

What I would tell parents in my own practice: First of all, circumcision is one of those procedures that has been done routinely and that nobody stopped and asked, "Why?"

It's helpful to know the history and religious roots of circumcision. Although circumcision is mentioned in the Bible, it began for non-Jewish families in England in the late 1800s, during the Victorian age. The idea was that boys who were circumcised would masturbate less.

Years later, the rationale was that it was more hygienic to circumcise boys. More recently, the rationale for circumcision was about decreasing the risk of penile cancer or cervical cancer in partners. None of these reasons have been scientifically validated.

What is true: circumcision hurts. The infant has *no say* in what's happening, bringing up the issue of lack of informed consent. Circumcision removes the most sensitive part of a boy's body. Currently, most places require anesthetic agents but the babies still cry from the needle used.

It is painful after the anesthetics wear off. Some say, "Yeah the babies scream, but it's quick." What they don't realize in the first couple of weeks in life, every time a baby needs to pee their penis is raw.

The foreskin of the penis functions the same way like an eyelid does for the eye. It has the highest density of nerve endings in a male body. Removing the foreskin exposes the glans of the penis to air. The glans becomes "keratinized" (the skin becomes thicker and dry rather than moist). Can you imagine what would happen to your eye if you removed your eyelid? You might see out of it, but it would become scarred and cloudy. You'd lose visual sensitivity. Studies of men who have been circumcised as adults have shown that they lose about 80 percent of their sensitivity. If you have been circumcised as an infant, you don't know any better because you've not experienced anything differently.

The American Academy of Pediatrics no longer recommends routine circumcision. It was thought at one time that urinary tract infections decreased among boys who were circumcised. These studies were done using inner city indigent populations and did not translate to the middle class clientele. But why are you doing something to prevent a urinary tract infection, which is *rare* to begin with in boys? There are rare medical reasons for circumcision such as scarring known as phimosis.

If circumcision is something you feel strongly about, why can't your son make the choice when he grows up? He can have it done, if he chooses, with an anesthetic agent.

The Procedure

When a doctor performs a circumcision, there are adhesions that stick the foreskin to the glands. A small metal tool is used to first break down the adhesions, then pull back the foreskin. A little device is inserted—it's either called a "Plastibell" or a "Gomco"—that locks around the penis. With the Plastibell, you pull the foreskin back over the area and tie a string around it and pull it tight. That's when the babies will scream. A scalpel is used to cut the foreskin off.

It has been shown in a position statement by the National Organization of Circumcision Information Resources Center (NOCIRC) that babies' sleep patterns are disrupted, as well as their nursing patterns.

Certainly when this happens to young girls and women in the Third World, it's called female genital mutilation. It has been condemned by the U.S. and other First World countries.

To me one of the concerns has to do with introducing *trauma* at such an early age. What are we doing to these baby's immune systems? To their nervous systems? Are we sensitizing them already to inflict sexual harm?

I heard Bethany Hayes, M.D. (Dr. Christiane Northrup's former partner) say, "One reason it was done in the 1960s had to do with the fact that a lot of young men went to the Korean War and got 'Jungle Rot,' a fungal infection. When they came back, they decided that their sons needed circumcision." But my question is, this: do you circumcise the baby because when they grow up, they *might* go off to war in a jungle and might get a fungal infection?

How many parents would participate in the circumcision to comfort their newborn? A few were brave enough, but most weren't.

I refuse to do it anymore. I send parents to a urologist or one of my colleagues, a pediatrician. "You might want to think about circumcision," I tell them. "That's socially accepted and done here, but you might want to ask *why* if it hurts the baby and there's no medical indication for it."

"I want my son to look like me," is one argument I hear from men. My counter to that is, "They aren't going to look like you until they are 17 years old. By that time, you are probably not going to compare them."

"What about all the other guys in the locker room?" is the other argument. I hope that we are raising our children in a way that they would understand differences. We have different hair colors, skin colors, and eye colors. We look different *everywhere*.

I did not circumcise my two sons. Even my mom agreed with me. Interestingly enough, one of the reasons has to do with my dad, who is European. European men don't get circumcised. They think it's ridiculous that we do in the U.S.

When my Polish father was seventeen, he was arrested by the Nazis. He was in Auschwitz and then Mauthausen (another concentration camp) for two years. My father was not gassed when he was in Auschwitz because he wasn't circumcised. They knew he was not Jewish.

My three brothers were not circumcised, either. They were among the few who weren't in the 1960s. None of them ever had a problem with it.

As global citizens, we need to recognize that around the world, 90 percent of men are not circumcised. Even *bris*, a Jewish celebration, can be done without circumcision.

Postpartum Depression (PPD)
Ann Dunnewold, Psychologist and Mother

I trained as a counseling psychologist. Early on in my training, I worked for Dallas Child Guidance Clinic with a great number of very young children, mostly three years of age and under. I began to realize what an intense transition that was, having a new baby, and how difficult that was for many women.

Then I had my first child. I didn't have postpartum depression per se, but at the time I thought I did. It's such an upheaval. People say, "You never know how much your life will change." There isn't any way you can know that ahead of time.

It's more difficult than anybody can imagine. When I had my babies, I worked part-time, but had no support. I experienced social isolation that many women do of not having a support group, no moms on my street, not knowing anybody else with a baby. One neighbor had a baby, but she was going back to work full-time. There was no one else to be with. All day long it was just my baby and me.

Defining Postpartum Depression

PPD is mainly a misnomer because most women have much more *anxiety* than depression. Some women do become tearful, fatigued, and withdrawn. But what's more common is for women to become riddled with anxiety and guilt—worrying if they are going to be a good mom, second guessing their abilities, and that sort of thing.

In *What to Expect When You are Expecting* by Heidi Murkoff, Arlene Eisenberg and Sandee Hathaway, the authors describe postpartum depression. Women may read it and think, *that's not what I have*...there must be something *really* wrong with me.

Sleep deprivation contributes to PPD; getting sleep helps recovery. It's actually postpartum anxiety.

Symptoms to Know if You Need Help
- Sleep disturbance: Can't go back to sleep after you've fed the baby.
- Processing such intense worries about the baby's well being to the point where you can't function well.
- Difficulty with normal activities of life: unable to eat, unable to keep anything down, not taking showers or getting dressed.
- Hallucinations or delusions.

The typical woman I see is someone accustomed to accomplishing lots of things, is a go-getter, and has no history of anxiety or depression. She suddenly finds that with a baby, she can no longer control her life the way she did before.

About fifty percent to eighty percent of new mothers have some negative feelings. It's when the balance shifts, when she has *more* negative feelings than positive feelings, that you need to pay attention. If you have negative feelings postpartum, it doesn't mean you have depression. It means you are normal. It's the question of balance: when there's more bad days than good days.

Exercise One—
Value What You Are Doing

You may find it difficult to adjust to motherhood because our society values *results* such as, "What did you do all day?" We measure our value with what we have accomplished. With a new baby, though, your accomplishment is taking care of the baby. You are making a contribution. *Taking care of the baby is why you are home.* I have women write down everything they did with the baby for one day:

1. Fed the baby
2. Burped the baby
3. Cleaned up the spit up
4. Changed the baby's clothes
5. Fed the baby
6. Rocked the baby
7. Walked with the baby
8. Changed the baby's diaper and more....

Fill up a whole page. Tally each time you do something. Put that up on the frig and say, "Oh, look I *did* do something today." Leave it up for a couple of weeks, because it's not going to change much. Take credit for what you *are* doing.

Exercise Two—
Renew Yourself with Small Bits of Time

We're all like a pitcher of water, and particularly new mothers who are home with small children. You keep pouring out, pouring out, pouring out. You may be taking care of the baby, you may be taking care of other children, you may be taking care of your husband, and you think you should be taking care of the house, or paying the bills. Perhaps you are also trying to work in a home business or returning to work. If you don't do something to fill up the pitcher again, you're going to be running on empty. Most women agree, "Yes, that's what I'm doing."

Fill the pitcher up again by doing *small* things for yourself. Take five minutes out of each hour, just to sit down and breathe. Sit down and read a magazine article. Break things into small manageable pieces. Do three- to five-minute exercises that renew *you*.

Cleaning

If you *must* clean when the baby naps, divide the time in half. If the baby sleeps for 20 minutes, 10 minutes for you and 10 minutes for the house. If the baby sleeps two hours, an hour for you and an hour for the house. You must replenish yourself.

Find Social Support

It helps to have neighbors with small children on your block. You can walk out your door and there's another mother you can talk to about your frustrations. You can watch her interacting with her child. You see that she's having trouble with that two-year-old, too. It's important to get vali-dation and support.

If you don't have neighbors, you have to look around for support:
- Early Childhood PTA
- Postpartum exercise classes
- La Leche League Groups
- New Parent Support Groups (sometimes at hospitals)
- Mothers of Preschoolers (MOPS)
- Gymboree
- Little Gym

Baby-proofing Your Marriage

Time with your spouse needs to be much more scheduled. Some cou-ples call it "couch time"—ten minutes to sit down on the couch together in the evenings. Some people make that clear to their children, if they have older children, from day one. "This is mom and dad's time, you go play." Or you do it when all the kids are in bed. But you have to make some time. It's sacrosanct. You can feel that there is more connection other than, "Hey, the baby spit up. Can you hand me a towel?"

We're a society that believes that if you put on a happy face, you'll feel happy. Husbands often fall into what I call the "bootstrap approach." They think she should be able to be happy. They ask, "What's the matter? You're able to stay home. You wanted a child. Be happy with what you have." This discounts the fact that the life you chose can still be taxing, demanding and hard.

A woman needs to negotiate a schedule with her husband so that *each* has breaks. Can *she* have ten minutes to go for a walk or take a shower while he watches the baby? If she is taking care of herself during the day, it is not going to be as big of a deal.

Mother's Helpers

I'm a big believer in "Mother's Helpers." They can be as young as ten if they have experience with young children. A Mother's Helper is *not* someone you would leave the house while they're there. They can simply entertain the baby. You can start the dinner. You're a little bit off-duty. Some ten-year-olds would be thrilled with $1 an hour. It doesn't cost you much.

Practicing Psychology While Shielding the Emotions of Clients

I have to be good about practicing what I preach:
- Drawing boundaries
- Taking care of myself
- Exercising regularly
- Using my social support network
- Taking breaks

I'm certainly affected by my work. When someone is having a difficult time, I think about them outside of work a lot. It's hard not to. I practice part-time which helps. I don't work any evenings because my family time is important to me.

For more information:
Postpartum Support International: www.postpartum.net,
Mother-to-Mother Postpartum Depression Support Book by Sandra Poulin

Baby Care and Safety Checklist

Newborn care

- After birth, place a cap on baby's head to prevent hypothermia. Newborns lose heat quickly.
- Wrap baby in dry towel and hold to your chest, skin-to-skin.
- Umbilical cord care: keep clean and dry. Avoid pulling the cord off. Avoid baths. Sponge bathe until the cord falls off in 8–10 days. Keep diapers below the baby's navel. If an odor or pus forms, use a cotton swab dipped in alcohol.
- Learn first aid and CPR

Baby-proof your home

- Cover electrical outlets and get rid of toxic house plants such as Dieffenbachia, Philodendron and Oleander. Purchase only non-toxic plants.
- Keep cleaning supplies and firearms locked away.

Protect baby's brain

- Never shake a baby because it could cause brain damage.

Take your baby out of the car

- Never ever leave baby in the car, an oven deathtrap. Keep purse or cell phone next to infant—a reminder when an infant seat is turned toward the back and the baby is sleeping or silent.
- Do not leave baby in a running car. An unlocked car with keys in the ignition could invite car theft.

Prevent choking

- Prevent small items like toys and food that cannot be chewed.
- Clear airway: Support infant's head and neck, turn infant face down on your arm—head lower than body, use heel of your other hand between the infant's shoulder blades and deliver 5 sharp, rhythmic forceful blows. Turn infant face up—head lower than body and use two fingers on the infant's chest (like CPR) to deliver 5 chest thrusts.
- Keep the cords of blinds, any wires, ribbons or plastic bags out of reach.

Prevent drowning

- Never leave your baby in a tub unattended or alone.
- Watch and block crawling babies and toddlers to keep them from entering pools, lakes and other water areas on their own.

Prevent falls, fire, burns and more

- Changing tables should be sturdy and use the safety strap. Never turn your back on a baby strapped to a changing table.
- Double-check latches on crib railings and use safety straps on high-chairs every time.
- Install smoke alarms and carbon monoxide detectors and keep batteries fresh.
- Keep baby away from fires, grills and ovens and other hot items that could burn such as curling irons, hot beverages or soups.
- Be aware of baby product recalls: www.recalls.gov

ACKNOWLEDGMENTS

Thank you to Margaret Christensen, M.D., my midwife, Susan Akins, and my doula Mara Black, Christiane Northrup, M.D. for her foreword and all of those who believed, shared their time, resources and stories—the mothers and fathers, midwives, physicians, nurses, therapists, anthropologists, doulas, educators and authors in this book.

To George Getschow, Kitty Ernst, CNM, MPH, and Audrey L. Graham, M.D. for reading the manuscript and sharing their feedback. To writing coach Jeff Davis, Suzanne Frank at SMU's Creative Writing Program, Larry Diana, M.D. and Dawn Patee, Pharmacist for the epidural information, photographers Steve Foxall and Neil Farris, and Tom Cellio for EMT training.

To Sarah Whyman at the Mayborn Literary Nonfiction Conference, Ron Chrisman, Director of UNT Press and the staff—Karen DeVinney, Managing Editor; Paula Oates, Marketing Manager; and Mary Young, Administrator. To authors Dan Burns and Susannah Charleson, wise counsel and mother-in-law Nell Jackson, Peggy Leeman, Yoka Bjeles, Jackie Burlingame, Virginia Brody, Ame Beanland, Julie Metz, Judith Rooks, Mindy Reed of Author's Assistant for indexing, Erika Liston and Jo Wharton for their help and support, and the kind words of those who gave their endorsement—Sheila Kitzinger, Dr. John F. Demartini, and Victoria Moran and Dr. Northrup.

To the "sisters of the sea"—the authors and facilitators of birth who encouraged the early conception of this book during a dolphin trip in the Florida Keys including Rima Star, Roberta Scaer, and Suzanne Arms. Plus the synchronicity of holding onto an unsuspecting passenger during brief turbulence on the flight back, Ellen Kassing, R.N., of Sutter Davis Hospital's labor and delivery.

To my family—husband William Jackson and son William Franklin Jackson, V, parents Peter and Sheila Buschauer and the late Donald W. Naas, and my sisters Lisa Naas and Beth Hooper for their cheering on. To my grandmothers, Agnes J. Hanson Naas and Elizabeth Clark Padley, who both birthed naturally at home.

—Kalena

All the midwives at Ben Taub, Jefferson Davis and Parkland hospitals who opened my mind and heart. The work of pioneering midwives Kitty Ernst and Sister Angela Murdoch, also anthropologists Robbie Davis Floyd and Carolyn Sargent, and authors Diana Korte and Roberta Scaer of *A Good Birth A Safe Birth*, the work of Klaus and Kennell on mother-infant bonding.—Margaret

To Frances Oldham Kelsey, an FDA inspector who bravely *blocked* the sale of Thalidomide in the U.S., a drug which unfortunately caused birth defects when taken for nausea in pregnant women in the U.K. in the 1960s.

APPENDIX

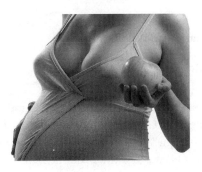

Nutrition

Creating the best environment for your baby to grow and develop in pregnancy means committing to a healthy lifestyle and eating foods with the most nutrition.

Ideally, plan to get your body ready *before* conception, eliminate unhealthy habits, cleanse or detox, and nourish. Women need folic acid—through food or with quality supplements—early in conception to help the baby form a strong spine.

Since almost half of U.S. pregnancies are not planned, be sure you are not pregnant before cleansing or detoxing because your fetus needs extra nutrition.

If you are already pregnant, supplement with a quality prenatal vitamin and a daily pharmaceutical grade fish oil supplement which helps your baby's brain to develop. DHA is very important. Also, take a high grade probiotic helps to prevent group B strep colonization and maintain optimal immune function of your gastrointestinal (GI) tract.

Begin adding from the list of superfoods and the top nutritional value foods for your meals. Buy and eat *organic* fruits and vegetables, whole grains, nuts and seeds, and quality protein—meat, fowl, fish or vegetarian forms of protein.

Get fresh air and sunshine, drink plenty of water, add snacks between meals or eat more frequently, adopt a moderate exercise routine, and get plenty of rest.

• AVOID AND ELIMINATE:

Alcohol

Caffeine: linked to miscarriage in the first trimester.

Smoking or second-hand smoke.

Drugs: illegal, prescriptions and over the counter drugs (OTC) including aspirin unless approved by your provider.

Other items: Inhalants, chemical fumes such as paints and varnishes, hair dyes, x-rays, cats, electromagnetic fields (EFMs) like microwaves and electric blankets.

Foods: Raw meat and raw eggs with risk of bacteria and salmonella. Deli meats, hotdogs, and soft cheeses because of the bacteria, Listeria, linked to miscarriage.

Fish: thick types of fish like tuna and swordfish because of potential mercury.

Foods of minimal nutritional value: empty calories or junk food such as sodas, candy, artificial sweeteners, preservatives, additives, flavor enhancers, and dyes.

• PRECONCEPTION CLEANSE OR DETOX:

Cleansing your colon and toning your organs is a good way to be ready for conception. Consult your provider on any program you are considering. Flush with clean water and juices and increase fiber by eating organic salads. Author Kalena Cook used Master Herbalist John Christopher's 3-day cleanse and prenatal formulation for the last six weeks of her pregnancy.

• WATER:

Drink filtered or distilled water, 64 oz. min/day (equal to two big 32 oz. bottles). Another easy way to figure the amount to drink is divide your weight in half and convert that number to ounces. Use glass, metal, or BPA-free containers. You need to flush waste out of your body continuously. Even though you need to use the restroom frequently, stay hydrated!

• PRENATAL VITAMINS:

Avoid synthetic vitamins coated with artificially dyed colors and synthetic iron. Instead, check the health food stores for a quality prenatal vitamin. Folic acid prevents birth defects.

Dr. Margaret Christensen recommends the Shaklee Vitalizer with iron strips as it has everything needed including fish oils and probiotics. She usually adds one extra Shaklee B to that because there is a huge need for all the B vitamins in our very stressed out, toxic environment which deplete B's (very important for birth defect prevention). She finds these strips are well tolerated. www.ChristensenCenter.com

There is a great chapter on vitamins and minerals in *The UltraMind Solution* by Mark Hyman, MD.

• PROTEIN:

In pregnancy, 60 grams of protein a day is needed for an average sized 5'3" woman weighing 135 pounds.

• SUPERFOODS: Foods packed with extra nutrition.

Acai - a dark purple fruit from the acai palm tree in Central South America that is high in antioxidents. Buy in health food stores versus online.

Almonds - not actually a nut, almonds are high in vitamin E, reducing cholesterol and the risk of heart disease.

Barley grass - eleven times more calcium than milk, five times more iron than spinach, and seven times more vitamin C than orange juice. Contains B_{12} and neutralizes heavy metals such as mercury in the blood.

Beets - high in foliate and prevent birth defects such as spinabifida.

Berries - blueberries' antioxidants destroy free radicals, help the brain and skin.

Black elderberry - antiviral qualities, short circuits the first sign of flu symptoms.

Broccoli - a good source of vitamin C and calcium.

Carrot juice - a source of beta-carotene, helpful for heart health and night vision.

Citrus fruits - high in vitamin C which protects the immune system

Echinacea - helpful as a tea or supplement at the onset of cold symptoms.

Eggs - fertile yard eggs, source of protein.

Flax - seeds are less likely to go rancid.

Ginger - soothes the intestinal tract and safely helps reduce nausea, grated in broth or to drink with water and lemon.

Goji berry - the dried berries are like raisins and more affordable than the juice, comes from China, Mongolia, and the Himalayas in Tibet. Contains antioxidants such as zeaxanthin, which helps protect the retina of the eye.

Noni - from areas such as Tahiti and Hawaii; the nutrients are found in the pulp powder versus the juice which only contains traces.

Kelp - the powder is an alternative to salt and contains over 70 minerals and trace elements.

Molasses - blackstrap molasses comes from the third boiling of sugar syrup made from sugar cane production. One tablespoon in water contains up to 20% of manganese, iron, calcium, potassium, magnesium, B_6 and selenium.

Olive Oil - a good fat that reduces cholesterol, lowers the risk of breast cancer, and helps the heart. An alternative to butter, use cold pressed virgin olive oil.

Omega 3s - found in flax and salmon.

Parsley - a great herb to sprinkle on meals after cooking. High in vitamin K.

Red Raspberry Leaf tea - tones female reproductive area with astringent quality. Helpful to drink tea after delivery to aid in breastmilk

Salmon - wild caught is preferred to farm raised.

Spinach - dark green leafy vegetable.

Spirulina - 70 percent protein.

Sweet Potatoes - high in vitamin A

Tumeric - used in Chinese and Indian medicine as an anti-inflammatory such as in the bowels, for arthritis and cystic fibrosis.

Wheat germ - contains vitamin E and folic acid, add to oatmeal or salads.

Wheatgrass - sprouted from the wheat seed without the gluten. Helps with live enzymes minerals and vitamins that immediately work in the bloodstream. Beneficial to mom and baby. Chase shot of wheatgrass with apple juice if needed to reduce the grassy taste.

Whole grains: amaranth, barley, buckwheat, oats, and quinoa are a few examples

Yogurt - organic source of calcium, protein and Lactobacillus casei, beneficial bacteria for the GI tract.

TOP FOODS FOR NUTRITIONAL VALUE

Folic Acid (organ meats & beans)

Chicken Liver 3.5 oz	770 Mcg
Chicken Giblets 3.5 oz	376 Mcg
Lentils 1C	358 Mcg
Turkey Giblets 3.5 oz	345 Mcg
Pinto beans 1C	294 Mcg
Garbanzo 1C	282 Mcg
Lima, Baby 1C	273 Mcg
Black Beans, cooked	256 Mcg
Navy Beans 1C	255 Mcg
Beef Liver 4 oz	245 Mcg
Yellow Beans cook 1C	143 Mcg
Spinach 1/2 C	131 Mcg
Soybean Sprouts, raw 1C	120 Mcg
Turnip Greens 1/2 C	107 Mcg
Asparagus	88 Mcg

Vitamin A

Organic Beef Liver 4 oz	40,436 IU
Carrot, raw, 1	20,253
Carrot, cooked 1/2C	19,152
Chicken Liver 3.5 oz	16,375
Mango, 1	8060
Chicken Giblet	7,431
Papaya 1	6,122
Cantaloupe 1C	5,158
Spinach Souffle 1 C	3,461
Pumpkin Pie 1/6 slice	3,700
Apricot Nectar	3,304
Persimmon	3,640

Vitamin C

In 1949, Fred. R. Klenner, M.D. recommended 10 grams of ascorbic acid for pregnancy for the healthy formation of the fetus and to protect against miscarriage.

Also found in citrus fruits, rose hips, acerola cherries, alfalfa seeds sprouted, black currants, guava, papaya, grapefruit, lemons, broccoli.

Vitamin E

Cold-pressed oils, wheat germ or olive oil, eggs, wheat germ, organ meats, molasses,sweet potato, leafy vegetables, sunflower seed, walnuts, peanuts

Calcium

Organic milk, yogurt, ricotta,parmesan, green leafy vegetables, collards, broccoli, tofu, soybeans, okra

Protein
  Meats

Lobster Newburg, 1 C.	46.3 Gm
Chuck roast, 4 oz.	35.2 Gm
Venison, 4 oz.	34.2 Gm
Leg of lamb, 4 oz.	32. Gm
Chicken, w/o skn, rstd.	30.9 Gm
Flounder, 3.5 oz.	30 Gm
Tenderloin	30 Gm
Goose egg, 1	20 Gm

Fish

Eat wild-caught salmon
Avoid steak types like swordfish and tuna because of possible higher mercury content

Vegetarian

Garbanzo beans, dry 1 C.	39 Gm
Soybeans, dry rstd 1/2 C.	34 Gm
Cottage cheese, 2%,, 1 C.	31 Gm

Vitamin K

Green leafy vegetables
Egg yolks
Safflower oil
Blackstrap molasses
Cauliflower
Soybeans

Top Foods Source: *Nutrition Almanac*: Fourth Edition, Gayla J. Kirschmann and John D. Kirschmann, 1996.

Exercise

What are Kegels?

Kegel exercises strengthen the pelvic floor muscles, aiding in delivery. They are the same muscles that cut the flow of urination. In fact, one way to begin practice is to urinate a little at a time, tablespoon by tablespoon, stopping the flow with strong contracting of your muscles.

1. Begin with 10 kegels per session.
2. Work up to 60, or 6 sets of 10, while driving. Use red lights as your time to begin.
3. Try the "elevator" kegel: contract up to the first level, go further up to the second and the strongest up the the third floor, then release.
4. The kegel "hold": contract a kegel and count to ten, gradually release.
5. In the bed: before sleep or upon waking, do your kegels.

Two other benefits of kegels are protecting against urinary stress incontinence and increasing sexual response.

Choose a moderate exercise routine daily—another key to vibrant health besides eating right. Remember to drink water during and after workouts. During pregnancy, exercise should never hurt or leave you totally exhausted.

- Walking
- Prenatal Yoga
- Stationary cycling
- Swimming
- Tai Chi

Epidural Ingredients

After you read the package insert warnings from the drug manufacturer, many women might rethink epidurals for routine use. The labels describe how epidurals fight the natural process and reveal the unintended effects that epidurals cause.

Bupivacaine and Fentanyl

1. **Bupivacaine** - an anesthetic which blocks the nerve impulses. Only in .25% and 0.5% are indicated for obstetrical anesthesia.

Warnings from the package insert: The 0.75% concentration of Bupivacaine Hydrochloride is *not recommended* for obstetrical anesthesia. There have been reports of *cardiac arrest* with difficult resuscitation or death during use of Bupivacaine Hydrochloride for epidural anesthesia in obstetrical patients. In *most* cases, this has followed use of the 0.75% concentration. Resuscitation has been difficult or impossible despite apparently adequate preparation and appropriate management. Cardiac arrest has occurred after convulsions resulting from systemic toxicity, presumably following unintentional intravascular injection. The 0.75% concentration should be reserved for surgical procedures where a high degree of muscle relaxation and prolonged effect are necessary.

There are no adequate and well-controlled studies in pregnant women of the effect of bupivacaine on the developing fetus.

Local anesthetics *rapidly cross the placenta*, and when used for epidural, caudal, or prudential block anesthesia, can cause varying degrees of maternal, fetal, and neonatal toxicity. Adverse reactions in the parturient (woman about to give birth), fetus, and neonate involve alterations of the central nervous system, peripheral vascular tone, and cardiac function.

Maternal hypotension (low blood pressure) has resulted from regional anesthesia. The fetal heart rate also should be monitored continuously and electronic fetal monitoring is highly advisable.

Epidural anesthesia has been reported to *prolong* the second stage of labor by removing the mom's urge to bear down or by interfering with motor function. The use of obstetrical anesthesia may increase the need for forceps assistance.

Nursing Mothers: Bupivacaine has been reported to be excreted in human milk suggesting that the nursing infant could theoretically be exposed to the drug. Because of the potential for serious adverse reactions in nursing infants, a decision should be made to *not* administer bupivacaine.

2. **Fentanyl Citrate** - an opioid, or narcotic, acting similar to morphine for analgesia and sedation.

Precautions: Fentanyl should be used with caution in patients with head injuries, brain tumors, impaired respiration, liver and kidney dysfunction, or cardiac bradyarrhythmias (slow irregular heartbeat).

Labor and Delivery: There is insufficient data to support the use of fentanyl in labor and delivery. *Therefore, such use is not recommended.*

Nursing Mothers: It is not known whether this drug is secreted in human milk. Because many drugs are excreted in breast milk, caution should be exercised when fentanyl citrate is administered to a nursing woman.

Adverse reactions: As with other narcotic analgesics, the most common serious adverse reactions reported to occur with fentanyl are respiratory depression, apnea, rigidity, and bradycardia (slow heart action). If these remain untreated, respiratory arrest, circulatory depression, or cardiac arrest could occur. Other adverse reactions that have been reported include hypertension, hypotension, dizziness, blurred vision, nausea, vomiting, laryngospasm (spasmodic closure of the larynx), and diaphoresis (profuse perspiration).

According to FDA estimates, more than half of the drugs approved every year that are likely to be used in children are not adequately tested or labeled for treating youngsters. Safety and effectiveness studies are is especially sparse for the over 7 million children under age 2.

Serious reactions in children include:

• seizures and cardiac arrest from the local anesthetic **bupivacaine**.

• withdrawal symptoms from the prolonged use of the painkiller **fentanyl**

"Protecting Pint-Sized Patients"
www.fda.gov/cder/about/whatwedo/testtube-13.pdf
Note: Italics added for emphasis and terms defined in parenthesis

Epidural Side Effects

Mother

- Increased length of first and second stage labor
- Requires an IV to reduce hypotension (drop in blood pressure)
- Increased use of oxytocin (known as Pitocin) to augment labor
- Urinary retention, requiring bladder catheterization
- Greater likelihood of fetal malposition and instrumental vaginal delivery
- Pruritus (itching due to the irritation of sensory nerve endings)
- Delayed respiratory depression in the mother
- Hypotension which may cause nausea
- "Walking" or "Light" epidurals have no ambulation (offer little mobility)
- Maternal fever, an allergic reaction, increasing if 6 hours on epidural
- Spinal Headache
- Shivering
- Localized short-term backache
- Loss of sensation in the legs
- Pushing ability diminished which increases the need for forceps or vacuum
- Use of instruments results in higher risk of deep episiotomy and vaginal lacerations
- Side effects may result in difficult mother-infant bonding
- Possible major complication risks, although rare
- Continuous monitoring

Newborn

- Epidural agents enter the maternal bloodstream, cross the placenta and have been found in the newborn's cord blood, confirming entry of chemicals into the baby.
- The fetus may suffer complications as a result of maternal effects (e.g. hypotension) or direct drug toxicity.
- Fetal monitor pierces baby's scalp in utero.
- Rapid heartbeat of baby or slowing down of heartbeat and drop in oxygen supply
- If instrument delivery is used, may bruise baby
- Unnecessary workup of infant for infections if mom developed a fever as a side effect
- Affects brain cells—dulls the senses and causes a stupor or sluggish behavior
- Newborn may be more prone to cry and to be inconsolable
- May have difficulty breathing
- May be less likely to be alert or less likely to breastfeed
- Interferes with mother-infant bonding
- Infant may have a poor state for up to 5 days
- Some studies question an increase possibility in drug addiction rates later if exposed to pain-relieving drugs in birth.

Little is known about the safety of epidural analgesia on the fetus and newborn.

Birthing Preferences

for Kalena Cook of "Baby Jackson"
Names: Boy–William Franklin Jackson, V or Girl–Britany Bergen Jackson

Prefer smooth admissions, waiving circumcision form, holding C-section form, natural vaginal delivery, least intervention as possible. Quiet, gently-lit room with *window* preferred, 6 hour stay in LDR and release to home, no separation from baby. Movement for mother and use of warm water in tub for laboring in.

Birth Team: Midwife, Husband/Coach, Doula, Pediatrician

Caring and respectfully cooperative nurse, when needed

LABOR

1. Wish for normal and natural vaginal delivery. Avoid C-section if at all possible.
2. If C-section is absolutely necessary, want to be awake with my husband
3. No routine drugs
   * No inducement or speeding up with Pitocin   * Want to avoid forceps
   * Guided imagery if needed
   * Going to try without an epidural   * Want to avoid episiotomy
4. Don't want my water broken. Avoid pelvic exams last 3 months to avoid PROM*
5. Limited EFM**: Wish to walk, position and work with body for contractions, shower, etc.
   * Drink liquids if needed
6. Sonograms only for emergency. Do not wish to know sex.

DELIVERY

7. Cord - cut cord after pulsating stops versus right away
   * Let my side drain into bowl, unclamped – shortens time to deliver placenta, prevents back-up of blood

BABY CARE

8. Baby rooms-in with me full-time
   * Bonding 1st hour to 1 1/2 after birth, no separation, clean and check baby *in my room, father is with baby at all times if not with mother.* Staying in LDR until pediatrician comes to release within 6 hrs. to go home

   Minimalize pokes, irritations —
   * Refusing eye drops. Blood tests show I have no chlamydia or gonorrhea
   * No PKU test – will have done at pediatrics office first week
   * Waive Vitamin K
   * Wish to breastfeed: no sugar water, no formula, no bottles, no pacifiers
   * No vaccinations or antibiotics after birth, plan to wait for PD
9. If boy, no circumcision. This is painful and unnecessary. (See resources)

* Premature rupture of membranes

** Electronic Fetal Monitor

Note: The risk of a C-section seems to be in proportion to the length of the birth plan. Focusing on what's important. Keep your birth plan to one page. You don't know what will happen. Have flexibility built in and an attitude to engage cooperation versus a militant approach.

Bereavement

Brooke Arnold, Midwife

I see natural births and I usually see things go right. However, if some-one experiences the loss of a child, the power of words is very important. In medical textbooks, for example, a miscarriage is called a "missed abor-tion." For someone who has just lost a baby, that term is the *last* thing they want to hear. To plan and want a child, then lose it is one of the saddest events a person has to deal with in life.

Some parents experience premature births, birth defects, or a still-born baby. You'd be surprised the things people say trying to be helpful, but they end up hurting the parent. "You can always have another one. You have a healthy child at home, be thankful for that. It is God's will."

Instead, they should simply *validate* their loss with empathy saying, "I'm so sorry."

If the baby didn't make it, the parents' experience is like they were launched into something wonderful, only to get it yanked away.

Our society says, particularly if the baby is stillborn, "Well, you know, you can have another one." We're not very good at proper responses. Don't say to a mother who lost a baby, "It was only a baby. You really never got to know them." It's not even really helpful to say, "It was God's will." That's a very offensive thing to many parents. How could God have want-ed them to go through this?

Instead, a very helpful response to loss is, "Oh, how horrible, and yes, you need to cry. And yes, you've got to take care of yourself. I'm so sorry. That must hurt so much." Just *validate* where they are and listen. Often, grieving is a part of postpartum depression, even if there *isn't* a neonatal loss. You grieve the loss of your lifestyle, the loss of the job that was impor-tant to you. There are all kinds of grief that women have to deal with.

Get help through social support groups and people who have been through what you are experiencing. Hospitals know of Infant Loss Groups. It takes time to cry, go to the grave, plant a tree, write a letter to the baby, whatever works. Churches can help, too.

Birth with Demise in a Hospital

1. In a hospital, a yellow rose symbol placed on the door of the moth-er's room signifies that there has been a loss and to be respectful. Usually the protocols are in place and the staff (LDR, NICU nurses, Postpartum and ER) goes through Sensitivity Training for a minimum of five hours.

2. The staff encourages the mom to hold her baby and offers a baptism to the family. They recommend to name, dress and take photos of the baby.

3. The mom feels scared. In disbelief, she wonders why this terrible thing happened. Instead of being taken to the cheerful postpartum mother-baby floor, the mom goes to the gynecological floor where she is taken care of without having to hear crying babies.

The way we practiced is based on a hospital-founded program called Resolve Through Sharing (RTS). The people in RTS visit hospitals' staff teaching the stages of bereavement and the grieving process. It is founded on research. One could even buy the materials, handouts, and packets. (See BereavementServices.org.)

There are laws on how you bury babies. If under 20 weeks of age, you don't have to go through a formal funeral home burial. Over 20 weeks, or over 350 grams of weight, there's a birth certificate, a death certificate, and the funeral home comes for cremation or burial.

It's not how old the baby was, it is how invested you were. Whether you told family or not. If not, you may be grieving silently. Processing through your feelings is not linear, like every day gets better. There are ups and downs, and time does help.

A mom once said, "It's been six weeks. I gave myself a limit and I'm still not feeling better." Or, two years later, you could still cry.

There is grieving with issues other than miscarriage or death. For example, a birth mother may grieve the loss of her child in an adoption. There may be grief when a birth does not go the way one planned, like a home birth ending up as a hospital C-section.

A lot of people who have the support of family and friends are able to talk about it and tell their story. Bereavement is a process. Know that men and women will grieve differently. You may experience some marital issues. Dealing with friends having children, attending baby showers, and going back to work can be challenging, as well.

I tell clients from the beginning, "Birth is totally unpredictable. You know what you want and you strive for it, but nature happens. You can't write your birth before it takes place. Of course, you always hope for the best."

You have many choices. Take a step and get the help you need.

Note: Brooke worked in a hospital helping patients deal with bereavement. She has experience with pastoral care and was a doula prior to becoming a midwife.
A Piece of My Heart: Living Through the Grief of Miscarriage, Stillbirth, or Infant Death by Molly Fumia (Conari Press, 2000)
Resources: PerinatalHospice.org, March of Dimes

Resources

PRACTIONERS
Midwives
- American Association of Birth Centers (AABC), www.birthcenters.org 215-234-8068 or 866-54-BIRTH
- American College of Nurse-Midwives (ACNM), midwife.org, MyMidwife.org 240-485-1800
- BabyOhm.com
- BetterBirthAmerica.com
- BirthPartners.com
- Citizens for Midwifery cfmidwifery.org, 888-CfM-4880
- FoundationForMidwifery.org
- MidwiferyToday.com FindaMidwifeToday.com/birthmarket
- Midwives Alliance of North America mana.org, 888-923-MANA (6262)
- MothersNaturally.org
- MyBirthTeam.com

- Canadian Association of Midwives canadianmidwives.org
- CappaCanada.ca
- International Alliance of Midwives midwiferytoday.com/international

Physicians
- American Academy of Family Physcians aafp.org, familydoctor.org
- American College of Obstetricians and Gynecologists, ACOG.com
- American Oesteopathic Association (Doctor of Osteopathic Medicine, DO) osteopathic.org

TOPICS
Birth & Advocacy
- Baby Friendly Hospitals by UNICEF/WHO, babyfriendlyusa.org
- TheBigPushforMidwives.org
- BirthNetwork.org 888-452-4784
- BirthPyschology.com
- BirthingProjectUSA.org for women of color
- BirthWorks.org
- TheBusinessofBeingBorn.com +DVD
- ChildbirthConnection.com 212-777-5000
- Childbirth.org
- ChoicesinChildbirth.org 212-983-4122
- Coalition for Improving Maternity Services, motherfriendly.org 919-863-9482
- GivingBirthNaturally.com
- Perinatal Education Associates BirthSource.com
- VBAC.com

- AIMS.org.uk

Breastfeeding
- BreastfeedingCafe.com
- Breastfeeding.com (videos)
- FitPregnancy.com
- Gotmom.org
- Human Milk Banking Association of North America, hmbana.org
- La Leche League International www.lalecheleague.org

Childbirth Education
- BirthingFromWithin.com 805-964-6611
- The Bradley Method of Natural Childbirth BradleyBirth.com, 800-4-A-BIRTH
- HypnoBabies.com, 714-952-2229
- HypnoBirthing.com, 603-798-3286
- International Cesarean Awareness Network (ICAN)

- International Childbirth Education Association, ICEA.org
- Lamaze.org, 800-368-4404
- SheilaKitzinger.com - Author and birth expert
- HenciGoer.com

Circumcision
- Circumcision.org
- Icgi.org
- NoCirc.org

Children
- Alliance for Transforming the Lives of Children, atlc.org
- Environmental Working Group ewg.org/childrenshealth
- Healthy Child, Healthy World Educating about chemicals and green, non-toxic steps
- Holistic Pediatric Association hpakids.org
- LoveandLogic.com for parenting
- Mindful-Mama.com

Down Syndrome
- National Down Syndrome Congress 800-232-6372 (770) 604-9500 ndsccenter.org
- National Down Syndrome Society 800-221-4602 (212) 460-9330 ndss.org

Doulas
- Association of Labor Asst. and Childbirth Educators alace.org, 888-222-5223
- Childbirth and Postpartum Professional Association, cappa.net, 888-My-CAPPA
- Doulas of North America dona.org, 888-788-DONA (3662)

- DoulaNetwork.com

Nutrition
- *Fast Food Nation* (book) and *Food, Inc.* (movie)
- FoodMatters.tv
- Naturalpedia.com
- Organicconsumers.org
- Whfoods.org

Loss
CompassionateFriends.org
Healing Hearts, babylosscomfort.com
Nationalshare.org

Postpartum
Postpartum.net
DepressionAfterDelivery.com

Publications
- *Mothering* magazine, mothering.com

Training & Accreditation
- Birth Arts International, BirthArts.org
- Midwifery Education Accreditation Council, MEACSchools.org
- The North American Registry of Midwives, narm.org

Twins
- MotherofTwins.com
- National Organization of Mothers of Twins Clubs, nomotc.org

Waterbirth
- BirthWorks.org, 888-TO-BIRTH
- Waterbirth.org

Note: names that are followed by .org, .com, .tv are websites.

Stations of the Baby

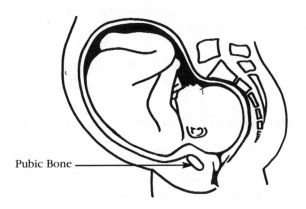

Pubic Bone

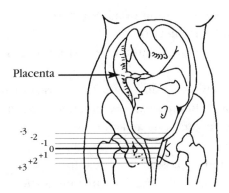

Placenta

-3
-2
-1
0
+1
+2
+3

Stations of fetal descent is like a reversed thermometer, starting at -3 as the highest station to 0 then to +3 as a baby begins to crown.

GLOSSARY

Active labor:The period of time when the cervix dilates between four and eight centimeters. Contractions usually come between three and five minutes apart, dilating the cervix one centimeter per hour.

Afterbirth:The placenta that is expelled after the birth of a newborn.

Albumin:A protein which if found in a pregnant woman's urine can be a sign of pre-eclampsia.

Alpha fetoprotein: A substance produced by the fetus. High levels in a mother's blood can indicate a neural tube defect, Down Syndrome, or multiple pregnancy.

Amino acid:A building block of protein which the body uses to build muscle and other tissue.

Amniocentesis:A prenatal test in which a small amount of amniotic fluid is removed from the uterus for analysis.

Amniotic fluid:The fluid that surrounds a developing fetus in utero.

Amniotic sac: The bag which holds the fetus and amniotic fluid in the womb.

Anesthesia: Using medicine to induce loss of sensation. General anesthesia involves the entire body, and local anesthesia involves only a specific area.

Anomaly:Abnormality or malformation of a body part.

Antibiotic:A drug used to fight infection.

Antibody:A protein produced by the immune system to destroy foreign substances in the body.

Apgar scoring system: A way of evaluating a baby's health immediately after birth. A score 0, 1 or 2 (being best) are given for appearance, pulse rate, grimace, activity and respirations at 1 minute and at 5 minutes after birth. A score of 10 is ideal.

Apnea:A temporary involuntary cessation of respiration.

Areola:The pink or brown area of skin that surrounds the nipple of the breast.

Aspirate: To breathe liquid into the lungs, or to remove liquid from the lungs by suction.

Bilirubin: Pigment in the blood, urine, and bile that comes from the normal breakdown of hemoglobin in the red blood cells.

Birthing ball: A large rubber ball used during labor. The woman can sit, rock, or bounce on the ball to ease labor.

Bloody show: Mucus from the vagina that is tinged with blood. This may mean that the mucus plug that has sealed off the cervix up has come out.

Braxton-Hicks contractions: "Practice" contractions that occur at various times during pregnancy, but usually increase in intensity during the last month.

Breech presentation: Fetal position in which the baby's head is up and the feet or buttocks are closest to the mother's cervix when labor begins. Complete Breech: the baby's buttocks are presenting at the cervix, but the legs are folded up "indian style." Footling Breech: the baby is presenting feet first. Frank Breech: the baby's buttocks are at the cervix and the legs extend up to the baby's head.

Catheter: A small, flexible tube commonly used in epidurals and when a woman cannot urinate (placed up the urethra and into the bladder).

Cervix: The lower part, or entrance to, the uterus.

Cesarean section: The baby is delivered through an incision in the abdominal and uterine wall.

Chromosomes: Long pieces of DNA found in the center of cells that contain the genes.

Circumcision: Removal of the foreskin from the penis by surgery.

Colostrum: The milk secreted shortly before and for several days after childbirth.

Congenital: Existing at birth.

Contraction: Periodic tightening and relaxing of the uterine muscle, working to dilate and efface the cervix to push the baby down the birth canal.

Crowning: The point in labor when the baby's head can be seen at the vagina and is ready to pass into the birth canal.

Dilation: The amount the cervix opens for childbirth, measured in centimeters. At ten centimeters, the mother is "fully dilated" and is ready to push.

Doppler: A machine that uses ultrasound to monitor the baby's heartbeat.

Down syndrome: A genetic disorder that results in mental handicap and medical problems.

Eclampsia: A serious pregnancy complication, characterized by high blood pressure and edema. It is the more severe form of preeclampsia, and is also known as pregnancy-induced hypertension or toxemia.

Ectopic pregnancy: Pregnancy in which the embryo grows outside the uterus, usually in one of the fallopian tubes.

Edema: Retention of fluid in body tissues resulting in swelling.

Effacement: Thinning and shortening of the cervix during labor in preparation for birth.

Electronic Fetal Monitoring (EFM): an external belt with sensors to track fetal heart rate in labor through ultrasound and produces a printed chart. Remote monitoring without wires, called telemetry permits free movement such as walking. Some feel continuous monitoring leads to more interventions. If internal monitoring is used, a wire is attached to the baby's scalp for continuous tracking. A stethoscope or periodic monitoring is also an option. Normal fetal heart rate should be 120 to 160 beats per minute.

Embryo: The name given to the developing fertilized egg until eight weeks after conception.

Endometriosis: A painful condition in which tissue that normally lines the uterus grows in another area of the body, usually the abdomen.

Epidural: A type of local anesthesia used to decrease or eliminate pain during delivery.

Episiotomy: An incision made to the perineum (area between the vagina and rectum) to widen the vaginal opening for delivery.

External version: Procedure in which the doctor/midwife manually attempts to move a breech baby into the head-down position for birth, usually done late in pregnancy.

Fallopian tubes: Two narrow tubes that extend from the ovaries to the uterus.

Fetus: The baby in utero from eight weeks until birth. The word fetus means "young one."

Fundus: The top of the uterus.

Gaskin maneuver: A birthing position in which the mother is on "all fours," used for the vaginal delivery of a baby with shoulder dystocia.

Gestational age: The fetus's age, measured from the first day of the last menstrual period.

Gestational diabetes: Diabetes that develops during pregnancy and usually subsides after delivery.

Group B Strep: A type of bacterial infection that affects 10–25% of all pregnant women and can cause serious health problems in a newborn, who contracts it during birth. The infection is usually treated with IV antibiotics.

Gynecologist: A physician who specializes in the health of the female reproductive system.

Hemorrhage: Loss of blood, either externally or internally.

Hormone: A chemical released by glands to stimulate certain activity in the body.

Induction: Artificial starting or accelerating of labor, usually though the use of Pitocin, placing prostaglandin gel on the cervix, or by rupturing the membranes.

Jaundice: A yellow discoloration of a newborn's eyes and skin caused by an excess of bilirubin, a substance produced by the normal breakdown of red blood cells.

Kegels: an exercise to strengthen the pelvic floor muscles, described in Appendix.

Labia: The inner and outer "lips," or skin folds at the opening of the vagina.

Lactation: Milk production by the breasts.

Lanugo: Fine, downy hair present on the body of a fetus.

Lightening: Also called "engagement," the time when the baby descends into the pelvic cavity in preparation for birth.

Lochia: Post-partum vaginal discharge including blood, mucus, and other fluids.

Meconium: The baby's first bowel movement, normally discharged shortly after birth.

Miscarriage: Spontaneous ending of the pregnancy prior to 24 weeks' gestation, before the fetus can survive outside the uterus; most common in the first trimester.

Mucus plug: A jellylike substance that seals off the cervix and is expelled before delivery.

Neonatal: Referring to a newborn infant.

Obstetrician: A doctor who specializes in the care of women through pregnancy and childbirth.

Ovulation: Release of a mature egg from the ovary.

Oxytocin: A hormone secreted by the pituitary gland during labor to stimulate contractions and milk production. It is sometimes administered in synthetic form, called Pitocin.

Pediatrician: A doctor who specializes in the medical care of infants, children, and adolescents.

Pelvic floor: The muscles that hold the pelvic organs in place.

Perineum: The muscle and tissue between the genitals and the anus.

Phenylketonuria (PKU): An inherited congenital disorder that can lead to mental retardation.

Pitocin: The synthetic form of the hormone oxytocin, used to stimulate labor.

Placenta: The tissue which connects the mother and fetus that transports nourishment and takes away waste during gestation.

Placental abruption: Premature separation of the placenta from the uterus prior to delivery, often causing bleeding and severe contractions; an emergency C-section would be required.

Placenta previa: A condition in which the placenta lies very low in the uterus and partially or completely covers the cervix, hindering vaginal delivery.

Postpartum: The period of time after birth.

Pre-eclampsia: A disorder of pregnancy characterized by high blood pressure, edema, and abnormal kidney function.

Presentation: The position of the baby before labor begins.

Prolapse of the cord: A situation during or before delivery in which the umbilical cord slips through the birth canal before the baby.

Quickening: When the mother first feels the fetus move, usually between 18–22 weeks.

Rh factor: A type of protein on the surface of red blood cells.

Rubella: A disease which, if contracted by a woman during pregnancy, can result in birth defects. It is also called German measles.

Show: The blood-stained mucus from the vagina, a sign that labor is about to begin.

Term: Referring to a full 40-week pregnancy.

Toxemia of pregnancy: Also called pregnancy-induced hypertension, it is a serious disorder of pregnancy in which poisonous compounds are present in the bloodstream. Symptoms may include elevated maternal blood pressure, edema, and protein in the urine.

Toxoplasmosis: An infection caused by a parasite found in cat feces.

Transverse presentation: Position in which the fetus is lying at right angles to, or across, the cervix when labor begins.

Trimester: One-third of a pregnancy, three months in each trimester.

Tubal pregnancy: Condition in which a fertilized egg begins to develop in the fallopian tube.

Ultrasound: The use of sonography to form visual images of the fetus.

Umbilical cord: The structure which carries blood, oxygen, and nutrients to the baby from the placenta during pregnancy.

Vacuum extractor: A medical instrument that attaches to the baby's head and helps guide it through the birth canal during delivery.

VBAC: Acronym for vaginal birth after cesarean.

Vernix: A white, waxy, cheese-like substance that covers and protects the fetus in the uterus and is present at birth.

NOTES

Introduction

1. World Health Organization, "Natural Childbirth Options," http://www.medicinenet.com /script/main/art.asp?articlekey=51188
2. Center for Disease Control Birth Statistics: www.cdc.gov
3. Natural birth may not be an option for "high-risk" women with health issues such as high blood pressure, known as hypertension or preeclampsia, diabetes, sexually transmitted diseases (STDs), kidney or urinary tract infection know as pyelonephritis, and genital tract abnormalities. These cases are referred to a Maternal-Fetal Medicine specialist.
4. CDC Birth Stats
5. The total number of midwives includes certified-nurse midwives and certified professional midwives.

Chapter 1

BirthQuest:

1. Diana Korte and Roberta Scaer, *A Good Birth, A Safe Birth* (Boston: Harvard Common Press, 1992): 38.

VBAC:

1. In Chapter 7—"Find Out How Birth Centers Bridge the Choice"- Elizabeth Gilmore, Midwife and Founder of Northern New Mexico Women's Health and Birth Center, Taos, NM.
2. In Chapter 5—"Know There's a Reason for the Squeezin'"—Dolphin Spirit.
3. In Chapter 2—"Get Informed and Shop Around"—See the CIMS Info and 10 Questions.
4. Robbie Davis-Floyd, *Birth as an American Rite of Passage* (Berkeley: University of California, 2004).

Chapter 2

1. Marsden Wagner, *Pursuing the Birth Machine: The Search for Appropriate Birth Technology* (ACE Graphics, 1994).
2. SB Barnett, Semin *Ultrasound CT MR* Oct. 23, 2002, 387-91 (from PubMed).
3. Newnham, J.P., Evans, S.F., Michael, C.A., Stanley, F.J., & Landau, L.I., *The Lancet*, 342 (Oct. 9, 1993): 887-891.
4. GJ Vella, VF Humphrey, FA Duck, SB Barnett, *Ultrasound Med Biol* 29 No. 8, (Aug. 2003): 1193-204.
5. D. Marinac-Dabic, C.J. Krulewitch, R.M. Moore Jr., *Epidemiology*, 2002 May; 13 (3 Suppl):S19-22. Center for Devices and Radiological Health, Food and Drug Administration, Rockville, MD 20850, USA.
6. Rob Edwards, "Shadow of a Doubt," *New Scientist,* June 1999.
7. Ian Sample, "Ultrasound Scans May Disrupt Fetal Brain Development," *New Scientist*, December 10, 2001. Journal reference: Epidemiology, Vol 12, p. 618.
8. Eugenie Samuel, "Fetuses Can Hear Ultrasound Examinations," *New Scientist*, December 4, 2001.
9. British Medical Ultrasound Society, BMUS Safety Guidelines, chaired by Francis Duck.

10. "Avoid Fetal 'Keepsake' Images, Heartbeat Monitors." *www.fda.gov./ForConsumers/ ConsumerUpdates/ucm095508.htm.* U.S. Department of Health & Human Services, FDA U.S. Food and Drug Administration, 2/19/2010. Online. 3/2/10.
11. European Federation of Societies for Ultrasound in Medicine and Biology, EFSUMB Clinical Safety Statement 2000.

Chapter 3
1. Melender, Hanna-Leenba, "Experiences of Fears Associated with Pregnancy and Childbirth: A Study of 329 Pregnant Women." *Birth* Vol 29, Number 2, June 2002.
2. Schmidt, Brad and Jeffrey Winters, "Anxiety After 9/11," *Psychology Today,* January 2002.

Chapter 5
1. Merlin Stone, *When God Was a Woman* (New York: Barnes & Noble Books, 1993).
2. Jeanne Achterberg, *Woman as Healer* (Boston: Shambhala, 1990).
3. Achterberg.
4. Achterberg.
5. Donald Caton, Michael Freolich, and Tammy Euliano. "Anesthesia for Childbirth: Controversy and Change." *American Journal of Obstetrics & Gynecology (AJOG)* Vol. 186, No. 5 (May 2002): S25-S30.
   OBSTETRIC Anesthesia, third edition, editor David Chesnut, Elsevier Mosby.
   Chapter 1 The history of Obstetric Anesthesia Donald Caton,
   Chapter 21 Epidural and Spinal Anesthesia part III: Effect on the progress of labor and method of delivery David Chesnut.
6. Suzanne Arms, *Immaculate Deception II* (Berkeley: Celestial Arts, 1994); Diana Korte and Roberta Scaer. *A Good Birth, A Safe Birth* (Boston: Harvard Common Press, 1992); Robbie Davis-Floyd, *Birth as an American Rite of Passage* (Berkeley: University of California, 2004).
7. Enkins.
8. E.D. Hodnett, "Pain and Women's Satisfaction with the Experience of Childbirth: A Systematic Review." *AJOG*, 186,5, 2002a, S160-172.
9. TR Marmor and David M. Krol, "Labor pain management in the United States: Understanding patterns and the issue of choice." *AJOG* 186, No 5 (2002): S173-180.

Epidurals:
1. LJ Mayberry, D. Clemmens, DE Anindya, "Epidural side effects, co-interventions and care of women during childbirth: A systematic review," *AJOG* 186, No 5 (2002): S81-S92.
2. Ibid.
3. Henci Goer, *Obstetric Myths vs Research Realities* (Westport: Bergin & Garvey, 1995).
4. Mayberry supplement.
5. Ellice Lieberman and Carol O'Donoghue, "Unintended effects of epidural analgesia during labor: A systematic review." *AJOG* 186, 5 (2002): S31-68.
6. "Pitocin Side Effects," http://www.drugs.com/sfx/pitocin-side-effects.html (accessed June 4, 2010).

7. Lieberman supplement; Barbara Leighton and Stephen H. Halpern, "The effects of epidural analgesia on labor, maternal, and neonatal outcomes: A systematic review," *AJOG* 186, 5 (2002): S69-77.
8. Lieberman.
9. Ibid.
10. Lieberman; Leighton.
11. Lieberman.
12. Lieberman; Leighton.
13. Leighton.
14. Leanne Bricker and Tina Lavender, "Parenteral opiods for labor pain relief: A systematic review," *AJOG* 186, 5 (2002): S94-109.
15. Lieberman.
16. Sepkowski et al "The effects of maternal epidural anesthesia on neonatal behavior during the first month." *Dev Med Child Neurol* 34 (1992): 1072-80.
17. Murray Enkin, "Effects of epidural anesthesia on newborns and their mothers," *Child Dev* 52 (1981): 71-82.
18. Bertil Jacobsen, "Obstetric care and proneness of offspring to suicide as adults: Case-control study," *BMJ* 317 (1998): 1346-49; K. Nyberg, et al. "Perinatal medication as a potential risk factor for adult drug abuse in a North American cohort," *Epidemiology* 11 (2000):715-6.
19. Lieberman, 175-176.
20. Bricker and Lavender.
21. Lieberman, 79, 117, 119, 143-146.
22. Lieberman, S56.
23. Ibid.
24. JD Traynor et al. "Is the management of epidural analgesia associated with an increased risk of cesarean delivery?" *AJOG* 182 No. 5 (May 2000): 1058-1062.

25. Verena Geissbyhler, "Waterbirths: A Comparative Study. A Prospective Study on More than 2,000 Waterbirths." Jakob Eberhard Clinic for Obstetrics and Gynecology, Thurgauisches Kantonsspital, Frauenfeld Switzerland *Fetal Diagnsosis and Therapy* 15:5 (2000): 291-300.

Chapter 7
1. 1989 *New England Journal of Medicine* report on the National Birth Center Study.
2. National Association of Childbearing Centers (NACC), Kate Bauer, Executive Director interview.

Chapter 9
1. The World Health Organization released a survey in January, 2010 that found while C-sections help reduce the risks of major complications, elective surgeries put mother and baby at greater risk.
Harmon, Katherine. "Elective cesarean sections are too risky, WHO study says." *Scientific American*, January 11, 2010, www.scientificamerican.com/blog/post.cfm?id= elective-cesarean-sections-are-too-21010-01-11&print=true

Chapter 10

1. F. Cardini and H. Weixin, "Moxibustion for correction of breech presentation: A randomized controlled trial." *JAMA* 280 18 (1998): 1580-84.

2. www.nichd.nih.gov/publications/pubs/downsyndrome.cfm

Chapter 11

1. The World Health Organization, http://whqlibdoc.who.int/publications/2006/924159084X_eng.pdf

Appendix

Nutrition
http://pregnancychildbirth.suite101.com/article.cfm/the_truth_about_caffeine_
http://www.americanpregnancy.org/pregnancycomplications/listeria.html
http://www.fns.usda.gov/cnd/menu/fmnv.htm

BIBLIOGRAPHY

Achterberg, Jeanne. *Woman as Healer.* Boston: Shambhala, 1991.

American Journal of Obstetrics and Gynecology (AJOG) General Books LLC, 2010.

Arms, Suzanne. *Immaculate Deception II.* Berkeley: Celestial Arts, 1994.

"Avoid Fetal 'Keepsake' Images, Heartbeat Monitors." *www.fda.gov./ForConsumers/ ConsumerUpdates/ucm095508.htm.* U.S. Department of Health & Human Services, FDA U.S. Food and Drug Administration, 2/19/2010. Online. 3/2/10.

Balaskas, Janet. *Active Birth.* Boston: Harvard Common Press, 1992.

Barnett, S.B. Semin Ultrasound CT MR Oct. 23, 2002 387-91 www.ncbi.nlm.nih.gov/ PubMed/

Birth: Issues in Preinatal Care, Hoboken: Wiley-Blackwell, quarterly.

Bradley, M.D., Robert. *Husband-Coached Childbirth.* New York: Bantam Dell, 2008.

Bricker, Leanne and Tina Lavender. "Parenteral opiods for labor pain relief: A systematic review." *AJOG* 186, 5 (2002): S94-109.

British Medical Ultrasound Society, BMUS. Safety Guidelines. www.bmus.org (2010)

Cardini, F. and H. Weixin. "Moxibustion for correction of breech presentation: A randomized controlled trial." *JAMA* 280 18 (1998): 1580-84.

Caton, Donald, Michael Freolich, and Tammy Euliano. "Anesthesia for Childbirth: Controversy and Change." *AJOG* 186, No. 5 (May 2002): S25-S30.

Center for Disease Control (CDC) Birth Statistics. http://www.cdc.gov/nchs/fastats/births.htm (accessed June 3, 2010).

Center for Disease Control Birth Statistics. www.cdc.gov

Christmas, Linda. *Birth.* poem.

Coalition for Improving Maternity Services (CIMS) www. motherfriendly.org/pdf/Having_a_Baby-English. pdf

Cochrane Library: Pregnancy & Childbirth www.thecochranelibrary.com

Davis-Floyd, Robbie. *Birth as an American Rite of Passage.* Berkeley: University of California, 2004.

Dew, M.D., Ronald. *Brushed by an Angel's Wings.* Privately published, 1992.

Dick-Reed, Grantly. *Childbirth Without Fear: The Principles and Practice of Natural Childbirth.* London: Pinter & Martin Ltd., 2005.

Edwards, Rob. "Shadow of a Doubt." *New Scientist,* June 12, 1999. http://www.newscientist.com/article/mg16221903.800-shadow-of-a-doubt.html

England, Pam. *Birthing From Within.* Albuquerque: Partera Press, 1998.

Enkin, Murray, Mark J.N.C. Keirse, et al., *A Guide to Effective Care in Pregnancy and Childbirth.* Oxford: Oxford University Press, 2000.

European Federation of Societies for Ultrasound in Medicine and Biology, EFSUMB Clinical Safety Statement 2000. www.efsumb.org/guidelines/2008safstat.pdf

Gaskin, Ina May. *Spiritual Midwifery.* Summertown: The Book Publishing Co., 2002.

Geissbyhler, Verena. "Waterbirths: A Comparative Study. A Prospective Study on More than 2,000 Waterbirths." Jakob Eberhard Clinic for Obstetrics and Gynecology, Thurgauisches Kantonsspital, Frauenfeld Switzerland *Fetal Diagnosis and Therapy,* Sep-Oct. 15, 2000, No. 5, 291-300. www.ncbi.nlm.nih.gov/pubmed/10971083 http://content.karger.com/ProdukteDB/produkte.asp?Aktion=ShowAbstract& ArtikelNr=21024&Ausgabe=225774&ProduktNr=224239

Goer, Henci. *Obstetric Myths vs Research Realities: A Guide to the Medical Literature.* Westport: Bergin & Garvey, 1995.

Goer, Henci. *The Thinking Woman's Guide to a Better Birth.* New York: Perigee, 1999.

Harmon, Katherine. "Elective cesarean sections are too risky, WHO study says." *Scientific American,* January 11, 2010, www.scientificamerican.com/blog/post.cfm?id=elective-cesarean-sections-are-too-21010-01-11&print=true

Harper, Barbara. *Gentle Birth Choices.* Rochester: Healing Arts Press, 2005.

Hodnett, Ellen D. "Pain and Women's Satisfaction with the Experience of Childbirth: A Systematic Review." *AJOG* 186, No. 5 Supplement (May 2002) S160-S172.

Jones, Carl. *Mind Over Labor.* New York: Penguin, 1988.

Kitzinger, Sheila. *The Complete Book of Pregnancy and Childbirth.* New York: Knopf, 2003.

Kitzinger, Sheila. *Rediscovering Birth.* New York: Pocket Books, 2001.

Klaus, Marshall H. and J. H. Kennel. *Maternal-Infant Bonding.* St. Louis: Mosby, 1983.

Klaus, Phyllis and Penny Simkin. *When Survivors Give Birth: Understanding and Healing the Effects of Early Sexual Abuse on Childbearing Women.* Seattle: Classic Day Publishing, 2004.

Korte, Diana and Roberta Scaer. *A Good Birth, A Safe Birth.* Boston: Harvard Common Press, 1992.

Lappe, Frances Moore. *You Have the Power: Choosing Courage in a Culture of Fear.* New York: Tarcher, 2005.

Leighton, Barbara and Stephen H. Halpern. "The effects of epidural analgesia on labor, maternal, and neonatal outcomes: A systematic review." *AJOG* 186, 5 (2002): S69-77.

Lieberman, Ellice and Carol O'Donoghue. "Unintended effects of epidural analgesia during labor: A systematic review." *AJOG* 186, 5 (2002): S31-68.

Marinac-Dabic D., Krulewitch C.J., Moore R.M. Jr. *Epidemiology,* 2002 May; 13 (3 Suppl): S19-22. Center for Devices and Radiological Health, Food and Drug Administration.

Marmor, Theodore and David M. Krol. "Labor pain management in the United States: Understanding patterns and the issue of choice." *AJOG* 186, No 5 (2002): S173-180.

Mayberry, Linda J., D. Clemmens, D.E. Anindya. "Epidural side effects, co-interventions and care of women during childbirth: A systematic review." *AJOG* 186, No 5 (2002): S81-S92.

Melender, Hanna-Leenba, RM, MNSc. "Experiences of Fears Associated with Pregnancy and Childbirth: A Study of 329 Pregnant Women." *Birth.* Vol. 29, No. 2, June 2002.

Mendelsohn, M.D., Robert. *Male Practice.* Chicago: Contemporary Books, 1982.

Mongan, Maria. *Hypnobirthing: The Mongan Method.* Deerfield Beach: Health Communications, Inc. 2005.

Mothering magazine

Moyers, Bill. *Healing and the Mind.* New York: Broadway Books, 2002.

Murray, John. "Effects of Epidural Anesthesia on Newborns and Their Mothers." *Child Dev* 1981, 52:71-82.

National Association of Childbearing Centers (NACC), Kate Bauer, Executive Director interview.

New England Journal of Medicine report on the National Birth Center Study. 1989.

Newnham, J.P., Evans, S.F., Michael, C.A., Stanley, F.J., & Landau, L.I. "Effects of Frequent Ultrasound During Pregnancy: A Randomized Controlled Trial." *The Lancet*, 342, 1993, 887-891.

Northrup, Christiane. *Mother-Daughter Wisdom*. New York: Bantam, 2006.

Northrup, Christiane. *Women's Bodies, Women's Wisdom*. New York: Bantam, 2006.

Nyberg K. et al. "Perinatal Medication as a Potential Risk Factor for Adult Drug Abuse in a North American Cohort." *Epidemiology* 2000;11:715-6.

ObGyn News Dec. 15, 1998 "Safe for Breech Presentations: Burning of Herbs Linked to Cephalic Version" Study published in *JAMA* (280 (18): 1580-84, 1998)

Odont, Michel. *Birth Reborn*. Medford: Birth Works, Inc., 1994.

Overend, Jenni. *Welcome With Love*. San Diego: Kane/Miller Book Pub, 1999.

Peterson, Gayle. *Birthing Normally: A Personal Growth Approach to Childbirth*. Berkeley: Shadow & Light Productions, 1984.

Pert, Candace and Deepak Chopra. *Molecules of Emotions: The Science Behind Mind-Body Medicine*. New York: Touchstone, 1999.

Pierce, Joseph Chilton. *Magical Child*. New York: Plume, 1992.

Ray, Sondra. *Ideal Birth*. Berkeley: Celestial Arts, 1995.

Redbook magazine, "Cindy Crawford: a revealing peek," March 2000.

Sample, Ian. "Ultrasound Scans May Disrupt Fetal Brain Development." *New Scientist*, December 10, 2001. Journal reference: *Epidemiology*, Vol 12, p. 618.

Samuel, Eugenie, "Fetuses Can Hear Ultrasound Examinations." *New Scientist*, December 4, 2001.

Schucman, M.D., Helen. *The Course in Miracles*. Mill Valley: Foundation for Inner Peace, 2007.

Sears, William. *The Birth Book: Everything You Need to Know to Have a Safe and Satisfying Birth*. Boston: Little, Brown and Company, 1994.

Sepkowski, et al. "The effects of maternal epidural anesthesia on neonatal behavior during the first month." *Dev Med Child Neurol* 1992;34:1072-80.

Star, Rima. *The Healing Power of Birth*. Austin: Star Publishing, 1986.

Stone, Merlin. *When God was a Woman*. Orlando: Harvest/Harcourt Brace, 1978.

Strong, Thomas H. Jr. *Expecting Trouble: What Expectant Parents Should Know About Prenatal Care in America*. New York: NYU Press, 2002.

Tew, Marjorie. *Safer Childbirth? A Critical History of Maternity Care*. London: Free Association Books, 1998.

Traynor, J.D., et al. "Is the Management of Epidural Analgesia Associated With an Increased Risk of Cesarean Delivery?" *AJOG* 1999;180:353-9.

Vella, G.J., Humphrey, V.F., Duck, F.A., Barnett, S.B., *Ultrasound Med Biol*, Aug; 29 (8): 1193-204.

Wagner, Marsden. *Pursuing the Birth Machine: The Search for Appropriate Birth Technology*. Sevenoaks, Kent: ACE Graphics 1994.

Wolf, Naomi. *Misconceptions: Truth, Lies, and the Unexpected on the Journey to Motherhood*. New York: Anchor, 2003.

World Health Organization, www.who.int/reproductivehealth/topics/maternal_perinatal/en/index.html.

INDEX

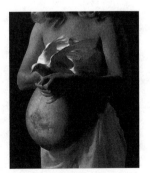

Posters & Baby Onesies at
www.naturalbirthsecrets.com